Neuroendocrinology of Aging

Neuroendocrinology of Aging

Edited by

Joseph Meites

Michigan State University
East Lansing, Michigan

Plenum Press • New York and London

Library of Congress Cataloging in Publication Data

Main entry under title:

Neuroendocrinology of aging.

Includes bibliographical references and index.
1. Neuroendocrinology. 2. Aging. 3. Endocrine glands—Diseases—Age factors.
I. Meites, Joseph, 1913–   . [DNLM: 1. Endocrine glands—Physiology. 2.
Nervous system—Physiology. WK 102 N4935]
QP356.4.N4835 1983   599'.0188   83-10937
ISBN 0-306-41310-8

©1983 Plenum Press, New York
A Division of Plenum Publishing Corporation
233 Spring Street, New York, N.Y. 10013

Printed in the United States of America

Contributors

Pierre Aschheim, Unité de Recherches Gérontologiques, INSERM U.118, 75016 Paris, France

Charles F. Aylsworth, Department of Anatomy, Michigan State University, East Lansing, Michigan 48824

James A. Clemens, Lilly Research Laboratories, Eli Lilly and Company, Indianapolis, Indiana 46285

Julian M. Davidson, Department of Physiology, Stanford University, Stanford, California 94305

Caleb E. Finch, Andrus Gerontology Center, Department of Biological Sciences, University of Southern California, Los Angeles, California 90007

Lloyd J. Forman, Department of Medicine, University of Medicine and Dentistry of New Jersey, Camden, New Jersey 08103

Paul E. Gottschall, Department of Physiology, Neuroendocrine Research Laboratory, Michigan State University, East Lansing, Michigan 48824

Gary D. Gray, Department of Physiology, Stanford University, Stanford, California 94305

Robert I. Gregerman, Gerontology Research Center, National Institute on Aging, NIH, Baltimore City Hospital, Baltimore, Maryland 21224

S. Mitchell Harman, Endocrinology Section, Clinical Physiology Branch, Gerontology Research Center, National Institute on Aging, NIH, Baltimore City Hospital, Baltimore, Maryland 21224

Henry H. H. Huang, Research Laboratory, Mercy Hospital and Medical Center, Chicago, Illinois 60616

Howard L. Judd, Department of Obstetrics and Gynecology, University of California at Los Angeles School of Medicine, Los Angeles, California 90024

John K. H. Lu, Departments of Obstetrics/Gynecology and Anatomy, University of California at Los Angeles School of Medicine, Los Angeles, California 90024

Joseph Meites, Department of Physiology, Neuroendocrine Research Laboratory, Michigan State University, East Lansing, Michigan 48824

Charles V. Mobbs, Andrus Gerontology Center, Department of Biological Sciences, University of Southern California, Los Angeles, California 90007

Ming-Tsung Peng, Department of Physiology, National Taiwan University Medical School, Taipei, Taiwan

Gail D. Riegle, Department of Physiology, Michigan State University, East Lansing, Michigan 48824

Dipak K. Sarkar, Department of Reproductive Medicine, University of California, San Diego, California 92093

James W. Simpkins, Department of Pharmaceutical Biology, College of Pharmacy, University of Florida, Gainesville, Florida 32610

Erla R. Smith, Department of Physiology, Stanford University, Stanford, California 94305

William E. Sonntag, Department of Physiology, Neuroendocrine Research Laboratory, Michigan State University, East Lansing, Michigan 48824

Richard W. Steger, Department of Obstetrics and Gynecology, University of Texas Health Science Center at San Antonio, San Antonio, Texas 78284

Paola S. Timiras, Department of Physiology–Anatomy, University of California, Berkeley, California 94720

Clifford W. Welsch, Department of Anatomy, Michigan State University, East Lansing, Michigan 48824

Contents

Chapter 3

Morphological Changes in the Hypothalamus and Other Brain Areas Influencing Endocrine Function during Aging

James A. Clemens

Chapter 4

Changes in Hypothalamic Hypophysiotropic Hormones and Neurotransmitters during Aging

James W. Simpkins

Chapter 5

Changes in Hormone Uptake and Receptors in the Hypothalamus during Aging

Ming-Tsung Peng

Chapter 6

Relation of Neuroendocrine System to Reproductive Decline in Female Rats

Pierre Aschheim

Chapter 7

Changes in Ovarian Function and Gonadotropin and Prolactin Secretion in Aging Female Rats

John K. H. Lu

Chapter 8

The Reproductive Decline in Male Rats

Richard W. Steger and Henry H. H. Huang

Chapter 9

Hormonal Influences on Hypothalamic Sensitivity during Aging in Female Rodents

Caleb E. Finch and Charles V. Mobbs

Chapter 10

Pathophysiology of Menopausal Hot Flushes

Howard L. Judd

Chapter 11

Relation of the Neuroendocrine System to Reproductive Decline in Men

S. Mitchell Harman

Chapter 12

The Sexual Psychoendocrinology of Aging

Julian M. Davidson, Gary D. Gray, and Erla R. Smith

Chapter 13

Regulation of Thyrotropin Physiology during Aging

Robert I. Gregerman

Chapter 14

Changes in Growth Hormone Secretion in Aging Rats and Man, and Possible Relation to Diminished Physiological Functions

William E. Sonntag, Lloyd J. Forman, and Joseph Meites

Chapter 15

Changes in Hypothalamic Control of ACTH and Adrenal Cortical Functions during Aging

Gail D. Riegle

Chapter 16

Relation of the Neuroendocrine System to the Development of Mammary Tumors in Rats during Aging

Clifford W. Welsch and Charles F. Aylsworth

Chapter 17

Relation of the Neuroendocrine System to Development of Prolactin-Secreting Pituitary Tumors

Dipak K. Sarkar, Paul E. Gottschall, and Joseph Meites

CHAPTER 1

Introduction

JOSEPH MEITES

The idea that the endocrine system is involved in aging processes is as old as the beginnings of endocrinology. The first endocrine experiment related to aging was reported by Brown-Séquard, who is usually regarded as the "father of endocrinology." In 1889, at the age of 72 years, he reported that he had succeeded in rejuvenating himself by injections of testicular extracts from dogs and guinea pigs. Although the favorable effects observed may have been due mainly to the powers of auto-suggestion, his reports created a considerable interest in endocrinology and its relation to aging, and eventually led to the use of estrogens for treating certain pre- and postmenopausal symptoms in women, and androgens for treating some symptoms in aging men. Up to about the 1960's, the relatively few studies on endocrine–aging relationships dealt mainly with changes in weight and histological appearance of endocrine organs in aging animals and human subjects, and included a limited number of measurements of endocrine function by bioassays and chemical (for steroids) procedures. Within these limitations, gerontological investigators were unable to establish any definite relationships between endocrine functions and aging processes, with the exception of the connection between reproductive decline and gonadal and pituitary activity.

The overriding importance of the brain, particularly its hypothalamic portion, in regulating pituitary and general endocrine activity, did not receive wide recognition among endocrinologists (and gerontological workers) until the publication in 1955 by Geoffrey Harris of his classic monograph, *Neural Control of the Pituitary Gland* (Arnold, London). Only in the 1960s did a few investigators begin to think about the possible involvement of the hypothalamus in aging processes. Among these were

JOSEPH MEITES • Department of Physiology, Neuroendocrine Research Laboratory, Michigan State University, East Lansing, Michigan 48824.

Aschheim in France; Frolkis and Dilman in the Soviet Union; Peng in Taiwan; Everitt in Australia; and Timeras, Finch, and our own laboratory in the United States. A marked upsurge in research on hypothalamic–aging relationships began in the second half of the 1970s, including research by many of the contributors to the present volume. An important factor in the increased research effort on this and other aspects of aging in the United States was the establishment of the National Institute on Aging in the mid-1970s and the funds it made available for these purposes.

The considerable amount of recent work on neuroendocrine–aging relationships has been done mainly on laboratory animals, particularly in the rat and mouse. This research has established that changes in neuroendocrine activity are responsible for many of the decrements seen in various body functions during aging. In old rats, for example, it has been shown by our laboratory and others that changes in neuroendocrine function are responsible for loss of estrous cycles in female rats, for development of mammary and pituitary tumors, and for the decline in secretion of growth hormone. In addition, it has been demonstrated that neuroendocrine intervention by direct manipulation of the hypothalamus or by use of central-acting drugs, can inhibit, halt, or even reverse some of the changes in body functions in old rats. Thus far, studies on possible neuroendocrine changes and their relation to aging decrements in elderly men and women have received little attention, but the knowledge gained from research on animal models provides at least some insight into the potential importance of the neuroendocrine system in aging processes. Indeed, it may even turn out that the endocrine system and the brain, the two great integrators of body functions, are the most important elements in determining aging processes.

The recent advances in knowledge of neuroendocrine–aging relationships were made possible, in part, by development of radioimmunoassays for accurately measuring hormones in the systemic circulation, in hypophysial portal blood, in endocrine glands, and in the hypothalamus. Also contributing were new methods for measuring neurotransmitters in the hypothalamus and other parts of the brain by histochemical, immunological, autoradiographic, and radioenzymatic techniques. Although none of these methods are without fault, they far exceed the technology that was available for the earlier endocrine studies. Other advances that have served to make neuroendocrine investigations related to aging more fruitful include improved methods for collecting blood from animals without stressing them; evidence that many, if not most, hormones are secreted in a pulsatile manner; that there are circadian, ultradian, and seasonal rhythms in hormone secretion; that there are changes in metabolism of hormones during aging; that hormone receptors must be present on tissues for hormones to act and that the number of receptors present in tissues may change during aging; and that environmental and nutritional factors can influence hormone secretion, etc. Some caution must be exercised in extrapolating observations made in one species to other species. Even in old rats and mice, it will be seen that some important differences have been uncovered in neuroendocrine functions.

This volume covers practically all of the important advances made on the neuroendocrinology of aging since inception of work in this area. Most of the leading investigators in this field are represented here. The topics covered include changes during aging in normal nuclei in the hypothalamus and elsewhere in the brain that help regulate pituitary hormone secretion; changes in hormone uptake and hormone receptors in the hypothalamus; the neurotoxic effects of some hormones on hypothalamic nuclei during aging; changes in neurotransmitters and hypophysiotropic hormone activity in the hypothalamus; the reproductive decline in rats, mice, men, and women, and associated changes in secretion of hypothalamic, pituitary, and gonadal hormones; alterations in reproductive behavior in animals and humans; relation of the neuroendocrine system to development of mammary and pituitary tumors; and alterations in secretion of growth hormone (GH), adrenocorticotropic hormone (ACTH)-adrenal cortical hormones, and thyrotropin (TSH)-thyroid function, and their significance in terms of body functions. This book will be of interest to investigators on aging, clinical gerontologists, neuroendocrinologists and endocrinologists in general, physiologists, pharmacologists, biochemists, biologists, brain scientists, and everyone interested in the phenomenon of aging, which, after all, is part of the life process we all share.

CHAPTER 2

Neuroendocrinology of Aging

Retrospective, Current, and Prospective Views

PAOLA S. TIMIRAS

1. Introduction

There was a time, not much more than ten years ago, when neuroen-docrinological theories of aging were almost totally ignored whenever aging theories were listed and discussed. Studies of cellular and molec-ular senescence focused primarily on the increase, with aging, in free radical reactions, lipid peroxidation, membrane damage, lysosomal leak-age and lipofucsin deposition, loss of cellular proliferative capacity, de-fective protein synthesis due to error-catastrophe or decline in DNA repair activity, and the cumulative damage (wear-and-tear theories) in-flicted on the organism by deleterious agents (Timiras, 1972; Rockstein *et al.*, 1974; Finch and Hayflick, 1977; Strehler, 1977; Schneider, 1978; Comfort, 1979; Kanungo, 1980; Masoro, 1981). None of these classical theories, however, was, or is now, sufficient to explain whether a change observed to occur with aging is simply the result of aging or whether it plays a causative role in the aging process. The same is true when these proposed mechanisms are categorized as "stochastic" (due to random chance events), or "programmed" (happening according to a definite plan), or both (e.g., programmed decline in the repair of stochastically generated damage). Likewise, the distinction of these mechanisms as "intrinsic" (built directly into the individual cells) and thereby capable of causing aging in the absence of outside influences, or "extrinsic" (imposed on the cell from the outside) and thereby assuming that aging is externally caused, begs, but does not resolve, the question of whether

PAOLA S. TIMIRAS ● Department of Physiology–Anatomy, University of California, Berkeley, California 94720.

a certain event is phenomenological or causal. While these theories continue to be prodded, new ones appear or prior theories, including neuroendocrinological ones, are returning or acquiring favor.

Neuroendocrinological theories of aging are derived from three major types of observations: (1) the well-demonstrated relationship between nervous and endocrine systems in the control of body functions, (2) the endocrine functions of the hypothalamus (particularly, the hypophysiotropic hormones) and their relation to neurotransmitters, and (3) the role played by the anterior pituitary and its target endocrines on key events of the life cycle, such as growth and sexual maturation. Much of the evidence offered in support of neuroendocrinological theories of aging is indirect, but, collectively, it is substantial and extends to all levels of control from molecular to organismic. The very fact that an entire book can be devoted to this field is evidence of its growth. In this chapter, theories will be examined first from a retrospective point of view, then some of the current information will be surveyed (with observations from our laboratory), and some future horizons will also be explored.

2. Retrospection

The concept that decrements in nervous and endocrine function are implicated phenomenologically or causally in the aging process was born simultaneously with the emergence of endocrinology as a separate biomedical field. In 1891, the French physiologist, Brown-Séquard and his assistant, d'Arsonval, suggested to the Society of Biology at Paris that potent substances they called "internal secretions" existed in animal tissues and that aging and disease probably resulted from their lack (Brown-Séquard and d'Arsonval, 1891). Organotherapy, that is therapy with tissue extracts, had originated in 1889, when Brown-Séquard, having postulated that "the feebleness of old men is in part due to the diminution of the function of the testicles" proceeded to administer testicular extracts to a number of old men (including himself) with positive results in terms of increased strength, vigor, and mental activity. In these early experiments, the relationship between internal secretions and the central nervous system was emphasized: "I have made this experiment (i.e., injections of testicular fluid) with the conviction that I would obtain with it notable augmentation of the powers of action of the nervous centers and especially the spinal cord" (Brown-Séquard, 1889). The fact that these attempts at rejuvenation did not completely fall into ridicule and disrepute but rather opened a vast scientific future is due to a series of subsequent clinical and experimental observations which clarified the physiologic basis for some of the diseases in question and the usefulness of the tissue extracts in their treatment. Thyroid extracts were found to be effective in the treatment of human and animal myxedema (as demonstrated by Murray in 1891), adrenal extracts to possess potent vasopressor activity (as demonstrated by the clinician Oliver and the physiologist Schäfer in 1893), and pancreatic grafts to prevent or ameliorate experimental diabetes in dogs (as demonstrated by von Mering and Minkowski in 1890; see the historical review by Borell, 1976). By confirming the existence of powerful extracts from specific tissues, these and other similar experiments focused scientific attention on internal secretions and, by the turn of the 19th century, the so-called "theory of internal secretions" came to represent a fruitful way of examining hitherto unexplored biomedical problems even though it had somewhat diverted from the original goal of finding a "cure for aging." In the next decade, two English physiologists, Bayliss and Starling, coined the word "hormone" and the direction of endocrinology changed from the study of the regulation of metabolism to that of cellular communication by means of chemical messengers.

It is not the purpose of this brief retrospection to review the many advances in endocrinology and neurobiology that have followed the early experiments described above. While both fields have progressed significantly and their interrelations have led to the recognition of the individual branch of neuroendocrinology, their impact on our understanding of the aging process remains uncertain and often controversial. For example, until the 1960s, research on the role of endocrines in aging did not consider central nervous system (CNS) interactions. The importance of hypothalamic regulation of pituitary function, although established by the work of Harris (1955) and others, had not yet aroused the interest of workers in the field of aging. Most of the observations reported were based either on gross, age-related, clinical alterations (e.g., the similarity between the signs and symptoms of aging and those of hypothyroidism, and/or hypogonadism), or on measurements of endocrine structure and function such as weight, gross and microscopic changes, levels of circulating hormones (first measured by bioassays and later by radioimmunoassays), secretory rates of the gland and response to exogenous stimulation or to tropic hormones, and sensitivity of target tissues to hormonal signals. Emerging from these observations was a discrepancy between the presence with progressive aging, of structural alterations and multiple signs of hormonal dysfunction and the apparent persistence of endocrine secretory competence well into old age (Vernadakis and Timiras, 1982). With the exception of the ovary, which exhausts its reproductive and endocrine functions at menopause, most endocrine glands continue to synthesize and release hormones, albeit at a somewhat altered level, until death. Such considerations remain valid even today with the increased sensitivity of diagnostic tests and with the increased awareness of the many variables which can particularly influence such organs as the endocrines, the primary function of which is responsiveness to the environment (Timiras, 1982a,b).

Beginning with a few studies in the 1960s and continuing with an increasing number in the 1970s, evidence has accumulated to indicate that aging may depend more on changes in the interrelationship between hormonal and neural signals than on isolated endocrine alterations. With the discovery of the neurosecretory activity of the hypothalamic cells, the identification of hypothalamic and hypophysiotropic hormones (Scharrer and Scharrer, 1963; Meites, 1970; Parsons, 1976; Guillemin, 1978; Schally, 1978) and with the knowledge that this secretory activity is regulated (or modulated) by neurotransmitters (the classical cholinergic, catecholaminergic, serotonergic, GABA—and the newer peptides), a neuroendocrinological approach to the clarification of aging mechanisms has proved to be more encouraging. Accordingly, much of the new information has derived from the study of the interrelations between neurotransmitters, neurohormones, and hormones, not only during steady-state conditions and in response to stimuli but also in terms of the cyclic, episodic, or tonic pattern of their release. This rhythmicity may be affected differentially by feedback control mechanisms (often situated in the hypothalamus), the sensitivity of which may change with increasing age. Indeed, several neuroendocrine processes contain within themselves some kind of intrinsic, timed mechanisms or "biological clocks" capable of determining the timetable of a number of biological events. The clock mechanism might be programmed to run from fertilization, when the genetic code is laid down, until death and signal an orderly sequence of changes characteristic of growth (e.g., fetal, postnatal), development (e.g., organogenesis, birth, puberty), and aging (e.g., cessation of reproductive function, decline of physiologic competence; Timiras, 1978). Alternatively, the program may extend only until reproductive maturity has been achieved and the continuation of the species assured; thereafter, in the absence of a program, the clock responsiveness to stochastic events would lead to failure of homeostasis with concomitant aging and finally death (Walker and Timiras, 1982). In either case, a "pacemaker" organ or "command" cells, possibly located in specific brain areas (e.g., hypothalamus, limbic system) would control the synchrony of the various clocks and eventually the nature of the neural signals responsible for hypothalamic neurosecretion, pituitary hormone secretions, and control of autonomic and sensorimotor functions. Two major

classes of pacemaker theories have been widely discussed in the gerontological literature; those discussed above, in which the pacemaker is
related to the brain, or more specifically to neuroendocrine control over
the anterior pituitary, and those in which the pacemaker is related to
the thymus gland or other aspects of the immune system.

The theories based on the view that aging may be due to the action
of a pacemaker, i.e., whether such a pacemaker follows a specific program for aging or becomes "disorganized" after adulthood has been
attained, and whether this pacemaker is located in specific brain areas
or in an endocrine gland (or in an organ of the immune system), need
to be verified by extensive experimentation and clinical observations.
They offer, however, some useful models on which to further study
aging processes in higher organisms and also provide some guidelines
for possible interventions. If further evidence can substantiate that aging
results from hormone-mediated disorganization of specific, neural, integrating centers, or, vice versa, that alterations in neural signals lead to
dysynchrony of endocrine functions, it may be possible in the future to
enhance adult vitality by stabilization or reduction of the rate of change
with age of these areas.

3. Current Neuroendocrine Theories of Aging

A defect produced at any level of the neuroendocrine pathways, or
in the target tissues (or cells or molecules) may be expected to produce
secondary aging changes. Several sites have been proposed where alterations which lead to aging may originate as well as mechanisms by which
they may act.

3.1. The Hypothalamic "Disregulation" Hypotheses

These hypotheses suggest that age-related changes in the hypothalamus are the cause of aging. In one view, aging of the hypothalamus
proceeds at a different pace in its various nuclei, the timetable of aging
varying in the hypothalamus, as is true for most body systems, from one
nucleus to another. Unequal changes in the numerous (endocrine, autonomic, and behavioral) functions of the hypothalamus would lead to a
breakdown of the synchronized (pacemaker?) communication within the
hypothalamic nuclei and between the hypothalamus and other neural
and endocrine centers.

Another view proposes that, with aging, the sensitivity of the hypothalamus to the negative feedback of hormones is decreased or lost

with consequent increase in the secretory rate of several endocrines and ensuing acceleration of aging phenomena (Dilman, 1976). One clear-cut example of increased hormonal secretion with aging is the high level of pituitary gonadotropins in women after menopause when the low estrogen levels in plasma can no longer inhibit the synthesis and release of hypothalamic gonadotropin-releasing hormone and of pituitary gonadotropins (see Chapters 6, 8, and 9). An age-related elevation of the hypothalamic threshold to negative feedback has also been reported for corticosteroids (Reigle, 1973) and gonadal steroids (Shaar *et al.*, 1975) in the rat. A third hypothesis, combining the foregoing, suggests that aging may be associated with a "shift" in the sensitivity of the hypothalamus to specific hormones, some nuclei becoming more, and others less, sensitive to the hormones. Such unequal and potentially discordant patterns of change, when associated with concomitant alterations in extrahypothalamic CNS areas and in endocrine functions, would be sufficient to account for the etiopathogenesis of aging processes.

Evidence in support of these theories derives from varied sources. Changes with aging in the morphology of the hypothalamus as well as in the secretion of hypophysiotropic hormones and in the uptake and binding of hormones from peripheral endocrines are presented in Chapters 3–5 and 13. For example, with respect to sex steroids, estradiol uptake and cytosol and nuclear binding are decreased in the hypothalamus with aging; these decreases show a regional specificity (greater in nuclei of anterior than posterior hypothalamus) and also sex specificity (decrease in female rats but not in males, in which a decrease in testosterone binding and uptake is reported; see Chapter 5). These alterations are associated with a loss of neurons and, in some of the remaining neurons, with a reduction in nuclear volume (similarly region- and sex-specific) as well as accumulation of lipofucsin (age pigments; Timiras, 1982a) and with a functional decline, as demonstrated by decreased induction of neurotransmitter (acetylcholinesterase) enzymes and decreased single unit activity in response to estrogens (Dudley, 1982). Corticosteroid uptake and receptor number (but probably not affinity) are significantly decreased in the cerebral cortex of rats (Roth, 1976) but not of mice (Nelson *et al.*, 1980), a difference which demonstrates species as well as regional and sex specificity for hormone brain receptors. Although systematic studies of corticosteroid receptor in the hypothalamus are not available (see discussion by Terry, 1980), the decreased sensitivity of the pituitary-adrenocortical axis to stimulation (e.g., stress) or to the inhibitory action of administered corticosteroids may be interpreted as due, at least in part, to alterations in neuronal uptake, binding, and/or metabolism of these hormones (see Chapter 13).

With respect to thyroid hormones, their role in many parameters of brain development is well known (Grave, 1977). Less understood is their role in the adult brain, although their influence on brain neurotransmitters and their enzymes and on behavior has been documented in several animals including man (Prange, 1974; Ito *et al.*, 1977; Vaccari *et al.*, 1977; Vaccari and Timiras, 1981). Receptors for thyroid hormones have been characterized in several brain areas, including the hypothalamus where they undergo changes during development and aging (Eberhardt *et al.*, 1976, 1978; Valcana and Timiras, 1978; Naidoo *et al.*, 1978; Valcana, 1979). With respect to the latter, the number and affinity of triiodothyronine (T_3) nuclear receptors are unchanged *in vitro* in whole brain (Cuttler, 1981) and cerebral hemispheres (Valcana 1979; Margarity *et al.*, 1981). However, some differences with aging are observed in *in vivo* experiments in which nuclear binding of T_3 in cerebral hemispheres appears higher in old than young rats (Margarity *et al.*, 1981; Timiras, 1982a). Increased nuclear T_3 binding *in vivo* and *in vitro* is also observed in the cerebral hemispheres and liver of rats made hypothyroid either neonatally or in adulthood (Valcana and Timiras, 1978, 1979) as well as in neuroblastoma and glioma cells cultured in the presence of very low thyroid hormone levels (Draves and Timiras, 1980). The increase in nuclear binding in these examples, represented by an increase in the number of receptors rather than their affinity, was interpreted as a compensatory response to the low circulating thyroid hormones. In the old rat, thyroxine (T_4) but not T_3, blood levels are significantly decreased, therefore the increase in neural receptor number may be viewed as compensatory to the age-related functional hypothyroidism (Cole *et al.*, 1982; Choy *et al.*, 1982; Timiras, 1982a).

In addition to the aging-associated changes shared by most neural cells in the senile brain (Timiras and Bignami, 1976; Barbagallo-Sangiorgi and Exton-Smith, 1980; Terry *et al.*, 1982), hypothalamic neurons, endowed with endocrine activity, also manifest their characteristic alterations in the synthesis and release of their products, the hypothalamic neuropeptides. While information on the structure and function of these neuropeptides is rapidly increasing, changes with aging have only begun to be investigated (see Chapter 4). The available studies show that hypothalamic levels of some of these peptides are higher in old than young animals (e.g., enkephalin, endorphin) others are lower (e.g., LHRH, somatostatin, vasopressin) and still others remain unchanged (e.g., TRH). The relation of the CNS aging, in general, to the aging of hypothalamic neurosecretion and vice versa, remains uncertain. Nevertheless, hypothalamic hormones have been empirically recommended and utilized in a number of mental disturbances including those of the aged. TRH, vasopressin and their analogs, and several other peptides (e.g., pituitary ACTH) have been administered to humans and other animals in an attempt to prevent or to arrest the decline in memory and cognitive functions and the appearance of behavioral impairment found sometimes in the normal elderly and always in those suffering with senile dementia (Crook and Gershon, 1981; Terry *et al.*, 1982). The results obtained so far with this growing group of compounds have been interesting and suggestive but no "magic bullet" has yet been identified. It is to be noted that several of the neuropeptides, such as TRH, are not limited to the hypothalamus but widely distributed throughout the brain and many possess, besides the hypophysiotropic function, other significant actions in the CNS. TRH, for example, potentiates the action of acetylcholine on cortical neurons (Breese *et al.*, 1975) perhaps by stimulating the receptor sensitivity (Yarbrough, 1976). The very idea that peptide hormones might be made anywhere in the brain besides the hypothalamus, and have other functions than the hormonal one, was astounding only a few years ago. Yet, the application of immunological and molecular biology techniques to the study of these peptide hormones has opened new avenues of investigation in the mechanism of action of these substances on neural and endocrine relations and their possible role in aging.

The use of specific complementary DNA (cDNA) to serve as a molecular probe to detect messenger RNA (mRNA) for peptide hormones has helped to determine that these hormones, or closely similar substances, are made by a variety of brain cells. The cDNA probes are also useful in identifying the sequences of hormone precursors, e.g., ACTH is derived from a large precursor mRNA containing sequences for four other hormones and enkephalins. Different cells cleave the precursor in different ways, thus, the hypothalamus produces enkephalins and the pituitary produces ACTH (Kolata, 1982a). With aging, changes in DNA, RNA, and enzyme activity may lead to modifications in the normal sequencing of the pro-hormone to the hormone, either quantitatively (e.g., accumulation of the less biologically active pro-hormone at the expense of the hormone) or qualitatively (e.g., failure of one or several hormones to be cleaved from the large precursor). Already in fetal and neonatal humans and mice, two to five mRNA for insulin types have been reported in the brain; they resemble, yet are different from, insulin and are not found in the adult brain (Kolata, 1982a). Whether further changes occur in aging is unknown. Inasmuch as these hormones have been suggested to have a role in neural growth (as is the case for insulin), or in specific sensory functions (e.g., endorphins with pain), or in intercellular communication, then alterations with aging in any of these functions can be the cause of or mediate changes in neuroendocrine (pacemaker?) control. If, as has been proposed (Roth *et al.*, 1982; Kolata, 1982b), cells contain many closely related genes for each hormone only one of which is ordinarily expressed in a particular cell, it may be possible to postulate that the hormone type expressed might also differ, among other variables, with the age of the cell. With aging, abnormalities in gene expression or the expression of specific genes for aging would be translated into any other type and level of organization. Hence, hormones, and neurotransmitters as well, would no longer be capable of, or would be delegated to functions other than regulation of growth and of adaptation and cell to cell communication.

3.2. The Neurotransmitter Hypotheses

These hypotheses implicate neurotransmitter excess or deficit, or imbalance among two or several neurotransmitters in discrete brain areas as being directly responsible for specific functional alterations. With aging, the selective vulnerability or resistance of relatively small populations of neurons possessing critical regulatory functions may delineate a pattern of neural and endocrine signals which dictate the functional characteristics of the senescent phenotype. Hence, major neurotransmitter losses need not be postulated with aging, and in fact, do not occur under physiologic conditions, rather, selective alterations (e.g., reduction of ACh in nucleus of Maynert, dopamine in substantia nigra, and norepinephrine in locus coeruleus) may be sufficient to desynchronize neurotransmitter balance and induce disorganization of the corresponding neural and endocrine signals which regulate homeostasis and adaptation (Enna *et al.*, 1981).

Current evidence (as discussed in Chapter 4), although still circumstantial, is indicative of a selective decrease with age in the number and function of catecholaminergic neurons (e.g., midbrain catecholaminergic nuclei in aged humans; Toffano *et al.*, 1982; Gottfries, 1982). Such loss may be ascribed to damage inflicted by free radicals (e.g., superoxide anions, hydrogen peroxide, derived hydroxyl radicals) in the neuron, and is illustrated indirectly by the intracellular presence of protective enzymes (e.g., superoxide dismutase, glutathione peroxidase, catalase) against such damage. Another hypothesis to explain this relative vulnerability is susceptibility to hypoxia, although definitive correlation has not been found between decreased catecholaminergic levels and cerebral atherosclerotic involvement.

In contrast to the selective vulnerability of the catecholaminergic systems, the serotonergic neurons are endowed with an apparent selective resistance (Calas and Van Den Bosch de Aguilar, 1980; Timiras and Hudson, 1980; Timiras, 1982a,b). Despite conflicting reports (e.g., decreased serotonin levels and turnover) (Meek *et al.*, 1977) our own studies in female Long–Evans rats indicate that serotonergic systems increase between birth and weaning (22 days of age in the rat), attain adult values by 40 days of age (age of sexual maturation) and remain essentially constant into old age (24 months and beyond). Inasmuch as catecholaminergic levels decrease in the same brain areas with aging, the ratio of serotonin to norepinephrine and to dopamine progressively increases. Thus, an imbalance between these neurotransmitter systems (and, eventually, other as yet incompletely known systems) may trigger those endocrine changes responsible for the passage from one life stage to another (e.g., puberty/menopause; growth/cessation of growth; adulthood/senescence; Müller *et al.*, 1977; Scapagnini *et al.*, 1980).

Another age-related change may involve neurotransmitter receptors and the interaction between neurotransmitter and receptor (Makman *et al.*, 1980). Neurotransmitter receptor functions have been examined at various ages by several investigators and in most studies the number of receptors decreased with age as do the hormone receptors. The picture that emerges from the currently reported studies is one of decreased neural cells responsiveness to chemical (transmitter or hormone) stimulation.

The known rhythmicity of neurotransmitter signals may also be altered with aging. For example, the characteristic circadian rhythm of serotonin, implicated in the regulation of several cyclic functions (e.g., sleep, locomotor activity, aggressive behavior, sex behavior, temperature regulation and regulation of hypophysiotropic hormones) changes with aging as do most of the associated functions. Similarly, catecholamine circadian rhythms in several brain areas (e.g., hypothalamic and pineal gland) may be altered by modifying the light/dark cycle, the diet, or by the administration of neurotropic drugs. In human beings as well as other animals and plants, certain time variations (e.g., daily, weekly, monthly, yearly) are maintained in the absence of any known environmental periodicity (e.g., circadian rhythms persist during flight in extraterrestrial space for the few weeks experienced so far) and their persistence may be due to the presence of an endogenous "synchronizer" acting through neural and endocrine signals (Halberg, 1982). With disease or environmental changes, some biologic frequencies best attuned to optimal health may shift, leading to deficits in physiologic performance and longevity. The circadian rhythm of urinary catecholamine in humans varies with age from 20 to 99 years, the greatest decrease in amplitude occurring after 65 years. Hormonal rhythms also show some shifts with aging (e.g., loss of GH peak during sleep in the elderly) perhaps in relation to neurotransmitter shifts. For example, a peak in the circadian serotonin cycle triggers the surge of LH preceding ovulation so that, given the proper hormonal (estrogen) environment, the actual levels of serotonin are less important for inducing the LH surge than a properly timed peak in the neurotransmitter (Walker *et al.*, 1980). Depression of the hypothalamic peak by the neonatal administration of serotonin inhibitors (e.g., parachlorophenylalanine, testosterone) or displacements of the peak (e.g., by altering light/dark cycles) will block the LH surge and alter the timetable of reproduction by accelerating both the onset of sexual maturation and that of sexual senescence (Walker and Timiras, 1980). Similarly, delaying brain maturation and, presumably, the maturation of serotonergic systems by neonatal hypothyroidism, alters the timetable of reproductive function (Walker and Timiras, 1981).

The proposition that CNS aging is associated with a progressive imbalance in neurotransmission resulting from differential changes in neurotransmitter levels, metabolism, receptors, and/or rhythmicity provides a rationale for proposing that aging may be amenable to neuropharmacological interventions (Ordy, 1979). Indeed, several reports show that the administration of certain centrally acting drugs (e.g., L-Dopa, iproniazid, lergotrile, bromocriptine), some of which are metabolic precursors, alters various aspects of aging (see Chapter 4). Other types of intervention include lowering serotonin levels in rat brain by restriction of the precursor, tryptophan, in the diet; or administration of the inhibitor parachlorophenylalanine either locally, in the hypothalamus, or systemically. In this manner, aging of reproductive function can be mimicked by local hypothalamic administration of the inhibitor (Walker *et al.*, 1980). In addition, prolonged dietary restriction of tryptophan initiated early in life, has been shown to retard growth and maturation as well as delay the onset of aging and possibly prolong the lifespan (Segall and Timiras, 1976; Segall *et al.*, 1978). With respect to the cholinergic system, although normal individuals show little change in acetylcholine and its metabolic enzymes in old age, in dementia (including Alzheimer's disease) the activity of choline acetyltransferase, the synthesizing enzyme of acetylcholine, is decreased in cortical (hippocampal) and subcortical (nucleus of Maynert) nuclei. In addition, several studies have shown that cholinergic dysfunction may be related to the memory impairment of old age and have suggested, at least as an empirical approach, that replacement therapy with choline or lecithin (its natural dietary source) or inhibition of the hydrolyzing enzyme by physostigmine might be beneficial in restoring or slowing down memory deficits. Although positive effects with dietary pharmacological replacement therapy have been reported in some elderly subjects and aged animals, these effects are relatively transient and inconsistent depending on the subject and the optimal doses (Roberts, 1981). Interesting and promising as these dietary and pharmacological interventions might be, additional clinical and experimental studies will have to be undertaken to take total advantage of their practical applicability as "anti-aging" agents.

3.3. The Pituitary Hypotheses

These hypotheses include some contrasting points of view. According to some investigators, severe hypofunction of the pituitary would induce involutional changes resembling those of old age; according to others, pituitary hormones would accelerate the aging process by causing (or contributing to) the pathology of senescence (Everitt and Burgess, 1976). The first hypothesis, based on hypopituitarism as a cause of aging, is supported by reports of senile changes occurring prematurely in a number of patients whose pituitaries had been destroyed by disease or are hypofunctioning due to unknown (genetic?) factors (Herman, 1976). In several cases, hypopituitarism symptoms can be corrected with appropriate hormonal replacement therapy, but whether or not the aging processes are slowed down as well, remains to be demonstrated. Evidence supportive of the second hypothesis derives from observations, primarily in rats, that drastic reduction in pituitary function by surgical, dietary, or pharmacological hypophysectomy, prolongs physiologic competence, inhibits the development of some diseases of old age, and delays the onset of aging but shortens the duration of life (Everitt and Burgess, 1976; Everitt, 1980).

Both quantitative and qualitative changes in pituitary secretion have been described with advancing age and have been reviewed recently by Meites (1981, 1982) as well as with respect to hypothalamic regulation (see Chapter 1). Information on aging of the various pituitary functions (secretions) is presented throughout this book and need not be repeated here except for those observations relevant to this discussion. In aged rats, the pituitary may secrete a factor (perhaps a new or transformed hormone?) which would reduce the responsiveness of peripheral tissues to the metabolic actions of thyroid hormones (Denckla, 1974). Although such a factor has not yet been characterized, the dramatic effects of hypophysectomy, combined with appropriate replacement therapy, in reducing tumor incidence, restoring a number of functions such as immunological function to their juvenile efficiency, and/or preventing age-related declines in old rats have been ascribed to the removal of this postulated inhibitory factor. Another mechanism by which qualitative changes may occur in pituitary secretion with aging involves alterations in the synthesis and metabolism of pituitary hormones (as discussed above for hypothalamic hormones), perhaps due to alterations in the activity of the enzymes assigned to cleave the hormones from larger precursor molecules (Segall, 1979). Most pituitary hormones show a certain polymorphism manifested by physicochemical differences (e.g., molecular weight, electrical charge) and reflected in different biological potency: so far, five forms of GH have been described, six forms of LH and five forms of TSH. Although such polymorphism is particularly evident at young ages, it seems to increase in old rats (Klug and Adelman, 1979). Similarly, a decline in carbohydrate content of glycoprotein hormones such as LH (Conn *et al.*, 1980) and TSH (Choy *et al.*, 1982) has been reported in rats with advancing age. What the functional significance of these abnormal forms is, remains to be clarified. The large LH form shows a slower metabolic rate than the major form, and the percentage of its secretion may be reduced by the administration of testosterone to old rats or may be increased by castration of young rats (Conn *et al.*, 1980). The only other hormone which has been studied in these terms is insulin. After glucose challenge, older subjects have a greater concentration of pro-insulin material in their circulation than younger subjects (Duckworth and Kitabchi, 1976). The reduced biological activity of pro-insulin as compared to insulin, may explain, at least in part, the high incidence of individuals with impaired glucose tolerance in the population aged 65 years and over (Cole *et al.*, 1982). Increased circulating levels of pro-insulin in older subjects have been related to the increased release of the "unfinished" hormone from the pancreas, although other factors (e.g., decreased renal clearance) may also be responsible.

A corollary to this theory is the "hypothyroid hypothesis," supported by the many signs and symptoms of altered thyroid state in the elderly, which suggest that thyroid hormones play a key role in the etiology of aging processes (Walker and Timiras, 1982; see also Chapter 11). Decrements in thyroid hormone levels, impaired conversion of T4 and T3, changes in receptor number, increased TSH polymorphism, and the appearance of an inhibitory factor with aging have all been considered as potentially operative in aging. Thyroid hormones are important in growth, maturation, and differentiation and may, perhaps in association with other hormones, similarly affect aging. An evolutionary precedent of interference with thyroid hormone action by a pituitary factor may be found in some anurans and uredels in which mammalian prolactin inhibits the developmental actions of thyroxine, perhaps by interfering with Na^+K^+-ATPase activity, a major target of thyroid action (Platt *et al.,* 1978). Growth, (GH) and thyroid hormones interact in growth processes in mammals. A factor similar to GH or prolactin, or a protein or peptide containing the same group of GH-related sequences, may modulate the developmental effects of thyroid hormones but exert an inhibitory action once maturity has been attained. Inasmuch as prolactin secretion is regulated by brain levels of dopamine (either directly or through the control of the hypothalamic prolactin-inhibiting hormone), the apparent decrease in brain dopaminergic activity with aging may be reflected in increased prolactin (and eventually of GH and related peptide) secretion and in alterations in their relationship to thyroid hormones. This occurs in the ob/ob mouse, currently a widely accepted model of maturity-onset diabetes, which shows a markedly altered control of GH and prolactin secretion and a selectively diminished Na^+K^+-ATPase response to thyroid hormones. The complexity of the endocrine alterations in this model points out that it may be unrealistic to ascribe aging to a single endocrine deficit such as hypothyroidism. Aging, rather, may result from multiendocrine disturbances.

3.4. Progeria and Progeroid Syndromes

These syndromes emphasize the role of genetic factors in determining the length of the lifespan and of genetic variants in determining accelerations or decelerations of changes in the senescent phenotype. Longevity is considered hereditary, at least in part, under stable environmental conditions (Martin, 1978). Progeria (premature old age) and progeroid (progerialike) syndromes resemble but do not quite duplicate the total pathophysiology of aging; each syndrome represents the acceleration of some characteristics, such as endocrine dysfunction, associated with normal aging. The etiology of these syndromes is obscure, but among the many causes proposed, neuroendocrinological dysfunction is supported by a number of alterations such as stunted growth.

3.5. The Stress Theory of Aging

This theory applies the cellular hypotheses of "wear and tear" and auto-intoxication to the organismic level and amalgamates them with neuroendocrinological theories of aging involving the hypothalamo-pituitary-adrenal axis. According to this theory, exposure to environmental stimuli, most often of a detrimental nature but also, in some cases, with a positive influence, may decrease and eventually exhaust the ability of the organism to maintain homeostasis.

Central to this concept, as first formulated by Selye (1950, 1974), is the role of the adrenal cortex. According to Selye's "adaptation syndrome," individuals are born with a fixed quantity of "adaptive energy" which is progressively reduced with each exposure to stress (the term stress being used to indicate both the stressing agent or stimulus and the response of the organism to it). The observation (now classic) that adrenocortical hormones (and particularly aldosterone) are necessary for survival and that hypophysectomized or adrenalectomized animals can survive only if kept under optimal environmental conditions but readily succumb to stress, forms the basis of the stress theory of aging. Exposure to a variety of stressors would induce a sequence of neural and endocrine events leading first to the activation of defense mechanisms necessary for survival (the so-called alarm reaction), followed by a period of enhanced adaptive capacity (the stage of resistance), and terminating with loss of the capacity to adapt (the stage of exhaustion). The passage from one stage to the other would be dictated by the efficiency of the hypothalamo-pituitary-adrenocortical axis in synchronizing: (1) nervous stimuli from the stress conditions, (2) hormonal secretions from the pituitary and the adrenals, and (3) the sensitivity of peripheral target tissues and cellular functions to the adrenocortical hormone levels and rhythmicity. The composite of these neuroendocrine reactions and their resulting cellular and tissular responses seems to resemble the timetable of the individual life; at an early age, adaptive capacity is not completely developed, with adulthood, resistance reaches an optimum, and thereafter, declines until death.

It is difficult to reconcile the stress theory, interesting as it may appear, with the apparent adequate adrenocortical function in old age both under basal and stress conditions or after ACTH administration. As discussed in Chapter 13 in more detail, even the decline with age in adrenocortical responses to injury appears slight. The age-related decline in resistance to stress may be dependent on qualitative rather than quantitative changes mentioned above with respect to the pituitary hormones and particularly ACTH. Indeed, it has been recently reported that aging causes a decrease in the ACTH precursor, pro-opiocortin, thereby lowering the availability of ACTH upon demand. However, contrary to what happens with TSH and LH, this decline is not accompanied by major changes in the processing of pro-opiocortin or in the physico-chemical forms of the hormone (Barnea *et al.*, 1982a,b). Other factors that may play a role in such "derailment" of normal adult physiological patterns are age-related changes in the sensitivity of target organs to adrenal hormones, in the efficiency with which the target organs can make the functional adjustments required for adaptation, in the articulation of neural and endocrine inputs in the optimal control of

these adjustments, or to a combination of all these factors. Equally un-
resolved is the suggestion that "diseases of adaptation" may ensue from
repeated exposure to stress. Such diseases, involving primarily the cir-
culatory (e.g., hypertension, atherosclerosis) and immune (e.g., arthritis,
autoimmune diseases) systems, are all commonly associated with old age.
The induction of disease by a variety of stresses in humans may contribute to aging; as in animals, exposure to stress induces "precocious
aging," i.e., a decrement in one or several functions at an earlier than
expected chronological age.

4. Outlook

In the previous section, we have often substituted the term "hypothesis" for "theory" to emphasize how incomplete our understanding
of neuroendocrine mechanisms in aging still is. Indeed, in the century
between the early work of Brown-Séquard and the current status of our
knowledge, a vast body of phenomenological information has accumulated and its evidence points to a critical role in aging processes for
endocrine and nervous functions and, perhaps more importantly, their
interactions. As reported by Adolph (1982), "life can maintain itself only
by a perpetual effort of defense and conquest." In this effort, success is
partially measured by longevity of the individual and depends to a large
extent on the integration of neuroendocrine controls. Any defect in these
controls may interfere with survival and result in a diminished expec-
tation of life duration. Conversely, a strengthening of these controls (or
reciprocally, a lowering of environmental demand) increases homeostatic
stability and promotes survival. Thus, neuroendocrine studies of aging
offer both theoretical and practical advantage which must be vigorously
pursued and for which private and public support must be forthcoming.
Such studies focus on two major control systems, closely connected, clearly
involved in the regulation of all body functions, and strongly implicated
in aging changes. The neuroendocrine approach also offers the possibility of intervening by various means (e.g., pharmacological, dietary)
either to prevent the aging process or delay its onset or restore normal
function. Continuing advances in the clarification of the mechanisms of
hormone, neurotransmitter, and neuropeptide actions and progress in
the synthesis of new agonists and antagonists provide a practical basis
to intervene in the aging process. Therefore, the number of investigators
interested in the neuroendocrinology of aging is rapidly growing and
their varied expertise has given impetus to research in this area. Several

avenues, briefly presented in Section 4 are currently being explored and are expected to yield significant new information.

4.1. Refinement in Detection of Neuroendocrine Changes with Aging

Improved techniques have made it possible, not only in laboratory animals but also in humans, to measure levels, metabolism, and receptors of hormones, neurotransmitters, and neuropeptides more accurately. While changes in some neurotransmitters with aging have been studied extensively (Crook and Gershon, 1981; Enna *et al.*, 1981; Terry *et al.*, 1982) and appropriate therapeutic regimens (e.g., single drug or drug "cocktail") have been tried, neuropeptides, other putative neurotransmitters, and/or neural modulators, have just begun to be identified (Snyder, 1980) and await further study in the adult and the elderly. Neuropeptides in brain (and other tissues) are being intensively investigated with more sensitive techniques in several laboratories; as "classic" neurotransmitters have not yet provided a definitive and exclusive link between neural stimulation and endocrine secretion, the search for new agents of cell communication goes on. Probably, more fruitful for the identification of the mechanism of aging, no matter how sophisticated our techniques may become, is not the study of the endocrine function *per se*, but rather the neural (hypothalamic) control of endocrine function.

4.2. Comparative Aspects of Neuroendocrine Changes with Aging

While early studies were conducted primarily in animals, recent improvements in noninvasive methodology have provided more information from humans. Rats and mice have, so far, been the most utilized animals for studies of neuroendocrine aging because of the wealth of available information on their endocrine function during development and adulthood. Nevertheless, they are unique and observations reported in these species cannot be safely extrapolated to others. By comparing neuroendocrine processes within these species and those of other animals, including humans, one might single out those universal changes that transect species characteristics. The universality of aging processes, even in neuroendocrine terms, is supported by the finding that unicellular organisms produce hormonal peptides which may act as intracellular messenger molecules, heralding their intercellular communicating role in vertebrates (Roth *et al.*, 1982).

Along these lines, tissue culture studies (e.g., cultured hypothalamus, pituitary, target tissue), by eliminating some of the complexity of the environmental and metabolic variables, offer the possibility of singling out intrinsic changes in neuroendocrine function with aging. Techniques are now becoming available for accelerating aging of neural (and other) cells in culture, permitting the telescoping of aging changes and allowing a rapid response to interventive measures, an important advantage when viewing the normal time span of aging in intact animals.

4.3. Relations between Neuroendocrine and Immune Controls in Aging

Another integrating system often implicated in the etiopathology of aging is the immune system. The response of the immune system to hormones (e.g., immunosuppressive effects of adrenal and sex hormones, increased incidence with aging of autoimmune diseases of endocrines) is well known in descriptive but not mechanistic terms. The thymus, one of the major organs of the immune system, has often been considered as an endocrine gland and thymosin identified as a hormone (Goldstein *et al.*, 1979). Recently, thymosin has been shown to stimulate LHRH secretion in the hypothalamus and, secondarily, LH from the pituitary (Rebar *et al.*, 1981). These data provide evidence of a direct effect of the "endocrine" thymus on the hypothalamus and suggest an important role for thymic peptides in reproduction. Whether these actions of the thymus are direct on the hypothalamus, and eventually adjacent brain nuclei such as the hippocampus and the amygdala, remains controversial (Cross *et al.*, 1982). Almost completely ignored until a few years ago were the relations between the immune system and the brain. The validity of such a relationship is becoming more apparent in recent studies in which brain and behavior were shown to influence several immune (humoral) responses (and vice versa) probably through hypothalamic mediation (Stein *et al.*, 1976). A still not completely identified substance, cortisin, has been extracted from the mouse brain and has been compared for its control of immune reactions to thymosin (Belokrylov, 1978). Lesioning of cerebral cortex induces a decrease in the T-cell number and in cell-mediated immune responses (Renoux *et al.*, 1980). The importance of the immune system to the body defense as a whole, the integrative actions of the system, the changes that this system undergoes with aging, the evidence that it interacts with the nervous and endocrine systems presage the value of continuing and initiating studies of immune-neuroendocrine relations in aging. With the refinement of our investigative techniques and the growing interest in these relations, such studies should advance rapidly.

4.4. Molecular Biology of Brain Hormones and of Hormonal Actions on Brain

We have emphasized the crucial role of the hypothalamus on the regulation of pituitary function with aging. Other areas which have already shown significant and rapid contributions, and promise yet more, are those utilizing methods from molecular biology leading to a better understanding of the transcription and translation of peptide hormones, the role of hormones in protein synthesis, and the manifestation of these effects in different target cells including neurons. Also worthy of further investigation is the effect of hypothalamic and peripheral hormones on neural cells, both neurons and glia. These effects have been studied extensively with respect to gross brain excitability and behavior and their structural and neurochemical correlates (see also Chapter 16). While hormone receptors have been identified and shown to be responsive to metabolic conditions and age, the exact site, mechanisms, and consequences of binding need further clarification. In view of the many behavioral changes with aging, the possibility of modifying behavior by hormonal manipulation might prove useful in restoring, at least partially, normal behavior in those elderly individuals afflicted with behavioral disturbances.

4.5. Changes with Aging in Hormone Metabolism and Tissue Responses

Another question which needs answering refers to the metabolism of hormones with aging. We have already discussed above, possible alterations in cleavage of peptide hormones from the pro-hormone and the increased incidence of polymorphic forms during development and in aging. Other changes might involve the conversion of one hormone to the other (e.g., T_4 to T_3) not only in the brain but also the liver and other tissues. Inasmuch as the varied hormonal forms and the hormones themselves also have different biological potency, the study of hormone metabolism may contribute to understanding the altered target tissue responses to neuroendocrine stimuli. Another reason for the altered tissular responsiveness with aging may lie in the intrinsic age-related changes in tissues, cells, and intracellular molecules themselves. Research in this area has only started and needs to be vigorously pursued.

4.6. Oxidative Cell Damage with Aging and Actions of Hormones

As part of their metabolic actions, hormones may influence the generation of free radicals which increases progressively with aging. Unstable chemical compounds with unpaired electrons and free radicals react with many types of biological molecules to produce substances (e.g., hydrogen peroxide, superoxide anions, derived hydroxyl radicals) highly toxic to the cell. With aging, increasing amounts of free radicals result from normal metabolic events and from continuing exposure to toxic environmental influences, either man-made (e.g., air pollutants, food additives), naturally occurring (e.g., animal and vegetable toxins), and/ or from the decline in the efficiency of the defensive mechanisms (e.g., lysosomes, enzymes) to guard against such damage (Harman, 1981). Inasmuch as it is impossible to eliminate adequately the many endogenous and exogenous sources of free radicals, current efforts are directed to the identification of substances such as vitamin E, beta-carotene, ascorbic acid, and more recently, uric acid, which act as scavengers of oxygen radicals (Ames *et al.*, 1981). Hormones may influence the formation of free radicals by accelerating cell metabolism, including oxidative reactions (e.g., thyroid hormones), by generating superoxide anions (e.g., corticosteroids), or by autoxidation (e.g., the estrogen metabolites, catecholestrogens; Nelson *et al.*, 1976; Ball and Knuppen, 1980). These metabolic actions have been demonstrated in several tissues, including brain where they may cause selective cell degeneration (shown in the hippocampus by Landfield *et al.*, 1978a,b) or selective autoxidation of neurotransmitters (suggested for dopamine). On this basis, the beneficial effects of hypophysectomy or thyroidectomy in delaying aging and prolonging lifespan could be ascribed to a slowdown of oxidative processes in the absence of the corresponding hormones. However, hormones may also enhance the natural defense mechanisms which metabolize intracellular peroxides and other free radical products. These natural mechanisms consist primarily of three enzyme systems, catalase, glutathione peroxide, and superoxide dismutase. While these enzymes are primarily substrate inducible, they may also be influenced by such regulatory factors as hormones. Thus, hormones might both protect from, or induce the generation of free radicals. The end result of these actions, whether beneficial or detrimental, depends on still unknown factors. Systematic studies of the relationship between hormones and protective enzymes for oxidative processes, especially in the nervous tissue, appear reasonable and may prove valuable in strengthening the natural defenses of the body and thereby delay the onset of age-related degenerative processes.

5. Summary and Conclusions

Several neuroendocrine hypotheses for aging have been presented here, but which of them is correct remains to be verified. In fact, all theories of aging await verification. The concept of pacemaker or "command" cells, possibly situated in the hypothalamus, and acting through neural and hormonal signals provides a useful model for further experimentation. Identification of the responsible signals may lead to a better understanding of the aging processes and their causes. More importantly, perhaps, are the rapid advances in recent years in endocrinology and neuropharmacology which make it possible to modify the signals, and hence, perhaps to influence the aging process. Thus, a defect produced at any level of the functional neuroendocrine pathways may be expected to produce aging changes which can be appropriately prevented or attenuated by specific interventions.

6. References

Adolph, E. F., 1982, Physiological integrations in action, *The Physiologist* (Suppl.) **25**:1–67.

Ames, B. N., Cathcart, R., Schwiers, E., and Hochstein, P., 1981, Uric acid provides an antioxidant defense in humans against oxidant- and radical-caused aging and cancer: A hypothesis, *Proc. Natl. Acad. Sci. USA* **78**:6858–6862.

Ball, P., and Knuppen, R., 1980, Catecholoestrogens (2- and 4- Hydroxyoestrogens): Chemistry, biogenesis, metabolism, occurrence and physiological significance, *Acta Endocrinologica* (Suppl. 232) **93**:1–27.

Barbagallo-Sangiorgi, G., and Exton-Smith, A. N. (eds.), 1980, *The Aging Brain: Neurological and Mental Disturbances,* Plenum Press, New York.

Barnea, A., Cho, G., and Porter, J. C., 1982a, A reduction in the concentration of immunoreactive corticotropin, melanotropin and lipotropin in the brain of the aging rat, *Brain Res.* **232**:345–354.

Barnea, A., Cho, G., and Porter, J. C., 1982b, Molecular-weight profiles of immunoreactive corticotropin in the hypothalamus of the aging rat, *Brain Res.* **232**:355–363.

Belokrylov, G. A., 1978, Tissue of the syngeneic brain cortex as an immunogenesis stimulant in thymectomized mice, *Biull. Eksper. Biol. Medit.* **86**:327–330.

Borell, M., 1976, Organotherapy, British physiology, and discovery of the internal secretions, *J. Hist. Biol.* **9**:235–268.

Breese, G. R., Cott, J. M., Cooper, B. R., Prange, A. J., Jr., Lipton, M. A., and Plotnikoff, N. P., 1975, Effects of thyrotropin-releasing hormone (TRH) on the actions of pentobarbital and other centrally acting drugs, *J. Pharmacol. Exp. Ther.* **193**:11–22.

Brown-Séquard, C.-E., 1889, Seconde note sur les effects produits chez l'homme par des injections sous-cutanées d'un liquide retiré des testicules frais de cobaye et de chien, *Compt. Rend. Soc. Biol.* (9th Ser.) **1**:420.

Brown-Séquard, C.-E., and d'Arsonval, A., 1891, De l'injection des extraits liquides provenant des glandes et des tissues de l'organisme comme methode therapeutique, *Compt. Rend. Soc. Biol.* (9th Ser.) **3**:248–250.

Calas, A., and Van Den Bosch de Aguilar, P., 1980, Comparative radioautographic study of serotonergic neurons in young and senescent rats, in: *The Psychobiology of Aging: Problems and Perspectives* (D. G. Stein, ed.), Elsevier-North Holland, Amsterdam, pp. 59–80.

Choy, V. J., Klemme, W. R., and Timiras, P. S., 1982, Variant forms of immunoreactive thyrotropin in aged rats, *Mech. Ageing Dev.* **53**:572–581.

Cole, G. M., Segall, P. E., and Timiras, P. S., 1982, Hormones during aging, in: *Hormones in Development and Aging* (A. Vernadakis and P. S. Timiras, eds.), SP Medical and Scientific Books, New York, pp. 477 550.

Comfort, A., 1979, *The Biology of Senescence,* Elsevier, New York.

Conn, P. M., Cooper, R., McNamara, C., Rogers, D. C., and Shoenhardt, L., 1980, Qualitative change in gonadotropin during normal aging in the male rat, *Endocrinology* **106**:1549–1553.

Crook, T., and Gershon, S. (eds.), 1981, *Strategies for the Development of an Effective Treatment for Senile Dementia,* Mark Powley Associates, New Canaan, Connecticut.

Cross, R. J., Brooks, W. H., Roszman, T. L., and Markesbery, W. R., 1982, Hypothalamic-immune interactions: Effect of hypophysectomy on neuroimmunomodulation, *J. Neurol. Sci.* **53**:557–566.

Cuttler, R. G., 1981, Thyroid hormone receptors in the brain of rat as a function of age and hypophysectomy, in: *Aging,* Vol. 17, *Brain Neurotransmitters and Receptors in Aging and Age-Related Disorders,* (S. J. Enna, T. Samorajski, and B. Beer, eds.), Raven Press, New York, pp. 117–132.

Denckla, W. D., 1974, Role of the pituitary and thyroid glands in the decline of minimal O_2 consumption with age, *J. Clin. Invest.* **53**:572–581.

Dilman, V. M., 1976, The hypothalamic control of aging and age-associated pathology. The elevation mechanism of aging, in: *Hypothalamus, Pituitary and Aging* (A. V. Everitt and J. A. Burgess, eds.), Charles C. Thomas, Springfield, Illinois, pp. 634–667.

Draves, D. J., and Timiras, P. S., 1980, Thyroid hormone effects in neural (tumor) cell culture; Differential effects on triiodothyronine nuclear receptors, Na^+K^+ ATPase activity and intracellular electrolyte levels, in: *Tissue Culture in Neurobiology* (E. Giacobini, A. Vernadakis, and A. Shahar, eds.), Raven Press, New York, pp. 291–301.

Duckworth, W. C., and Kitabchi, A. E., 1976, The effect of age on plasma proinsulinlike material after oral glucose, *J. Lab. Clin. Med.* **88**:359–367.

Dudley, S. D., 1982, Responsiveness to estradiol in central nervous system of aging female rats, *Neurosci. Biobehav. Rev.* **6**:39–45.

Eberhardt, N. L., Valcana, T., and Timiras, P. S., 1976, Hormone-receptor interactions in brain: Uptake and binding of thyroid hormone, *Psychoneuroendocrinology* **1**:399–409.

Eberhardt, N. L., Valcana, T., and Timiras, P. S., 1978, Triiodothyronine nuclear receptors: An *in vitro* comparison of the binding of triiodothyronine to nuclei of adult rat liver, cerebral hemisphere and anterior pituitary, *Endocrinology* **102**:556–561.

Enna, S. J., Samorajski, T., and Beer, B. (eds.), 1981, *Aging,* Vol. 17, *Brain Neurotransmitter and Receptors in Aging and Age-Related Disorders,* Raven Press, New York.

Everitt, A. V., 1980, The neuroendocrine system and aging, *Gerontology* **26**:108–119.

Everitt, A. V., and Burgess, J. A. (eds.), 1976, *Hypothalamus, Pituitary and Aging,* Charles C. Thomas, Springfield, Illinois.

Finch, C. E., and Hayflick, L. (eds.), 1977, *Handbook of the Biology of Aging,* Van Nostrand Reinhold, New York.

Goldstein, A. L., Thurman, G. B., Low, T. L. K., Trivers, G. E., and Rossio, J. L., 1979, Thymosin: The endocrine thymus and its role in the aging process, in: *Physiology and*

Cell Biology of Aging (A. Cherkin, C. E. Finch, N. Kharasch, T. Makinodan, F. D. Scott, and B. S. Strehler, eds.), Raven Press, New York, p. 51–59.

Gottfries, C. G., 1982, Brain, monoamines and aging, in: *Neural Aging and Its Implications in Human Neurological Pathology, Aging,* Vol. 18 (R. D. Terry, C. L. Bolis, and G. Toffano, eds.), Raven Press, New York, pp. 161–168.

Grave, G. D. (ed.), 1977, *Thyroid Hormones and Brain Development,* Raven Press, New York.

Guillemin, R., 1978, Peptides in the brain: The new endocrinology of the neuron, *Science* **202:**390–402.

Halberg, F., 1982, Biological rhythms, hormones and aging, in: *Hormones in Development and Aging* (A. Vernadakis and P. S. Timiras, eds.), SP Medical and Scientific Books, New York, pp. 451–476.

Harman, D., 1981, The aging process, *Proc. Natl. Acad. Sci. USA* **78:**7124–7128.

Harris, G. W., 1955, *Neural Control of the Pituitary Gland,* Arnold, London.

Herman, E., 1976, Senile hypophyseal syndromes, in: *Hypothalamus Pituitary and Aging* (A. V. Everitt and J. A. Burgess, eds.), Charles C. Thomas, Springfield, Illinois, pp. 157–170.

Ito, J. M., Valcana, T., and Timiras, P. S., 1977, Effect of hypo- and hyperthyroidism on regional monoamine metabolism in the adult brain, *Neuroendocrinology* **24:**55–64.

Kanungo, M. S., 1980, *Biochemistry of Aging,* Academic Press, New York.

Klug, T. L., and Adelman, R. C., 1979, Altered hypothalamic-pituitary regulation of thyrotropin in male rats during aging, *Endocrinology* **104:**1136–1142.

Kolata, G., 1982a, Molecular biology of brain hormones, *Science* **215:**1223–1224.

Kolata, G., 1982b, New theory of hormones proposed, *Science* **215:**1383–1384.

Landfield, P. W., Lindsey, J. D., and Lynch, G., 1978a, Apparent acceleration of brain aging pathology by prolonged administration of glucocorticoids, *Soc. Neurosci. Abst.* (Abst. No. 350) **4:**118.

Landfield, P. W., Waymire, J. C., and Lynch, G., 1978b, Hippocampal aging and adrenocorticoids: Quantitative correlations, *Science* **202:**1098–1102.

Makman, M. H., Gardner, E. L., Thal, L. J., Hirschhorn, I. D., Seeger, T. F., and Bhargava, G., 1980, Central monoamine receptor systems: Influence of aging, lesion and drug treatment, in: *Neural Regulatory Mechanisms During Aging* (R. C. Adelman, J. Roberts, G. T. Baker, III, S. I. Baskin, and V. J. Cristofalo, eds.), Alan R. Liss, New York, pp. 91–127.

Margarity, M., Veskoukis, M., Matoskis, N., Valcana, T., Miller, C., and Timiras, P. S., 1981, Changes with aging in serum thyroid hormone levels and thyroid hormone binding in brain tissue, The Endocrine Society, 63rd Annual Meeting, June 17–19, Cincinnati, Ohio, Abstract No. 1136, p. 366.

Martin, G. M., 1978, Genetic syndromes in man with potential relevance to the pathobiology of aging, in: *Genetic Effects on Aging* (D. Bergsma, D. E. Harrison, and N. W. Paul, eds.), Alan R. Liss, New York, pp. 5–39.

Masoro, E. J. (ed.), 1981, *CRC Series Handbook of Physiology in Aging,* CRC Press, Boca Raton, Florida.

Meek, J. L., Bertilsson, L., Cheney, D. L., Zsilla, C., and Costa, E., 1977, Aging-induced changes in acetylcholine and serotonin content of discrete brain nuclei, *J. Gerontol.* **32:**129–131.

Meites, J. (ed.), 1970, *Hypophysiotropic Hormones of the Hypothalamus,* Williams and Wilkins, Baltimore.

Meites, J., 1981, Changes in hypothalamic regulation of pituitary function in aging rats, in: *Brain Neurotransmitters and Receptors in Aging and Age Related Disorders, Aging,* Vol. 17 (S. J. Enna, T. Samorajski, and B. Beer, eds.), Raven Press, New York, pp. 117–132.

Meites, J., 1982, Changes in neuroendocrine control of anterior pituitary function during aging, *Neuroendocrinology* **34:**151–156.

Müller, E. E., Nistico, G., and Scapagnini, U. (eds.), 1977, *Neurotransmitters and Anterior Pituitary Function*, Academic Press, New York.

Naidoo, S., Valcana, T., and Timiras, P. S., 1978, Thyroid hormone receptors in the developing rat brain, *Am. Zool.* **18:**522–545.

Nelson, S. D., Mitchell, J. R., Dybing, E., and Sasame, H. A., 1976, Cytochrome P-450-mediated oxidation of 2-hydroxyestrogens to reactive intermediates, *Biochem. Biophys. Res. Commun.* **70:**1157–1165.

Nelson, J., Felicio, L., Sinha, Y. N., and Finch, C. E., 1980, Ovarian hormones and the etiology of reproductive aging in mice, in: *Aging—Its Chemistry* (A. A. Deitz, ed.), Am. Soc. Clin. Chemists., Washington, D.C., pp. 64–81.

Ordy, J. M., 1979, Geriatric psychopharmacology: Drug modification of memory and emotionality in relation to aging in human and non-human primate brain, in: *Brain Function in Old Age* (F. Hoffmeister and C. Muller, eds.), Springer-Verlag, Berlin, pp. 435–455.

Parsons, J. A., 1976, *Peptide Hormones*, Macmillan, New York.

Platt, J. E., Christopher, M. A., and Sullivan, C. A., 1978, The role of prolactin in blocking thyroxine-induced differentiation of tail tissue in larvae and neotenic Ambystoma tigrinum, *Gen. Comp. Endocrinol.* **35:**402–408.

Prange, A. J., Jr. (ed.), 1974, *The Thyroid Axis, Drugs, and Behavior*, Raven Press, New York.

Rebar, R. W., Miyake, A., Low, T. L. K., and Goldstein, A. L., 1981, Thymosin stimulates secretion of luteinizing hormone-releasing factor, *Science* **214:**669–671.

Reigle, G. D., 1973, Chronic stress effects on adrenocortical responsiveness in young and aged rats, *Neuroendocrinology* **11:**1–10.

Renoux, G., Biziere, K., Renoux, M., Gyenes, L., Degenne, P., Guillemin, J. M., Bardos, P., and Lebranchu, Y., 1980, Effects of the ablation of the left cerebral cortex on T-cell number and cell mediated responses in the mouse, *Int. J. Immunopharmacol.* **2:**156.

Roberts, E., 1981, A speculative consideration on the neurobiology and treatment of senile dementia, in: *Strategies for the Development of an Effective Treatment for Senile Dementia* (T. Crook and S. Gershon, eds.), Mark Powley Associates, New Canaan, Connecticut, pp. 247–320.

Rockstein, M., Sussman, M. L., and Chesky, J. (eds.), 1974, *Theoretical Aspects of Aging*, Academic Press, New York.

Roth, G. S., 1976, Reduced glucocorticoid binding site concentration in cortical neuronal perikarya from senescent rats, *Brain Res.* **107:**345–354.

Roth, J., LeRoith, D., Shiloach, J., Rosenzweig, J. L., Lesniak, M. A., and Havrankova, J., 1982, The evolutionary origins of hormones, neurotransmitters, and other extracellular chemical messengers: Implications for mammalian biology, *N. Engl. J. Med.* **306:**523–527.

Scapagnini, U., Canonico, P. L., Drago, F., Amico-Roxas, M., Toffano, G., Valeri, P., and Angelucci, L., 1980, Neuroendocrinology and aging of the brain, in: *The Aging Brain: Neurological and Mental Disturbances* (G. Barbagallo-Sangiorgi and A. N. Exton-Smith, eds.), Plenum Press, New York, pp. 33–49.

Schally, A. V., 1978, Aspects of hypothalamic regulation of the pituitary gland: Its implications for the control of reproductive processes, *Science* **202:**18–28.

Scharrer, E., and Scharrer, B., 1963, *Neuroendocrinology*, Columbia University Press, New York.

Schneider, E. L. (ed.), 1978, *The Genetics of Aging*, Plenum Press, New York.

Segall, P. E., 1979, Interrelations of dietary and hormonal effects in aging, *Mech. Ageing Dev.* **9:**515–525.

Segall, P. E., and Timiras, P. S., 1976, Pathophysiologic findings after chronic tryptophan deficiency in rats: A model for delayed growth and aging, *Mech. Ageing Dev.* **5:**109–124.

Segall, P. E., Ooka, H., Rose, K., and Timiras, P. S., 1978, Neural and endocrine development after chronic tryptophan deficiency in rats, I. Brain monoamine and pituitary responses, *Mech. Ageing Dev.* **7:**1–17.

Selye, H., 1950, *Stress—The Physiology and Pathology of Exposure to Stress*, Acta Inc. Medical Publishers, Montreal, Quebec.

Selye, H., 1974, *Stress Without Distress*, J. B. Lippincott, Philadelphia.

Shaar, C. J., Euker, J. S., Riegle, G. D., and Meites, J., 1975, Effects of castration and gonadal steroids on serum LH and prolactin in old and young rats, *J. Endocrinol.* **66:**45–51.

Snyder, S. H., 1980, Brain peptides as neurotransmitters, *Science* **209:**976–983.

Stein, M., Schiavi, R. C., and Camerino, M., 1976, Influence of brain and behavior on the immune system, *Science* **191:**435–440.

Strehler, B. L., 1977, *Time, Cells, and Aging*, 2nd Ed., Academic Press, New York.

Terry, R. D., 1980, Some biological aspects of the aging brain, *Mech. Ageing Dev.* **14:**191–201.

Terry, R. D., Bolis, C. L., and Toffano, G. (eds.), 1982, *Neural Aging and Its Implications in Human Neurological Pathology, Aging*, Vol. 18, Raven Press, New York.

Timiras, P. S., 1972, *Developmental Physiology and Aging*, Macmillan, New York.

Timiras, P. S., 1978, Biological perspectives of aging: In search of a master plan, *Am. Sci.* **66:**605–613.

Timiras, P. S., 1982a, Neuroendocrine theories of aging: Homeostasis and stress, in: *Hormones in Development and Aging* (A. Vernadakis and P. S. Timiras, eds.), SP Medical and Scientific Books, New York, pp. 551–586.

Timiras, P. S., 1982b, Physiology of aging: Aspects of neuroendocrine regulation, in: *Textbook of Geriatric Medicine* (M. S. J. Pathy, ed.), John Wiley and Sons, New York (in press).

Timiras, P. S., and Bignami, A., 1976, Pathophysiology of the aging brain, in: *Special Review of Exp. Aging Research Progress in Biology* (M. F. Elias, B. E. Eleftheriou, and P. K. Elias, eds.), EAR, Bar Harbor, Maine, pp. 351–378.

Timiras, P. S., and Hudson, D. B., 1980, Changes in neurohumoral transmission during aging of the central nervous system, in: *Neural Regulatory Mechanisms During Aging* (R. C. Adelman, J. Roberts, G. T. Baker, III, S. I. Baskin, and V. J. Cristofalo, eds.), Alan R. Liss, New York, pp. 25–51.

Toffano, G., Calderini, G., Battistella, A., Scapagnini, U., Gaiti, A., Ponzio, F., Algeri, S., and Crews, F., 1982, Biochemical changes related to neurotransmission in the aging brain, in: *Aging*, Vol. 18, *Neural Aging and Its Implications in Human Neurological Pathology*, (R. D. Terry, C. L. Bolis, and G. Toffano, eds.), Raven Press, New York, pp. 119–128.

Vaccari, A., and Timiras, P. S., 1981, Alterations in brain dopaminergic receptors in developing hypo- and hyperthyroid rats, *Neurochem. Int.* **3:**149–153.

Vaccari, A., Valcana, T., and Timiras, P. S., 1977, Effects of hypothyroidism on the enzymes for biogenic amines in the developing rat brain, *Pharmacol. Res. Commun.* **9:**763–780.

Valcana, T., 1979, The role of triiodothyronine (T3) receptors in brain development, in: *Neural Growth and Differentiation* (E. Meisami and M. A. B. Brazier, eds.), Raven Press, New York, pp. 39–57.

Valcana, T., and Timiras, P. S., 1978, Nuclear triiodothyronine receptors in the developing rat brain, *Mol. Cell. Endocrinol.* **2**:31–41.

Valcana, T., and Timiras, P. S., 1979, Changes in rat liver nuclear triiodothyronine receptors with age and thyroid activity, in: *Hormones and Development* (L. Macho and J. Strbak, eds.), Slovak Academy of Sciences, Bratislava, pp. 47–75.

Vernadakis, A., and Timiras, P. S. (eds.), 1982, *Hormones in Development and Aging,* SP Medical and Scientific Books, New York.

Walker, R. F., and Timiras, P. S., 1980, Loss of serotonin circadian rhythms in the pineal gland of androgenized female rats, *Neuroendocrinology* **31**:265–269.

Walker, R. F., and Timiras, P. S., 1981, Serotonin in development of cyclic reproductive function, in: *Advances in Experimental Biology and Medicine,* Vol. 133 *Serotonin: Current Aspects of Neurochemistry and Function,* (B. Haber, S. Gabay, M. R. Issidorides, and S. G. A. Alivisatos, eds.), Plenum Press, New York, pp. 515–539.

Walker, R. F., and Timiras, P. S., 1982, Pacemaker insufficiency and the onset of aging, in: *Cellular Pacemakers,* Vol. 2 (P. Carpenter, ed.), Wiley Interscience, New York, pp. 396–425.

Walker, R. F., Cooper, R. L., and Timiras, P. S., 1980, Constant estrus: Role of rostral hypothalamic monoamines in development of reproductive dysfunction in aging rats, *Endocrinology* **107**:249–255.

Yarbrough, G. G., 1976, TRH potentiates excitatory actions of acetylcholine on cerebral cortical neurons, *Nature* **263**:523–524.

CHAPTER 3

Morphological Changes in the Hypothalamus and Other Brain Areas Influencing Endocrine Function during Aging

JAMES A. CLEMENS

1. Introduction

Morphological alterations or nerve cell loss in neuroendocrine regulatory areas represent a convenient explanation for the demise of neuroendocrine function which accompanies aging. Biochemical evidence and lesion experiments support the idea that morphological changes in the brain may be responsible for the age-related changes in estrous cycles and hormone secretory patterns. In addition, the feedback of target organ hormones has been proposed to accelerate neuronal degeneration in neuroendocrine regulatory areas. However, while several lines of evidence are suggestive of the occurrence of morphological changes in neuroendocrine regulatory areas with aging, little neuroanatomical data is presently available to support the existence of such changes. The purpose of this chapter is to rcview the available evidence for morphological changes in brain areas influencing endocrine function.

2. Nerve Cell Loss

Cell loss in the central nervous system (CNS) during aging is well documented. However, to imply that cell loss occurs throughout the

JAMES A. CLEMENS • Lilly Research Laboratories, Eli Lilly and Company, Indianapolis, Indiana 46285.

brain is incorrect, because neuronal decreases occur only in certain areas. Morphological studies have shown age-related cell loss from the cerebral cortex of man (Henderson *et al.*, 1975), rhesus monkey (Brizzee *et al.*, 1976), and the rat (Brizzee, 1973). Purkinje cells are lost from the cerebellum (Hall *et al.*, 1975), and dopamine neurons are lost from the substantia nigra (McGeer *et al.*, 1977). A dramatic drop in number of neurons was found in the human visual cortex during aging (Devaney and Johnson, 1980). The decrease in neuron population density was as great as 50%. Although the neuronal cell loss in the areas mentioned probably has little impact on neuroendocrine aging, it serves to demonstrate that loss of neurons does occur in several different brain areas. In addition to neuronal cell loss, neuronal perikaryon size and shape changes occur with aging (Shulz and Hunziker, 1980).

Neuronal cell loss has also been reported in brain areas that are involved in neuroendocrine control mechanisms. However, a certain degree of caution must be used when interpreting these studies. The degree of cell loss or whether or not any cell loss occurs with aging seems to depend on the species studied, and within the species loss varies. Hsu and Peng (1978) found age-related changes in neuron numbers in the medial preoptic, anterior hypothalamic, and arcuate nuclei in rats. Their findings are of great interest, because the decline in the hypothalamo-pituitary-ovarian axis could be explained by alterations in these areas. Sabel and Stein (1981) have reported a marked loss of neurons in a number of different subcortical regions such as the ventromedial and lateral hypothalamic nuclei, the substantia nigra, the septum, reticular formation, and regions of the amygdala in the aged rat. In addition to cell loss, neuronal shrinkage was observed. In contrast, Lamperti and Blaha (1980) reported that no difference exists in the number of neurons in hypothalamic nuclei of young vs. reproductively senescent female golden hamsters; however, the oldest animals in their study were 15–18 months old. Others have reported that most brainstem nuclei appear to maintain stable neuronal populations with age (Brody and Vijaya-shanker, 1977).

The hypothalamus receives massive afferent tracts from various limbic structures, some of which show significant age-related changes. The modulation of endocrine function by limbic structures has been established (Carrillo *et al.*, 1977). The hippocampus exhibits decreased neuronal density during aging in humans (Ball, 1977), monkeys (Brizzee *et al.*, 1980), and rats (Landfield *et al.*, 1981). The hippocampal pyramidal cells appear to be most affected by the aging process. Loss of hippocampal neurons may influence some of the rhythmic neuroendocrine processes.

The hypothalamus receives its noradrenergic input from brainstem structures. An abundance of evidence exists supporting the view that norepinephrine neurons are stimulatory to the release of LH (Sawyer *et al.*, 1978; Clifton and Sawyer, 1979). The locus coeruleus has been identified as an important source of forebrain norepinephrine (Palkovitz *et al.*, 1980). The locus coeruleus in the human has been reported to show cell loss with aging (Vijayashankar and Brody, 1979). However, in the rat locus coeruleus no cell loss could be found (Goldman and Coleman, 1981). The source of the forebrain norepinephrine neurons that regulate LH release is not clear, but some evidence exists that the locus coeruleus may not be the source (Hancke and Wuttke, 1979).

In summary, not enough evidence is available to generalize that nerve cell loss is a primary factor that contributes to the senescence of the neuroendocrine system in all species. In addition, it is difficult to ascertain the functional significance of small amounts of neuronal loss. For example, a greater than 90% destruction of dopamine nerve terminals in the striatum is needed in order to produce a supersensitivity or contralateral turning behavior after dopamine agonists (Heikkila *et al.*, 1981). As a result of the vast number of studies utilizing electrolytic brain lesions or hypothalamic deafferentations, it is common knowledge that many animals with significant but incomplete lesions or cuts appear no different from controls. Further definitive studies of cell loss as a cause of neuroendocrine dysfunction are needed.

3. Other Morphological Changes

While cell loss alone may or may not contribute significantly to the age-related changes in the endocrine system, a multitude of other slow, progressive, insidious changes are occurring, that when viewed together, could easily account for the observed functional alterations. The elegant Golgi studies of Machado-Salas *et al.* (1977) demonstrated that there was a progressive disruption of hypothalamic architecture in mice, paralleled by deterioration and loss of dendritic surface in most areas involved with neuroendocrine control. They reported a high incidence of neuropathology in the anterior hypothalamus and especially in the preoptic area. In the suprachiasmatic nucleus there was somatic distortion, swelling of dendritic stalks, and decreased dendritic arborization. A similar spectrum of change was found in all neurosecretory nuclei.

Similar changes have been described in other brain areas. Scheibel (1979) reported a loss of dendritic spines, swelling of cell bodies and dendrite complexes, and progressive destruction of the dendritic domain with aging in the hippocampus. Other studies have demonstrated synaptic atrophy in the hippocampus (Bondareff, 1979) and loss of axosomatic synapses in the dentate gyrus of rats (Geinisman, 1979). Not only is there dendritic atrophy and a loss of synapses with aging, but the brain tends to lose its ability to form new synapses (Cotman and Scheff, 1979).

In summary, neuronal cell loss in areas regulating neuroendocrine processes may not be great, but neuronal connections in several areas are lost. In essence, the neurons become "deafferented" to a great extent and become incapable of responding appropriately to stimuli provided by external sources, hormones, or other neurons.

4. Hormones as Causative Factors in the Neuronal Degenerative Processes

A growing body of evidence is gradually implicating steroid hormones as being causative factors in the neuronal degenerative processes in certain brain areas. Several brain areas may be involved.

4.1. Estrogens, Prolactin, and the Arcuate Nucleus

Administration of estrogens to young cycling female rats induces neuronal degeneration with astrocytic and microglial hyperactivity in the hypothalamic arcuate nucleus (Brawer et al., 1978, 1980a). The arcuate degeneration appeared to be associated with a reduction in the LH surge after stimulation of the preoptic area (Brawer et al., 1980b). Schipper et al. (1981) reported that gliosis occurs spontaneously in the aging arcuate nucleus and its development is primarily dependent on estradiol. Ovariectomy at two months of age significantly suppressed gliosis in old female rats and mice. Thus, assuming that gliosis is an accurate index of neuronal degeneration, it would appear that the continuous exposure of the brain to estrogens (or perhaps to other steroids as well) results in degeneration of the arcuate nucleus of the hypothalamus.

Casanueva et al. (1982) reported that chronic estradiol valerate treatment caused lesions in the arcuate nucleus and also produced extremely high serum prolactin levels. Measurement of dopamine in the median eminence showed the presence of progressively decreasing dopamine levels. Since such high prolactin levels are obtained after estradiol treatment, perhaps prolactin may have participated in the neurotoxic action of estradiol.

4.2. Glucocorticoids and the Hippocampus

In a similar system Landfield *et al.* (1978) reported that long-term adrenalectomy significantly reduced age-related glial activity in the rat hippocampus. Conversely, the pathological changes in the hippocampus were enhanced in rats receiving corticosterone. Interestingly, Landfield *et al.* (1981) reported that the aging changes in the hippocampus could be antagonized by chronic treatment with ACTH (4–9) and by pentylenetetrazole. In support of Landfield's adrenocortical hypothesis of hippocampal aging, Cotman and Scheff (1979) found that hydrocortisone administration inhibited formation of new synapses in the hippocampus after partial denervation.

The arcuate nucleus and hippocampus both have high concentrations of steroid receptors, and it may be attractive to conclude that only areas with steroid receptors will be sensitive to the neurotoxic effects of the steroids. However, this has not yet been established.

4.3. Estrogens, Prolactin, and Nigrostriatal Neurons

Estrogens and prolactin seem to be involved in some manner with the development of dopaminergic supersensitivity after neuroleptic treatment. Hruska and Silbergeld (1980) reported that estradiol increased dopamine receptor supersensitivity after chronic haloperidol treatment. Furthermore, they attributed the formation of neuroleptic-induced dopamine receptor supersensitivity to the high prolactin levels that result from estradiol treatment (Hruska *et al.*, 1980). Tardive dyskinesia results from chronic neuroleptic treatment and may be due to supersensitive dopamine receptors. Since this condition becomes permanent, the causative factors (prolactin, neuroleptics) must have induced some pathological change.

In contrast, Gordon *et al.* (1980) reported that estradiol reduces the ability of haloperidol to produce a dopamine receptor supersensitivity. Also, the lack of tardive dyskinesia or other motor impairments in patients with chronic hyperprolactinemia casts doubt on the hypothesis that prolactin is involved in modification of striatal dopaminergic function. This area needs further clarification.

5. Brain Lesions That Mimic Age-Related Changes

An additional line of evidence that is supportive of the hypothesis that pathological alterations in the CNS lead to the neuroendocrine dysfunction associated with aging is the work done with brain lesions. All of the abnormal secretory patterns of hormones encountered in the old rat can be duplicated in the young adult rat by placement of specific brain lesions. For example, Clemens and Bennett (1977) induced repeated pseudopregnancies in young rats by placing electrolytic lesions in the medial preoptic area. Constant vaginal estrus was observed when the lesions extended into the anterior hypothalamic area or suprachiasmatic nucleus.

Perhaps the irregular, repeated pseudopregnancies observed in many old rats are due to an age-related morphological alteration in the preoptic area. The A14 group of dopamine neurons might be involved because the dopamine agonist, lergotrile mesylate, was found to induce normal estrous cycles in both the young rats with medial preoptic area lesions and in the 2-year-old rats.

When the anterior connections to the hypothalamus are severed, rats enter a state of constant estrus (Halasz and Gorski, 1967). Constant estrus is also produced in rats with damage to the anterior hypothalamic area or suprachiasmatic nucleus. Rats with suprachiasmatic lesions resemble old constant estrous rats in many ways. Estrous cycles and ovulation can be reinstated in both groups (Clemens *et al.*, 1969; Barraclough, 1963) by treatment with progesterone. Thus, since discrete brain lesions can produce, in young rats, endocrine alterations similar to those observed in senile rats, the hypothesis that the endocrine disturbances that occur during aging result from alterations in brain function seems reasonable.

6. Biochemical Evidence for Age-Induced Morphological Changes

Biochemical changes with aging such as changes in transmitters, receptors, and hormones will not be elaborated upon here, because they are dealt with in detail in other chapters of this volume. It is important to mention, however, that the alterations in neurotransmitter concentrations and turnover, and the changes in receptors that have been reported with advancing age are additional although indirect supportive evidence for the occurrence of morphological alterations. A decrease in receptors and neurotransmitter levels in certain areas is highly compatible with a loss of dendrites and synapses.

7. General Summary

Morphological alterations as a result of aging do occur in areas concerned with neuroendocrine regulation. Cell loss appears not to be very significant in neuroendocrine regulatory areas. However, when cell loss is combined with the loss of dendrites and synapses, and possible damage resulting from the action of steroid hormones, the total amount of pathological alterations in the neuroendocrine regulatory areas of the aging brain may be substantial.

8. References

Ball, M. J., 1977, Neuronal loss, neurofibrillary tangles and granulovacuolar degeneration in the hippocampus with aging and dementia: A quantitative study, *Acta Neuropathol.* **37**:111–121.

Barraclough, C. A., 1963, Secretion and release of LH and FSH: Discussion, in: *Advances in Neuroendocrinology* (A. V. Nalbandov, ed.), University of Illinois Press, Urbana, pp. 224–233.

Bondareff, W., 1979, Synaptic atrophy in the senescent hippocampus, *Mech. Ageing Dev.* **9**:163–171.

Brawer, J. R., Naftolin, F., Martin, J., Sonnenschein, C., 1978, Effects of a single injection of estradiol valerate on the hypothalamic arcuate nucleus and on reproductive function in the female rat, *Endocrinology* **103**:501–512.

Brawer, J. R., Ruf, K. B., and Naftolin, F., 1980a, The effects of estradiol-induced lesions of the arcuate nucleus on gonadotropin release in response to preoptic stimulation in the rat, *Neuroendocrinology* **30**:144–149.

Brawer, J. R., Schipper, H., and Naftolin, F., 1980b, Ovary-dependent degeneration in the hypothalamic arcuate nucleus, *Endocrinology* **107**:274–279.

Brizzee, K. R., 1973, Quantitative histological studies on aging changes in cerebral cortex of rhesus monkey and albino rat with notes on effects of prolonged low-dose ionizing irradiation in the rat, *Prog. Brain Res.* **40**:141–160.

Brizzee, K. R., Ordy, J. M., Hansche, J., and Kaack, B., 1976, Quantitative assessment of changes in neuron and glia cell packing density and lipofuscin accumulation with age in the cerebral cortex of a non-human primate (Macaca mulatta), in: *Aging: Neurobiology of Aging* (R. D. Terry and S. Gershon, eds.), Raven Press, New York, pp. 229–244.

Brizzee, K. R., Ordy, J. M., and Bartus, R. T., 1980, Localization of cellular changes within multimodal sensory regions in aged monkey brain: Possible implications for age-related cognitive loss, *Neurobiol. Aging* **1**:45–52.

Brody, H., and Vijayashankar, N., 1977, Anatomical changes in the nervous system, in: *Handbook of the Biology of Aging* (C. E. Finch and L. Hayflick, eds.), Van Nostrand-Reinhold, New York, pp. 241–254.

Carrillo, A. J., Rabii, J., Carrer, H. F., and Sawyer, C. H., 1977, Modulation of the proestrous surge of luteinizing hormone by electrochemical stimulation of the amygdala and hippocampus in the unanesthetized rat, *Brain Res.* **128:**81–92.

Casanueva, F., Cocchi, D., Locatelli, V., Flauto, C., Zambotti, F., Bestetti, G., Rossi, G. L., and Mueller, E., 1982, Defective central nervous system dopaminergic function in rats with estrogen-induced pituitary tumors, as assessed by plasma prolactin concentrations, *Endocrinology* **110:**590–599.

Clemens, J. A., and Bennett, D. R., 1977, Do aging changes in the preoptic area contribute to loss of cyclic endocrine function? *J. Gerontol.* **32:**19–24.

Clemens, J. A., Amenomori, Y., Jenkins, T., and Meites, J., 1969, Effects of hypothalamic stimulation, hormones, and drugs on ovarian function in old female rats, *Proc. Soc. Exp. Biol. Med.* **132:**561–563.

Clifton, D. H., and Sawyer, C. H., 1979, LH release and ovulation in the rat following depletion of hypothalamic norepinephrine: Chronic vs. acute effects, *Neuroendocrinology* **28:**442–449.

Cotman, C. W., and Scheff, S. W., 1979, Synaptic growth in aged animals. in: *Physiology and Cell Biology of Aging* (A. Cherkin, ed.), Raven Press, New York, pp. 109–120.

Devaney, K. O., and Johnson, H. A., 1980, Neuron loss in the aging visual cortex of man, *J. Gerontol.* **35:**836–841.

Geinisman, Y., 1979, Loss of axosomatic synapses in the dentate gyrus of aged rats, *Brain Res.* **168:**485–492.

Goldman, G., and Coleman, P. D., 1981, Neuron numbers in locus coeruleus do not change with age in Fischer 344 rat, *Neurobiol. Aging* **2:**33–36.

Gordon, J. H., Borison, R. K., and Diamond, B. I., 1980, Modulation of dopamine receptor sensitivity by estrogen, *Biol. Psychiat.* **15:**389–396.

Halasz, B., and Gorski, R., 1967, Gonadotropic hormone secretion in female rats after partial or total interruption of neural afferents to the medial basal hypothalamus, *Endocrinology* **80:**608–622.

Hall, T. C., Miller, A. K. H., and Corsellis, J. A. N., 1975, Variations in the human purkinje cell population according to age and sex, *Neuropathol. Appl. Neurobiol.* **1:**267–292.

Hancke, J. L., and Wuttke, W., 1979, Effects of chemical lesions of the ventral noradrenergic bundle or of the medial preoptic area on preovulatory LH release in rats, *Exp. Brain Res.* **35:**127–134.

Heikkila, R. E., Shapiro, B. S., and Duvoisin, R. C., 1981, The relationship between loss of dopamine nerve terminals, striatal [^{3}H]spiroperidol binding and rotational behavior in unilaterally 6-hydroxy-dopamine-lesioned rats, *Brain Res.* **211:**285–292.

Henderson, G., Tomlinson, B. E., and Weightman, D., 1975, Cell counts in the human cerebral cortex using a traditional and an automatic method, *J. Neurol. Sci.* **25:**129–144.

Hruska, R. E., and Silbergeld, E. K., 1980, Increased dopamine receptor supersensitivity after estrogen treatment using the rat rotation model, *Science* **208:**1466–1468.

Hruska, R. E., Ludmer, L. M., and Silbergeld, E. K., 1980, Hypophysectomy prevents the striatal dopamine receptor supersensitivity produced by chronic haloperidol treatment, *Eur. J. Pharmacol.* **65:**455–456.

Hsu, H. K., and Peng, M. T., 1978, Hypothalamic neuron number of old female rats, *Gerontologist* **24:**434–440.

Lamperti, A., and Blaha, G., 1980, The numbers of neurons in the hypothalamic nuclei of young and reproductively senescent female golden hamsters, *J. Gerontol.* **35:**335–338.

Landfield, P. W., Waymire, J. C., and Lynch, G., 1978, Hippocampal aging and adrenocorticoids: Quantitative correlations, *Science* **202:**1098–1102.

Landfield, P. W., Baskin, R. K., and Pitler, T. A., 1981, Brain aging correlates: Retardation by hormonal-pharmacological treatments, *Science* **214:**581–584.

Machado-Salas, J., Scheibel, M. E., and Scheibel, A. B., 1977, Morphologic changes in the hypothalamus of the old mouse, *Exp. Neurol.* **57:**102–111.

McGeer, P. L., McGeer, E. G., and Suzuki, J. S., 1977, Aging and extrapyramidal function, *Arch. Neurol.* **34:**33–35.

Palkovitz, M. L., Zaborsky, L., Feminger, A., Mezey, E., Fekete, M. I. K., Herman, J. P., Kanyicska, B., and Szabo, D., 1980, Noradrenergic innervation of the hypothalamus: Experimental biochemical and electron microscopic studies, *Brain Res.* **191:**161–171.

Sabel, B. A., and Stein, D. G., 1981, Extensive loss of subcortical neurons in the aging rat brain, *Exp. Neurol.* **73:**507–516.

Sawyer, C. H., Radford, H. M., Krieg, R. J., and Carter, H. F., 1978, Control of pituitary-ovarian function by brain catecholamines and LH-releasing hormone, in: *Brain-Endocrine Interaction III, Neural Hormones and Reproduction*, 3rd International Symposium, Karger, Basel, pp. 263–273.

Scheibel, A. B., 1979, Organizational patterns in health and senescence, *Mech. Ageing Dev.* **9:**89–102.

Schipper, H., Brawer, J. R., Nelson, J. F., Felicio, L. S., and Finch, C. E., 1981, Role of the gonads in the histologic aging of the hypothalamic arcuate nucleus, *Biol. Reprod.* **25:**413–419.

Shulz, V., Hunziker, O., 1980, Comparative studies of neuronal perikaryon size and shape in the aging cerebral cortex, *J. Gerontol.* **35:**483–491.

Vijayashankar, N., and Brody, H., 1979, A quantitative study of the pigmented neurons in the locus coeruleus and subcoeruleus in man as related to aging, *J. Neuropathol. Exp. Neurol.* **38:**490–496.

CHAPTER 4

Changes in Hypothalamic Hypophysiotropic Hormones and Neurotransmitters during Aging

JAMES W. SIMPKINS

1. Introduction

It is well established that the central nervous system (CNS) regulates anterior pituitary (AP) function by the production of releasing hormones and release-inhibiting hormones from specialized neurosecretory cells in the hypothalamus. These neurohormones are secreted into the vicinity of the primary capillary plexus of the portal vascular system for delivery to the AP. These secretory neurons are, in turn, under the regulatory influence of afferent neuronal inputs to the hypothalamus and from peripheral hormones secreted by AP hormone target tissues.

The important role played by trophic hormones in homeostatic processes places the AP and its regulatory mechanism in a critical position in the hierarchy of the aging process. Indeed, several investigators have suggested that the neuroendocrine system is primarily responsible for the age-related decline in homeostatic capacity and perhaps for the aging of organisms (Dilman, 1971; Everitt, 1980). However, while the neuroendocrine system remains a primary focus of students of aging, there is at present insufficient evidence to establish a heirarchy of the aging process. Rather than attempt to support the plethora of theories as to the ultimate cause of the aging process, a more fruitful endeavor is to delineate the consequences of increasing age on the components of the CNS which influence AP function. In the present report we will attempt

JAMES W. SIMPKINS • Department of Pharmaceutical Biology, College of Pharmacy, University of Florida, Gainesville, Florida 32610.

to describe and evaluate the effects of increasing age on the function of neuronal systems, particularly hypothalamic afferents, which are critical to the regulation of AP hormone secretion.

While many brain substances have been classified as neurotransmitters and/or neuromodulators (Cooper *et al.*, 1978), relatively few have been studied in sufficient detail in the aging animal to warrant consideration here. Among these neuronal systems, primary consideration will be given to dopaminergic, noradrenergic, serotonergic, and opioid pathways for several reasons. First, each of these systems resides in or sends extensive terminal fields to the hypothalamus and associated ventral diencephalon. Second, these neuronal systems have been extensively studied in young animals and to a lesser extent in senescent animals. And finally, the evidence for a physiological role in AP hormone secretion has been documented for each of these neuronal systems.

2. Aging of Dopaminergic Neurons

The dopaminergic innervation of the hypothalamus appears to arise from multiple groups of dopaminergic perikarya located in several brain regions. Cell bodies of the tuberoinfundibular dopamine (TIDA) system originate in the arcuate nucleus (NA) and ventral periventricular nucleus (PVN) and provide the dopaminergic innervation of the external layer of the median eminence (ME) (Hökfelt and Fuxe, 1972a; Bjorklund *et al.*, 1973). A second component of this TIDA system innervates the infundibular stalk and the intermediary and posterior lobes of the pituitary (Bjorklund *et al.*, 1973). Since it is estimated that only 20% of the dopamine (DA) in the ME originates from the TIDA system (Moore and Bloom, 1978; Bjorklund *et al.*, 1973), terminal input to this region from the nigrostriatal (Kizer *et al.*, 1976) and incertohypothalamic (Bjorklund *et al.*, 1975) dopaminergic systems may be of considerable importance. The incertohypothalamic DA (IHDA) system has cell bodies in the zona incerta, candal hypothalamus, and PVN with nerve terminals primarily in the medial preoptic area, anterior hypothalamus, and dorsal medial hypothalamic nuclei, although projections of this system to the ME have been described (Bjorklund *et al.*, 1975). Finally, the periventricular DA (PVDA) system appears to innervate the ventral medial and dorsal medial nuclei of the hypothalamus from cell bodies in the periaquaductal gray and periventricular regions of the brain (Kizer *et al.*, 1976).

Thus, in the hypothalamus and its closely associated preoptic area, several neuronal systems contribute to the dopaminergic nerve terminal field. This heterologous dopaminergic input into several regions of the ventral diencephalon, while indicating the complexity of the DA neuronal function in the hypothalamus, may provide a partial explanation for the apparent differential rate of age-related alteration in hypothalamic dopaminergic activity considered below.

The most frequently and consistently observed age-related changes in DA concentrations occur in the ME of the medial basal hypothalamus (MBH), in the neurointermediary lobes of the pituitary and in the striatum. By two years of age, a 25–40% decline in hypothalamic DA concentrations is observed in male rats (Estes and Simpkins, 1980; Demarest et al., 1980; Wilkes et al., 1979), female rats (Estes and Simpkins, 1981, 1982; Demarest et al., 1981) and male C57BL/6J mice (Finch, 1973). A decline of similar magnitude has been described for the MBH of two-year-old rats (Simpkins et al., 1977) and ME of male mice (Finch, 1979). Histofluorescence studies have revealed DA loss from nerve terminals in the ME (Hoffman and Sladek, 1980) and reductions of DA concentrations in portal blood (Gudelsky et al., 1981) in two-year-old male rats. This latter observation strongly suggests that the decline in ME DA concentration observed in old male rats is of significance since considerably less DA reaches the AP gland.

Interestingly, while ME DA concentrations are substantially decreased, DA levels in the arcuate nucleus showed a modest decline in male rats (Estes and Simpkins, 1980) and did not change substantially through two years of age in female rats (Estes and Simpkins, 1981). The maintenance of NA DA levels, in the face of decreasing ME DA, appears to be the result of DA accumulation in NA cell bodies. In young animals, the DA is transported to terminals in the ME (Hoffman and Sladek, 1980).

In other nuclei of the MBH, DA is decreased by 50% in old male and female rats in the area retrochiasmatica (ARC; Estes and Simpkins, 1980, 1981), by 50% in suprachiasmatic nucleus (Estes and Simpkins, 1981), and by 25–40% in the TIDA projection to the neurointermediary lobes of the pituitary (Demarest et al., 1980, 1981; Estes and Simpkins, 1981).

Of the ventral diencephalonic areas innervated by the IHDA system, only the preoptic area medialis (POAm) and anterior hypothalamic nucleus (AH) have been examined for age-related alterations. In male rats, the POAm and AH show dramatic increases in DA concentrations with age (Estes and Simpkins, 1980), while in the female rats, few age-related alterations are observed (Estes and Simpkins, 1981). Although the cause of these sex-related differences in the effects of age on IHDA nerve terminals are not known, Masuoka et al., (1979) have observed intensely fluorescing catecholamine accumulation in old male mice in the same region in which we have observed DA accumulation with age in male rats. Thus, DA accumulation in the rostral diencephalon of old male rats may represent axonal catecholamines storage subsequent to the degeneration of nerve terminals.

Recently, Steger *et al.* (1980a,b) demonstrated that in the white-footed mouse, hypothalamic DA concentrations remain unchanged through 48 months of age. This strain of mouse has a mean lifespan which is greater than that of the laboratory mouse (Sacher and Hart, 1978) and maintains reproductive capacity until late in life. Thus, the maintenance of reproductive capacity and long life is associated with the maintenance of normal brain catecholamine levels. This concept is consistent with the observation that dietary supplementation of the catecholamine (CA) precursor L-dopa in rats (Clemens *et al.*, 1979) significantly increases mean lifespan.

Tyrosine hydroxylase, the rate-limiting enzyme in catecholamine biosynthesis, exhibits decreased activity with increasing age, in the substantia nigra, putamen, and caudate nucleus in non-parkinsonian patients (Ordy *et al.*, 1975; Cote and Kremzner, 1975) and rats (McGeer *et al.*, 1971; Reis *et al.*, 1977), but not in CB6F1 mice (Reis *et al.*, 1977).

A significant decline in DA turnover has been demonstrated in the whole hypothalamus of the male rat and mouse (Finch, 1973; Ponzio *et al.*, 1978), the MBH and ME of the male rat (Simpkins *et al.*, 1977; Demarest *et al.*, 1980), and ME of the constant estrous female rat (Demarest *et al.*, 1981). In contrast, in the old repeated pseudopregnant (PP) female rat, while DA turnover is decreased in the NA and in several POA nuclei, DA turnover is accelerated in the ventromedial hypothalamic nucleus (NVM) and in the ME (Estes and Simpkins, 1981).

While the complex differential response of central dopaminergic neurons to increasing age does not permit simple conclusions as to the cause or effect of the observed alterations, several important concepts emerge from the studies. First, the multiple DA inputs to the hypothalamus and POA likely contribute to the differential rate at which subpopulation of dopaminergic neurons age. Second, in male rats and constant estrous female rats, for which a decline in ME DA concentrations and turnover rates has been clearly documented, the commonly observed age-related elevation in serum prolactin concentrations is likely a direct consequence of the dysfunction in this TIDA system (for Review see Meites *et al.*, 1978). However, in the PP female rat, which we have extensively studied (Estes and Simpkins, 1981), accelerated DA turnover in the TIDA system is associated with the hyperprolactinemia of aging. In view of the extensive literature which has shown that elevation in serum prolactin enhances the turnover of TIDA neurons (Hökfelt and

Fuxe, 1972b; Olson *et al.*, 1972; Gudelsky *et al.*, 1976; Hohn and Wuttke, 1978; Selmonoff, 1981; Kalra *et al.*, 1981; Annunziato and Moore, 1978; Perkins *et al.*, 1979; Morgan and Herbert, 1980), it would appear that in the PP rat, alterations in DA metabolism which accompany increasing age are a consequence of, rather than the cause of the hyperprolactinemic state.

Relevant to this latter point is the possibility that for dopaminergic neurons in general, age-related alterations in serum hormone levels may contribute to their rate of aging. All four major central dopaminergic neuronal systems have now been shown to respond to elevated serum prolactin concentrations (Hökfelt and Fuxe, 1972b; Perkins and Westfall, 1978; Fuxe *et al.*, 1977; Kalra *et al.*, 1981). Further, chronic elevations in serum prolactin levels in young animals cause depletion of MBH and POA DA concentrations which are remarkably similar to those observed in senescent rats (Simpkins *et al.*, 1982). Thus, it is possible that the chronic hyperprolactinemia of old rats, by virtue of persistent stimulation of central DA neurons, causes their age-related dysfunction. Consistent with this proposal is the recent observation that in several brain regions (including the ME) of the PP Fischer 344 rat, a decline in DA concentration is associated with enhanced DA turnover (Estes and Simpkins, 1981). In these PP Fischer 344 rats, normal estrous cycles are maintained until late in life whereupon animals enter a PP state (Saiduddin and Zassenhaus, 1979; Estes and Simpkins, 1981). Thus, hyperprolactinemia has a late onset in these old PP rats. In contrast, in male rats (Sakensa and Lau, 1979) and constant estrous female rats (Everett, 1939; Huang *et al.*, 1976a), chronically elevated serum prolactin is established relatively early in life and presumably, as a consequence, dopaminergic neuronal function is more severely affected by age.

3. Aging of Noradrenergic Neurons

The noradrenergic innervation of the hypothalamus and POA is from perikarya located in the locus coerulius (LC) and subcoerulial areas of the midbrain. The LC projections to the hypothalamus travel as part of the dorsal noradrenergic bundle and terminate largely in the peri- and paraventricular nuclei of the hypothalamus. The noradrenergic component of the remaining hypothalamic and POA nuclei arises from subcoerulial areas and travels rostrally via the ventral noradrenergic bundle (see Moore and Bloom, 1979 for review).

Norepinephrine (NE) levels have been reported to decrease with increasing age in the hypothalamus and hindbrain of human and nonhuman primates (Robinson *et al.*, 1972; Samorajski, 1975), the rat hypothalamus (Miller *et al.*, 1976; Simpkins *et al.*, 1977; Huang *et al.*, 1977), and the MBH of rats (Simpkins *et al.*, 1977). In microdissected regions of the ventral diencephalon, NE concentrations are reduced by 20–30% in the ME, NA, and POAm of old male rats (Estes and Simpkins, 1980; Wilkes *et al.*, 1979), and by 40–70% in several hypothalamic regions of female rats including the NA, AH, ARC, and suprachiasmatic nucleus (SCN). Thus, in discrete regions located along the extent of the preoptico-tuberal pathway, a significant decline in NE levels occurs in old rats. In contrast to these alterations in NE concentrations in man, monkeys, and rats, NE concentrations appear to be very stable in brain regions of old male mice (Samorajski *et al.*, 1971; Finch, 1973, 1979; Steger *et al.*, 1980a,b).

In both the mouse and rat, NE turnover is substantially decreased in senescent animals (Finch, 1973; Simpkins *et al.*, 1977; Ponzio *et al.*, 1978; Huang *et al.*, 1977; Estes and Simpkins, 1982). Further, the normally observed acceleration in NE turnover induced by ovariectomy is absent in the old constant estrous rat (Huang *et al.*, 1977). In the rat, but not the mouse, dopamine-β-hydroxylase activity is decreased with advanced age (Reis *et al.*, 1977).

Evaluation of regional alterations in NE turnover revealed that of six hypothalamic nuclei which showed an age-related decline in NE concentration, five of these regions exhibited extremely high NE turnover in middle-aged animals (Estes and Simpkins, 1981). Further, in nuclei which showed stable NE concentrations with increasing age, no preceding hyperactivity of noradrenergic neurons was observed in middle-aged rats. These data suggest that the loss of noradrenergic function in senescent rats may be subsequent to a period of excessive NE hyperactivity and subsequent neuronal exhaustion. This exhaustion hypothesis is consistent with the observation that overstimulation of neurons with glutamic acid analogues lead to the destruction of neurons with glutamate receptors (Kizer *et al.*, 1978). Whether this phenomena applies to strains of rats other than Fischer 344 strain and to other species, remains to be documented.

While the decline in NE activity in senescent animals is likely to contribute to the age-related decline in the efficiency of numerous autonomic control mechanisms, its involvement in the impairment of the secretion of several AP trophic hormones is likely profound. For example, the loss of cyclic preovulatory surges of LH and the attenuated postcastration gonadotropin secretion are probably direct consequences of the age-related decline in NE neuronal activity (Sharr *et al.*, 1975;

Huang *et al.*, 1976b, 1978, 1980a; Howland, 1976; Lu *et al.*, 1977, 1980, 1981; Peluso *et al.*, 1977; Estes *et al.*, 1980; Wilkes and Yen, 1981). Also, the diminution in episodic growth hormone secretion (Sonntag *et al.*, 1980) may be a consequence of the effects of age on NE function.

4. Aging of Serotonergic Neurons

Two groups of serotonergic perikarya are found in the central nervous system. The primary serotonergic cell bodies are located in the dorsal and ventral raphé nuclei of the upper brainstem (Dahlstrom and Fuxe, 1964). Axons from the ventral raphé nuclei appear to provide a major serotonergic input to the hypothalamus, and in particular the SCN. A second group of serotonergic perikarya has recently been localized within the dorsal medial nuclei of the hypothalamus. This appears to represent an intrahypothalamic serotonergic neuronal system (Beaudet and Descarries, 1979). The role of the latter serotonergic system in neuroendocrine function is not known.

Studies of serotonin (5-HT) concentrations in samples taken from senescent animals and man have yielded equivocal results. In human subjects and the rhesus monkey, 5-HT concentrations decrease with age (Bertler, 1961; Samorajski and Rolsten, 1973), but hindbrain 5-HT levels in human patients are reported to be unchanged (Robinson *et al.*, 1972). In the senescent rat, decreases in 5-HT concentrations in the hypothalamus have been observed (Simpkins *et al.*, 1977; Meek *et al.*, 1977). In the mouse, whole brain 5-HT levels are reported to be stable (Finch, 1973) or slightly decreased with age (Samorajski *et al.*, 1971). Recently, Walker (1980) has observed that while mean hypothalamic 5-HT concentrations are not altered by age in constant estrous female rats, the circadian variation in hypothalamic 5-HT is absent in the old rats. This absence of rhythmic alterations in 5-HT levels in old rats may play a role in the alteration in the circadian variation of many parameters of autonomic function.

Estimates of serotonergic neuronal activity have not been successful in delineating the effects of age on this neuronal system. The activity of tryptophan hydroxylase, the rate-limiting enzyme in 5-HT biosynthesis, has been reported to decrease in the raphé nuclei, the septum, and hippocampus of old Sprague–Dawley rats (Meek *et al.*, 1977), but is not changed in the raphé nuclei of old Fischer 344 rats (Reis *et al.*, 1977). In rat whole brain and human cerebrospinal fluid, 5-hydroxyindolacetic acid (5-HIAA, the major 5-HT metabolite) levels are elevated with age

(Bowers and Gerbode, 1968; Gottfries *et al.*, 1971; Simpkins *et al.*, 1977). In male rats, the accumulation of 5-HT following the blockade of monoamine oxidase is greater in the hypothalamus, but not the whole brain of old vs. young animals. This suggests a higher activity of serotonergic neurons (Simpkins *et al.*, 1977). However, based upon the limited data available and the relatively small magnitude of alteration in 5-HT concentrations and turnover observed in old animals, it is not possible, at present, to make definitive conclusions as to the effects of age on 5-HT metabolism.

5. Aging of Opioid Neurons

Acute morphine treatment (Barraclough and Sawyer, 1955) as well as narcotic addiction (Santen *et al.*, 1975) has long been known to exert profound effects on neuroendocrine functions. The more recent discovery of a family of brain peptides which possess opioid activity and that appear to function as neurotransmitters and/or neuromodulators (Hughes *et al.*, 1975; Simantov and Snyder, 1976; Bradbury *et al.*, 1976; Guillemin *et al.*, 1976) initiated an intense effort to elucidate the role of these peptides in many neuroendocrine states (Meites *et al.*, 1979).

The three primary opioid peptides in the brain, methionine (Met-) enkephalin, leucine (Leu-) enkephalin and β-endorphin occur in relatively high concentrations in the hypothalamus and appear to have separate but overlapping distributions (Uhl *et al.*, 1978; Bloom *et al.*, 1978; Larsson *et al.*, 1979). Also, there is substantial opioid activity in the pituitary gland which likely represents β-endorphin and the newly discovered opioid peptide, dynorphin (Guillemin *et al.*, 1976; Goldstein *et al.*, 1979; Synder, 1980).

Efforts to assess the influence of increasing age on opioid neurons are hampered by the lack of an effective means of measuring the turnover rates of these and other peptides. Nonetheless, several studies have attempted to assess indirectly the influence of increasing age on opioid activity. Age-related elevations in met-enkephalin levels in the hypothalamus (Kumar *et al.*, 1980; Steger *et al.*, 1980c) and anterior pituitary gland (Kumar *et al.*, 1980) have been reported. Gambert *et al.* (1980) and Forman *et al.* (1981) observed increased pituitary and decreased hypothalamic β-endorphin levels in old male rats. Regional analysis of β-endorphin concentrations in the brains of two-year-old male rats revealed that except for the ME there was a 50% decrease in β-endorphin concentrations in all POA and hypothalamic regions examined (Barden *et al.,* 1981). Additionally, a threefold increase in plasma β-endorphin was observed in old male rats (Forman *et al.,* 1981).

While estimates of opioid peptide concentrations alone do not clarify the direction of the alterations in opioid neuronal activity, several lines of evidence support the hypothesis that hyperactive opioid neurons are present in old animals. First, many reports indicate that senescent animals are less sensitive to painful stimuli than their younger counterparts (Nicak, 1971; Nilsen, 1961; Pare, 1969; Hess *et al.,* 1981), although reports of no change (Lippa *et al.,* 1980) and increased sensitivity (Gordon *et al.,* 1978) in old animals have appeared. In view of this apparent decline in pain sensitivity and the observation of reduced brain opioid receptor concentrations in several brain regions (Messing *et al.,* 1980, 1981; Hess *et al.,* 1981), a plausible explanation suggested by Hess *et al.* (1981) is that the decline in opioid receptor number occurs secondary to a hyperactivity of opioid neurons. Finally, the observation by Steger *et al.* (1980c) that following administration of the opioid receptor antagonist, naloxone, serum LH, and testosterone levels increased acutely, suggests that the hyperactivity of opioid neurons may contribute to reproductive senescence. A further evaluation of the age-related changes in opioid neuronal activity is likely to lead to a better understanding of the aging process.

6. Aging of Luteinizing Hormone-Releasing Hormone (LHRH) Neurons

The decapeptide, LHRH, is the primary brain neurohormone responsible for the regulation of luteinizing hormone (LH) and follicle-stimulating hormone (FSH) secretion. Thus, LHRH neurons may play a key role in the age-related decline in gonadotropin secretion and reproductive senescence. Numerous studies have attempted to evaluate the activity of these neurons in senescent rats. However, for LHRH, like brain opioids, there is not an effective means of directly monitoring the activity of this peptide. As a consequence, LHRH concentrations coupled with ongoing secretory rates of gonadotropins have been employed to estimate age-related changes in LHRH neuronal activity.

Initial studies using bioassay procedures to estimate releasing factor activity in hypothalamic tissue reported elevated follicle stimulating hormone-releasing activity in old constant estrous female rats (Clemens and Meites, 1971) and no change in luteinizing hormone-releasing activity in old constant estrous female or male rats (Riegle *et al.,* 1977; Miller and Riegle, 1978). The later development of antibodies to LHRH permitted the use of sensitive radioimmunoassays and immunocytochemical procedures in the evaluation of LHRH levels in old animals. In constant estrous female rats, hypothalamic LHRH concentrations are reduced and these old rats fail to show the normal castration-induced decline in hypothalamic LHRH levels (Wise and Ratner, 1980; Steger et al., 1979). A similar age-related decline in LHRH concentrations in male rats has been observed in the ME, NA, and organum vasculosum of the lamina terminalis (OVLT; Simpkins et al., 1979) and in the ME by immunocytochemical methods (Hoffman and Sladek, 1980). One report of increased hypothalamic LHRH concentrations associated with a significant alteration in the intraneuronal distribution of this peptide has appeared (Barnea et al., 1980).

The close association between LHRH function and reproductive status of old animals is indicated by the observation that animals which maintain normal gonadotropin secretory capacity with age, also maintain LHRH neuronal function. Thus, the PP rat, which exhibits relatively normal gonadotropin secretion in response to steroid treatment (Lu et al., 1980) and acute ovariectomy (Estes et al., 1981; Huang et al., 1976a), also maintains normal levels of LHRH in the hypothalamus (Estes et al., 1981; Steger et al., 1979) and POA (Estes et al., 1981) and exhibit a post-castration depletion of LHRH stores (Wise and Ratner, 1980; Estes et al., 1981). Further, the white footed mouse, which maintains reproductive capacity through its third year of life, likewise exhibits normal LHRH concentrations through 3–4 years of age (Steger et al., 1980a,b).

Collectively, these data indicate that the rate of aging of LHRH neurons may determine the time of reproductive senescence in rodents. In turn, the aging of LHRH neurons may be a consequence of the preceding alteration in catecholamine, indoleamine, and/or opioid neurons. A wide variety of drugs whose common CNS action is the enhancement of central catecholamine activity, can reinitiate estrous cycles in old rats (Everett, 1940; Clemens et al., 1969; Quadri et al., 1973; Huang and Meites, 1975; Huang et al., 1976b; Linnoila and Cooper, 1976; Clemens and Bennett, 1977; Cooper et al., 1979; Forman et al., 1980). Presumably, by restoring normal catecholamine activity, these drugs enhance the release of LHRH. However, whether activation of catecholamine neurons can restore LHRH concentrations to levels found in young animals remains to be demonstrated. Additionally, the possibility that chronic alterations in serum levels of gonadal steroids and/or prolactin contribute to the dysfunction of LHRH neurons in old rats has been suggested (Lu et al., 1981; Simpkins et al., 1982).

7. Aging of Somatostatin Neurons

The effects of age on somatostatin (growth hormone-inhibiting factor) containing neurons has received relatively little attention. Only two reports estimating somatostatin activity in hypothalamic tissues have been published. Sonntag *et al.* (1980) reported a decline in caudal, but not rostral, hypothalamic somatostatin content associated with a decline in the amplitude of growth hormone (GH) pulses in old male rats. Hoffman and Sladek (1980) observed decreased somatostatin concentrations in the ME of male rats by immunocytochemical methods. That the dampening of GH pulses in old rats may be due to an overactivity of somatostatin-containing neurons is suggested by the observation that passive immunization against somatostatin elevated GH more in old than in young rats (Sonntag *et al.*, 1981). Additionally, growth hormone-releasing factor (GRF) activity may be lower in the hypothalamus of old vs. young rats as was suggested by Pecile *et al.* (1965). Increased somatostatin and/or decreased GRF activity may account for the observation that old men and women show a depressed GH secretory response to stress, surgical trauma, exercise, and arginine treatment (Dudl *et al.*, 1973; Blichert-Toft, 1975; Bazzarre *et al.*, 1976) as well as an absence of sleep-induced GH secretion (Finkelstein *et al.*, 1972; Carlson *et al.*, 1972; Blichert-Toft, 1975). Finally, the observation that pulsatile GH secretion in the rat is dependent upon activity in central noradrenergic neurons (Durand *et al.*, 1977) suggests that the decline in noradrenergic activity in old animals contributes to the age-related alterations in somatostatin and/or GRF activity.

8. Aging of Thyrotropin-Releasing Hormone Neurons

In the absence of direct measurement of thyrotropin-releasing hormone (TRH) concentrations in the hypothalamus of old rats, estimates of TRH neuronal activity during aging have relied upon measurement of thyroid-stimulating hormone (TSH) responses to environmental and endocrine manipulations. Huang *et al.* (1980b) have demonstrated that the TSH secretory response to low ambient temperature or thyroidectomy is equal in young and old male rats. Further, basal TSH levels are normal in old male rats (Simpkins *et al.*, 1977). Thus, in old male rats TRH neurons can maintain normal TSH levels and respond normally to stimuli for TSH secretion. In contrast, the old male rat appears to lose the capacity to inhibit TSH secretion. Simpkins *et al.* (1978) observed that while several types of stresses produce a rapid decline in serum TSH in young animals, this response diminishes with age. Relevant to this observation is a report by Klug and Adelman (1979) that the loss of a circadian rhythm in serum TSH with age is due to the absence of a "dark phase" decline in TSH levels in old rats. Thus, while the secretory capacity of TRH neurons remains normal, the regulatory mechanism which mediates the cessation in TSH secretion is deficient in old animals.

9. Summary

While significant progress has been made in the description of differences in neuroendocrine capacity at the extremes of age (young vs. old), few studies have yet evaluated the chronological order of alterations in the components of the CNS during aging. Thus, the sequences of alterations in neurotransmitters and hypophysiotropic hormones which accompanies, and perhaps causes, the aging process is not known. In addition, the manner in which the aging of individual components of the CNS relate to the aging of other CNS components is at present uncertain. The most convincing evidence for a cause–effect relationship among CNS components is the dysfunction of the LHRH gonadotropins secretory system associated with a decline in noradrenergic activity (Meites *et al.*, 1978). Animal models which show severe norepinephrine (NE) deficiency also exhibit LHRH neuronal dysfunction, whereas old animals with relatively normal noradrenergic activity exhibit normal LHRH secretory responses. Additionally, drugs which apparently improve noradrenergic function restore, in part, normal patterns of LHRH release.

The importance of aging of central neuronal systems to the dysfunction in other hypophysiotropic hormones is less certain. While a decline in adrenergic tone may explain the relative absence of pulses of GH in old rats, it is uncertain whether this effect is exerted on somatostatin neurons or GRF-containing neurons. Interestingly, TRH neurons apparently maintain normal secretory capacity into late life, despite the decline in activity of NE, a neurotransmitter which clearly exerts a stimulatory influence on TSH secretion. Thus, TRH neurons appear to retain their secretory capacity despite age-related changes in neurotransmitter systems. Elucidation of the mechanism of this adaptation to a changing neuronal environment may add substantially to our understanding of the mechanism of CNS aging.

Finally, the contribution that peripheral hormones play in the rate of aging of various components of the CNS, has not been studied in detail. This gap in our understanding of the neuroendocrinology of aging is apparent when we consider that most hormones and/or their receptors have been observed in the CNS. Preliminary evidence for neurotoxic effects of estrogens, as well as the DA-depleting capacity of prolactin, suggest that chronic alterations in serum hormone concentrations or in their pattern of secretion may contribute to the age-related alterations in CNS function. The further documentation of peripheral hormone–CNS interaction is a promising area for new insights into the aging process.

ACKNOWLEDGMENT. Part of the work presented was supported by NIA grant AG 02021.

10. References

Annunziato, L., and Moore, K. E., 1978, Prolactin in CSF selectivity increases dopamine turnover in the median eminence, *Life Sci.* **22**:2037–2042.

Barden, N., Dupont, A., Labric, F., Merand, Y., Rouleau, D., Vandry, H., and Biossier, J. R., 1981, Age-dependent changes in the β-endorphin content of discrete rat brain nuclei, *Brain Res.* **208**:209–212.

Barnea, A., Cho, G., and Porter, J. C., 1980, Effect of aging on the subneuronal distribution of luteinizing hormone-releasing hormone in the hypothalamus, *Endocrinology* **106**:1980–1988.

Barraclough, C. A., and Sawyer, C. H., 1955, Inhibition of the release of pituitary ovulatory hormone in the rat by morphine, *Endocrinology* **57**:329–336.

Bazzarre, T. L., Johanson, A. J., Huseman, C. A., Varma, M. M., and Blizzard, R. M., 1976, Human growth hormone changes with age, in: *Growth Hormone and Related Peptides* (A. Pecile and E. E. Muller, eds.), Excerpta Medica, Amsterdam, pp. 261–270.

Beaudet, A., and Descarries, L., 1979, Radioautographic characterization of a serotonin-accumulating nerve cell group in adult rat hypothalamus, *Brain Res.* **160**:231–243.

Bertler, A., 1961, Occurrence and localization of catecholamines in the human brain, *Acta Physiol. Scand.* **51**:97–107.

Bjorklund, A., Moore, R. Y., Nobin, A., and Stenevi, U., 1973, The organization of tubero-hypophyseal and reticulo-infundibular catecholamine neuron systems in the rat brain, *Brain Res.* **51**:171–191.

Bjorklund, A., Lindvall, O., and Nobin, A., 1975, Evidence of an incertohypothalamic dopamine neuron system in the rat, *Brain Res.* **89**:29–42.

Blichert-Toft, M., 1975, Secretion of corticotrophin and somatotrophin by the senescent adenohypophysis in man, *Acta Endocrinol.* **78**:1–157.

Bloom, F., Battenberg, E., Rosier, J., Ling, N., and Guillemin, R., 1978, Neurons containing β-endorphin in rat brain exist separately from those containing enkephalin. Immunocytochemical studies, *Proc. Natl. Acad. Sci. USA* **75**:1591–1595.

Bowers, M. B., and Gerbode, R. A., 1968, Relationship of monoamine metabolites in human cerebrospinal fluid to age, *Nature* **219**:1256–1257.

Bradbury, A., Smyth, D. G., and Snell, C. R., 1976, The peptide hormones: Molecular and cellular aspects, *Ciba Found. Symp.* **41**:61–75.

Carlson, H. E., Gillin, J. C., Gorden, P., and Synder, F., 1972, Absence of sleep related growth hormone peaks in aged normal subjects and acromegaly, *J. Clin. Endocrinol. Metabol.* **34**:1102–1105.

Clemens, J. A., and Bennett, D. R., 1977, Do aging changes in the preoptic area contribute to loss of cyclic endocrine function? *J. Gerontol.* **32**:19–24.

Clemens, J. A., and Meites, J., 1971, Neuroendocrine status of old constant-estrous rats, *Neuroendocrinology* **7**:249–256.

Clemens, J. A., Amenomori, Y., Jenkins, T., and Meites, J., 1969, Effects of hypothalamic stimulation, hormones, and drugs on ovarian function in old female rats, *Proc. Soc. Exp. Biol. Med.* **132**:561–563.

Clemens, J. A., Fuller, R. W., and Owen, N. V., 1979, Some neuroendocrine aspects of aging, in: *Advances in Experimental Medicine and Biology,* Vol. 113, *Parkinson's Disease-II* (C. E. Finch, D. E. Potter, and A. D. Kenny, eds.), Plenum Press, New York, pp. 77–100.

Cooper, J. R., Bloom, F. E., and Roth, R. H., 1978, *The Biochemical Basis of Neuro-pharmacology,* 3rd Ed., Oxford University Press, New York.

Cooper, R. L., Brandt, S. J., Linnoila, M., and Walker, R. F., 1979, Induced ovulation in aged female rats by L-Dopa implants into the medial preoptic area, *Neuroendocrinology* **28**:234–240.

Cote, L. J., and Kremzner, L. T., 1975, Changes in neurotransmitter systems with increasing age in human brain, *Trans. Am. Soc. Neurochem.* **5**:83.

Dahlstrom, A., and Fuxe, K., 1964, Evidence for the existence of monoamine containing neurons in the central nervous system. I. Demonstration of monoamines in the cell bodies of brain stem neurons, *Acta Physiol. Scand. (Suppl. 232)* **62**:1–55.

Demarest, K. T., Riegle, G. D., and Moore, K. E., 1980, Characteristics of dopaminergic neurons in the aged male rat, *Neuroendocrinology* **31**:222–227.

Demarest, K. T., Moore, K. E., and Riegle, G. D., 1981, Aging influences tuberoinfundibular dopamine neurons and anterior pituitary dopamine content in the female rat, *Fed. Proc.* **40**:509A.

Dilman, V. M., 1971, Age-associated elevation of hypothalamic threshold to feedback control, and its role in development, aging and disease, *Lancet* **i**:1211–1219.

Dudl, R. J., Ensinck, J. W., Palmer, H. E., and Williams, R. H., 1973, Effect of age on growth hormone secretion in man, *J. Clin. Endocrinol. Metabol.* **37**:11–16.

Estes, K. S., and Simpkins, J. W., 1980, Age-related alterations in catecholamine concentrations in discrete preoptic area and hypothalamic regions in the male rat, *Brain Res.* **194**:556–560.

Estes, K. S., and Simpkins, J. W., 1981, Catecholamine levels and activity change at different rates in discrete brain regions of aging female rats, *Fed. Proc. (Abst.)* **40**:509.

Estes, K. S., and Simpkins, J. W., 1982, Catecholamine activities and concentrations within discrete brain regions are differently altered with advancing age in ovariectomized Long-Evans rats, Proc. 64th Annu. Meeting of the Endocrine Soc., San Francisco, Abstract No. 571.

Estes, K. S., Simpkins, J. W., and Chen, C. L., 1980, Alteration in pulsatile release of LH in aging female rats, *Proc. Soc. Exp. Biol. Med.* **163**:384–387.

Estes, K. S., Simpkins, J. W., and Kalra, S. P., 1981, Effects of advancing age and ovariectomy on LHRH concentrations in discrete preoptic area and hypothalamic regions of the rat, *Endocrinology* **109**:201A.

Everett, J. W., 1939, Spontaneous persistent estrus in a strain of albino rats, *Endocrinology* **25**:123–127.

Everett, J. W., 1940, The restoration of ovulatory cycles and corpus luteum formation in persistent-estrous rats by progesterone, *Endocrinology* **27**:681–686.

Everitt, A. V., 1980, The neuroendocrine system in aging, *Gerontology* **26:**108–119.

Finch, C. E., 1973, Catecholamine metabolism in the brains of aging male mice, *Brain Res.* **52:**271–276.

Finch, C. E., 1979, Age-related changes in brain catecholamines: A synopsis of findings in C57BL/6J mice and other rodent models, in: *Advances in Experimental Medicine and Biology, Parkinson's Disease-II,* Vol. 113 (C. E. Finch, D. E. Potter, and A. D. Kenny, eds.), Plenum Press, New York, pp. 15–40.

Finkelstein, J. W., Roffwarg, H. P., Boyer, R. M., Kream, J., and Hellman, I., 1972, Age-related change in the twenty-four-hour spontaneous secretion of growth hormone, *J. Clin. Endocrinol. Metabol.* **35:**665–670.

Forman, L. J., Sonntag, W. E., Miki, N., and Meites, J., 1980, Maintenance by L-Dopa treatment of estrous cycles and LH response to estrogen in aging female rats, *Exp. Aging Res.* **6:**547–554.

Forman, L. J., Sonntag, W. E., Van Vugt, D. A., and Meites, J., 1981, Immunoreactive β-endorphin in the plasma, pituitary and hypothalamus of young and old male rats, *Neurobiol. Aging* **2:**281–284.

Fuxe, K., Eneroth, P., Gustafason, L. A., and Skeet, P., 1977, Dopamine in the nucleus accumbens: Preferential increase of DA turnover by rat prolactin, *Brain Res.* **122:**177–182.

Gambert, S. R., Garthwaite, T. L., Pontzer, C. H., and Hagen, T. C., 1980, Age-related changes in central nervous system beta-endorphin and ACTH, *Neuroendocrinology* **31:**252–255.

Goldstein, A., Tachibana, S., Lowney, L. I., Humkapiller, M., and Hood, L., 1979, Dynorphin-(1-13), an extraordinary potent opioid peptide, *Proc. Soc. Natl. Acad. Sci. USA* **76:**6666–6670.

Gordon, W. C., Scobie, S. R., and Frankl, S. E., 1978, Age-related differences in electric shock detection and escape thresholds in Sprague-Dawley albino rats, *Exp. Aging Res.* **4:**23–25.

Gottfries, C. G., Gottfries, I., Johansson, R., Olsson, R., Persson, T., Roos, B. E., and Jostrom, R., 1971, Acid monoamine metabolites in human cerebrospinal fluid and their relations to age and sex, *Neuropharmacology* **10:**665–672.

Gudelsky, G. A., Simpkins, J. W., Mueller, G. P., Meites, J., and Moore, K. E., 1976, Selective actions of prolactin on catecholamine turnover in the hypothalamus and on serum LH and FSH, *Neuroendocrinology* **22:**206–215.

Gudelsky, G. A., Nansel, D. D., and Porter, J. C., 1981, Dopaminergic control of prolactin secretion in the aging male rat, *Brain Res.* **204:**446–450.

Guillemin, R., Ling, N., and Burgus, R., 1976, Endorphines, peptides, d'origine hypothalamique et neurophysaire activité morphinomimétique. Isolement et structure moléculaire de l'endorphin, *C. R. Acad. Sci. Ser. D* **282:**783–785.

Hess, G. D., Joseph, J. A., and Roth, G. S., 1981, Effects of age on sensitivity to pain and brain opiate receptors, *Neurobiol. Aging* **2:**49–55.

Hoffman, G. E., and Sladek, J. R., Jr., 1980, Age-related changes in dopamine, LHRH and somatostatin in the rat hypothalamus, *Neurobiol. Aging* **1:**27–37.

Hohn, K. G., and Wuttke, W. O., 1978, Changes in catecholamine turnover in the anterior part of the mediobasal hypothalamus and the medial preoptic area in response to hyperprolactinemia in ovariectomized rats, *Brain Res.* **156:**241–252.

Hökfelt, T., and Fuxe, K., 1972a, Brain endocrine interaction: On the morphology and the neuroendocrine role of hypothalamus catecholamine neurons, in: *Median Eminence, Structure and Function* (M. Knigge, E. E. Scott, and A. Weindle, eds.), Karger, Basel, pp. 181–223.

Hökfelt, T., and Fuxe, K., 1972b, Effects of prolactin and ergot alkaloids on the tubero-infundibular dopamine (DA) neurons, *Neuroendocrinology* **4:**100–122.

Howland, B. E., 1976, Reduced gonadotropic release in response to progesterone or gonadotropin releasing hormone (GnRH) in old female rats, *Life Sci.* **19:**219–224.

Huang, H. H., and Meites, J., 1975, Reproductive capacity of aging female rats, *Neuroendocrinology* **17:**289–295.

Huang, H. H., Marshall, S., and Meites, J., 1976a, Capacity of old vs. young female rats to secrete LH, FSH and prolactin, *Biol. Reprod.* **14:**538–543.

Huang, H. H., Marshall, S., and Meites, J., 1976b, Induction of estrous cycles in old non-cyclic rats by progesterone, ACTH, ether stress or L-DOPA, *Neuroendocrinology* **20:**21–34.

Huang, H. H., Simpkins, J. W., and Meites, J., 1977, Hypothalamic norepinephrine (NE) and dopamine (DA) turnover and relation to LH, FSH and prolactin release in old female rat, *Endocrinology (Suppl.)* **100:**331.

Huang, H. H., Steger, R. W., Bruni, J. F., and Meites, J., 1978, Patterns of sex steroid and gonadotropin secretion in aging female rats, *Endocrinology* **100:**1855–1859.

Huang, H. H., Steger, R. W., Sonntag, W. E., and Meites, J., 1980a, Positive feedback by ovarian hormones on prolactin and LH in old vs. young female rats, *Neurobiol. Aging* **1:**141–143.

Huang, H. H., Steger, R. W., and Meites, J., 1980b, Capacity of old vs. young male rats to release thyrotropic (TSH), thyroxine (T$_4$) and triiodothyronine (T$_3$) in response to different stimuli, *Exp. Aging Res.* **6:**3–12.

Hughes, J., Smith, T. W., Kosterlitz, W. H., Fothergill, L., Morgan, B. A., and Morris, H. R., 1975, Identification of two related pentapeptides from the brain with potent opiate agonist activity, *Nature* **285:**577–579.

Kalra, P. S., Simpkins, J. W., and Kalra, S. P., 1981, Hyperprolactinemia counteracts the testerone-induced inhibition of the preoptic area dopamine turnover, *Neuroendocrinology* **33:** 118–122.

Kizer, J. S., Palkovitz, M., and Brownstein, M. J., 1976, The projections of the A8, A9 and A10 dopaminergic cell bodies: Evidence for a nigro-hypothalamic-median eminence dopaminergic pathway, *Brain Res.* **108:**363–370.

Kizer, J. S., Memeroff, C. B., and Youngblood, W. W., 1978, Neurotoxic amino acids and structurally related analogs, *Pharmacol. Rev.* **29:**301–318.

Klug, T. L., and Adelman, R. C., 1979, Altered hypothalamic-pituitary regulation of thyrotropin in male rats during aging, *Endocrinology* **104:**1136–1142.

Kumar, M. S. A., Chen, C. L., and Huang, H. H., 1980, Pituitary and hypothalamic concentrations of met-enkephalin in young and old rats, *Neurobiol. Aging* **1:**153–155.

Larsson, L., Childers, S., and Synder, S. H., 1979, Met- and len-enkephalin immunoreactivity in separate neurons, *Nature* **282:**407–410.

Linnoila, M., and Cooper, R. L., 1976, Reinstatement of vaginal cycles in aged female rats, *J. Pharm. Exp. Ther.* **199:**477–482.

Lippa, A. S., Pelham, R. W., Beer, B., Critchett, D. J., Dean, R. L., and Bartus, R. T., 1980, Brain cholinergic dysfunction and memory in aged rats, *Neurobiol. Aging* **1:**13–19.

Lu, K. H., Huang, H. H., Chen, H. T., Kurtz, M., Mioduszewski, R., and Meites, J., 1977, Positive feedback by estrogen and progesterone on LH release in old and young rats, *Proc. Soc. Exp. Biol. Med.* **154:**82–85.

Lu, J. K. H., Damassa, D. A., Gilman, D. P., Judd, H. L., and Sayer, C. H., 1980, Differential patterns of gonadotropin responses to ovarian steroids and to LH-releasing hormone between constant-estrous and pseudopregnant states in aging rats, *Biol. Reprod.* **23:**345–351.

Lu, J. K. H., Gilman, D. P., Meldrum, D. R., Judd, H. L., and Saywer, C. H., 1981, Relationship between circulating estrogens and the central mechanism by which ovarian steroids stimulate luteinizing hormone secretion in aged and young female rats, *Endocrinology* **108**:836–841.

Masuoka, D. T., Jonsson, G., and Finch, C. E., 1979, Aging and unusual catecholamine-containing structures in the mouse brain, *Brain Res.* **169**:335–341.

McGeer, E. G., Fibiger, H. C., McGeer, P. L., and Wickson, V., 1971, Aging and brain enzymes, *Exp. Gerontol.* **6**:391–396.

Mek, J. L., Bertilsson, L., Cheney, D. L., Zsilla, G., and Costa, E., 1977, Aging induced changes in acetylcholine and serotonin content of discrete brain nuclei, *J. Gerontol.* **32**:129–131.

Meites, J., Huang, H. H., and Simpkins, J. W., 1978, Recent studies on neuroendocrine control of reproductive senescence in rats, in: *Aging,* Vol. 4, *The Aging Reproductive System* (E. L. Schneider, ed.), Raven Press, New York, pp. 213–235.

Meites, J., Bruni, J., Van Vugt, D. A., and Smith, A. F., 1979, Relation of endogenous opioid peptides and morphine to neuroendocrine function, *Life Sci.* **24**:1325–1336.

Messing, R. B., Vasquez, B. J., Spiehler, V. R., Martinez, J. L., Nensen, R. A., Rigter, H., and McGaugh, J. L., 1980, ^{3}H-dihydromorphine binding in brain regions of young and aged rats, *Life Sci.* **26**:921–927.

Messing, R. B., Vasquez, B. J., Samaniego, B., Jensen, R. A., Martinez, J. L., and McGaugh, J. L., 1981, Alterations in dihydromorphine binding in cerebral hemispheres of aged male rats, *J. Neurochem.* **36**:784–790.

Miller, A. E., and Riegle, G. D., 1978, Hypothalamic LH-releasing activity in young and aged intact and gonadectomized rats, *Exp. Aging Res.* **4**:145–155.

Miller, A. E., Shaar, C. J., and Reigle, G. D., 1976, Aging effects on hypothalamic dopamine and norepinephrine content in the male rat, *Exp. Aging Res.* **2**:475–480.

Moore, R. Y., and Bloom, F. E., 1978, Central catecholamine neuron systems: Anatomy and physiology of the dopamine system. *Annu. Rev. Neurosci.* **1**:129–169.

Moore, R. Y., and Bloom, F. E., 1979, Central catecholamine neuron systems: Anatomy and physiology of the norepinephrine and epinephrine systems, *Annu. Rev. Neurosci.* **2**:113–168.

Morgan, W. W., and Herbert, D. C., 1980, Early responses of the dopaminergic tubero-infundibular neurons to anterior pituitary homografts, *Neuroendocrinology* **31**:212–215.

Nicak, A., 1971, Changes of sensitivity to pain in relation to postnatal development in rats, *Exp. Gerontol.* **6**:111–114.

Nilsen, P. L., 1961, Studies on algesimetry by electrical stimulation of the mouse tail, *Acta Pharmacol. Tox.* **18**:10–22.

Olson, L., Fuxe, K., and Hökfelt, T., 1972, The effects of pituitary transplants on the tuberoinfundibular dopamine neurons in various endocrine states, *Acta Endocrinol.* **71**:233–244.

Pare, W. P., 1969, Age, sex, and strain differences in the aversive threshold to grid shock in the rat, *J. Comp. Physiol. Psychol.* **69**:214–218.

Pecile, A., Müller, E., Falconi, G., and Martini, L., 1965, Growth hormone releasing activity of hypothalamic extracts at different ages, *Endocrinology* **77**:241–246.

Peluso, J. J., Steger, R. W., and Hafez, E. S. E., 1977, Regulation of LH secretion in aged female rats, *Biol. Reprod.* **16**:212–215.

Perkins, N., and Westfall, T., 1978, Effects of prolactin on dopamine release from rat striatum and medial basal hypothalamus, *Neuroscience* **3**:59–63.

Perkins, N. A., Westfall, T. C., Paul, C. V., MacLeod, R., and Rogol, A. D., 1979, Effect of prolactin on dopamine synthesis in medial basal hypothalamus: Evidence for a short loop feedback, *Brain Res.* **160**:431–444.

Ponzio, F., Brunell, N., and Algeri, S., 1978, Catecholamine synthesis in the brain of aging rats, *J. Neurochem.* **30**:1617–1620.

Quadri, S. K., Kledzik, G. S., and Meites, J., 1973, Reinitiation of estrous cycles in old constant estrous rats by central acting drugs, *Neuroendocrinology* **11**:248–255.

Reis, D. J., Ross, R. A., and Joh, T. H., 1977, Changes in the activity and amounts of enzymes synthesizing catecholamines and acetylcholine in brain, adrenal medulla, and sympathetic ganglia of aged rat and mouse, *Brain Res.* **136**:465–474.

Riegle, G. D., Meites, J., Miller, A. E., and Wood, S. M., 1977, Effects of aging on hypothalamic LH-releasing and prolactin inhibiting activities and pituitary responsiveness to LHRH in the male laboratory rat, *J. Gerontol.* **32**:13–18.

Robinson, D. S., Nies, A., Davis, J M., Bunncy, W. E., Davies, J. M., Colburn, R. W., Bourne, H. R., Shaw, D. M., and Copper, A. J., 1972, Aging, monoamines and monoamine oxidase, *Lancet* **1**:290–291.

Sacher, G. A., and Hart, R. W., 1978, Longevity, aging and comparative cellular and molecular biology of the house mouse, *Mus imusculus* and the white-footed mouse, *Peromyscus leucopus*, *Birth Defects* **14**:71–96.

Saiduddin, S., and Zassenhaus, P., 1979, Estrous cycles, decidual cell response and uterine estrogen and progesterone receptors in Fischer 344 virgin aging rats, *Proc. Soc. Exp. Biol. Med.* **161**:119.

Sakensa, S. K., and Lau, I. F., 1979, Variations in serum androgens, estrogens, progestins, gonadotropins and prolactin levels in male rats from prepubertal to advanced age, *Exp. Aging Res.* **5**:179–194.

Samorajski, T., 1975, Age-related changes in brain biogenic amines, in: *Aging, Vol. I: Clinical, Morphological and Neurochemical Aspects in the Aging Central Nervous System* (H. Brody, D. Harman, and J. M. Ordy, eds.), Raven Press, New York, pp. 199–214.

Samorajski, T., and Rolsten, C., 1973, Age and regional differences in the chemical composition of brains of mice, monkeys and humans, in: *Progress in Brain Research, Vol. 40: Neurobiological Aspects of Maturation and Aging* (D. H. Ford, ed.), Elsevier Press, New York, pp. 253–265.

Samorajski, T., Rolsten, C., and Ordy, J. M., 1971, Changes in behavior, brain and neuroendocrine chemistry with age and stress in C57BL/10 male mice, *J. Gerontol.* **26**:168–175.

Santen, R. J., Sofsky, J., Bilic, N., and Lippert, R., 1975, Mechanism of action of narcotics in the production of menstrual dysfunction in women, *Fert. Ster.* **26**:538–548.

Selmonoff, 1981, The lateral and medial median eminence: Distribution of dopamine, norepinephrine and luteinizing hormone-releasing hormone and the effect of prolactin on catecholamine turnover, *Endocrinology* **108**:1716–1722.

Shaar, C. J., Euker, J. S., Riegle, G. D., and Meites, J., 1975, Effects of castration and gonadal steroids on serum luteinizing hormone and prolactin in old and young rats, *J. Endocrinol.* **66**:45–51.

Simantov, R., and Synder, S. H., 1976, Morphine-like factors in mammalian brain: Structure elucidation and interaction with opiate receptor, *Proc. Natl. Acad. Sci. USA* **73**:2515–2519.

Simpkins, J. W., Mueller, G. P., Huang, H. H., and Meites, J., 1977, Evidence for depressed catecholamine and enhanced serotonin metabolism in aging male rats: possible relation to gonadotropin secretion, *Endocrinology* **100**:1672–1678.

Simpkins, J. W., Hodson, C. A., and Meites, J., 1978, Differential effects of stress on release of thyroid-stimulating hormone in young and old male rats, *Proc. Soc. Exp. Biol. Med.* **157**:144–147.

Simpkins, J. W., Estes, K. S., Kalra, P. S., and Kalra, S. P., 1979, Age-related alterations in catecholamines and LHRH concentrations in brain nuclei of the male rate, in: *Endocrine Aspects of Aging* (S. G. Koreman, ed.), NIH Publication, Bethesda (Abst.).

Simpkins, J. W., Hodson, C. A., Kalra, P. S., and Kalra, S. P., 1982, Chronic hyperpro-lactinemia depletes hypothalamic dopamine concentrations in male rats, *Life Sci.* **30:**1349–1353.

Snyder, S. H., 1980, Brain peptides as neurotransmitters, *Science* **209:**976–983.

Sonntag, W. E., Steger, R. W., Forman, L. J., and Meites, J., 1980, Decreased pulsatile release of growth hormone in old male rats, *Endocrinology* **107:**1875–1879.

Sonntag, W. E., Steger, R. W., Forman, L. J., Meites, J., and Arimura, A., 1981, Effects of CNS active drugs and somatostatin on growth hormone release in young and old male rats, *Neuroendocrinology* **33:**73–78.

Steger, R. W., Huang, H. H., and Meites, J., 1979, Relation of aging to hypothalamic LHRH content and serum gonadal steroids in female rats, *Proc. Soc. Exp. Biol. Med.* **161:**251–254.

Steger, R. W., Peluso, J. J., Huang, H. H., Hodson, C. A., Leung, F. C., Meites, J., and Sacher, G., 1980a, Effects of advancing age on the hypothalamic-pituitary-ovarian axis of the female white-footed mouse *(Peromyscus leucopus)*, *Exp. Aging. Res.* **4:**329–339.

Steger, R. W., Huang, H. H., Hodson, C. A., Leung, F. C., Meites, J., and Sacher, G. A., 1980b, Effects of advancing age on hypothalamic-hypophysial-testicular function in the male white-footed mouse *(Peromyscus leucopus)*, *Biol. Reprod.* **22:**805–809.

Steger, R. W., Sonntag, W. E., Van Vugt, D. A., Forman, L. J., and Meites, J., 1980c, Reduced ability of naloxone to stimulate LH and testerone release in aging male rats: Possible relation to increase in hypothalamic metenkephalin, *Life Sci.* **27:**747–754.

Uhl, G. R., Childers, S. R., and Snyder, S. H., 1978, Opioid peptides and the opiate receptors, in: *Frontiers in Neuroendocrinology* (W. F. Ganong and L. Martine, eds.), Raven Press, New York, p. 289.

Walker, R. F., 1980, Serotonin circadian rhythm as a pacemaker for reproductive cycles in the female rat, in: *Progress in Psychoneuroendocrinology* (F. Brambilla, G. Racagni, and D. de Wied, eds.), Elsevier/North-Holland Biomedical Press, Amsterdam, pp. 591–600.

Wilkes, M. M., and Yen, S. S. C., 1981, Attenuation during aging of the postovariectomy rise in median eminence catecholamines, *Neuroendocrinology* **33:**144–147.

Wilkes, M. M., Lu, K. H., Fulton, S. L., and Yen, S. S. C., 1979, Hypothalamic-pituitary, ovarian interactions during reproductive senescence in the rat, in: *Advances in Experimental Medicine and Biology, Vol. 113: Parkinson's Disease-II* (C. E. Finch, D. E. Potter, and A. D. Kenny, eds.), Plenum Press, New York, pp. 127–148.

Wise, P. M., and Ratner, A., 1980, Effects of ovariectomy on plasma LH, FSH, estradiol and progesterone and medial basal hypothalamic LHRH concentrations in old and young rats, *Neuroendocrinology* **30:**15–20.

CHAPTER 5

Changes in Hormone Uptake and Receptors in the Hypothalamus during Aging

MING-TSUNG PENG

1. Introduction

With advancing age, female rats tend to show irregular vaginal estrous cycles. By 15–24 months of age, most female rats show a prolonged vaginal cornification, characterized by many well-developed and even cystic follicles, but no evidence of ovulation or formation of corpora lutea (designated as PVC). Some animals during this period show prolonged pseudopregnancies of up to 30 days duration or longer, with numerous corpora lutea (designated as PSP). The oldest rats, 2–3 years of age, often exhibit an anestrous state, characterized by atrophic ovaries with only small or primary follicles and an infantile-appearing uterus (designated as ANE; Aschheim, 1964; Huang and Meites, 1975; Lu *et al.*, 1979).

When the ovaries of old rats are transplanted to young ovariectomized rats, they can resume normal or near normal function, indicating that their functional capacity is not lost with aging (Aschheim, 1964; Peng and Huang, 1972). Deficiencies in the hypothalamic-pituitary axis of aging rats are suggested by Krohn (1955), Aschheim (1964), Zeilmaker (1969), and Peng and Huang (1972) on the basis of their observation that even after replacing the ovaries of old rats or mice with those from immature animals, vaginal cyclic activity could not be restored. By a more direct approach, Peng and Huang (1972) replaced pituitaries of

MING-TSUNG PENG • Department of Physiology, National Taiwan University Medical School, Taipei, Taiwan.

young female rats with pituitaries from old rats, grafted beneath the median eminence. In 10 out of 30 cases, there was a resumption of vaginal estrous cycles. Corpora lutea were observed in three rats, and one rat showed fertility. Thus, pituitaries from old rats can function normally in young females, but they do so much less frequently than pituitaries from young rats grafted beneath the median eminence of young recipients. Taken together, these results indicate that the ovaries of old rats retain considerable functional capacity throughout their lifespan, and the primary cause for cessation of estrous cycles lies in altered hypothalamic-pituitary function. After these pioneer observations, other neuroendocrine aspects of reproductive aging were studied more extensively.

Regulation of pituitary gonadotropic hormone output requires that the brain detect levels of gonadal steroids by receptors. The biological response of steroid-sensitive tissues such as the uterus, pituitary, and brain tissues also depends upon the formation of a complex between receptors and hormones that initiate a series of events at the molecular level. Steroids generally diffuse passively into cells and bind to soluble receptors in the cytoplasm. The receptor–hormone complex is translocated from the cytoplasm into the nucleus, where it binds to the chromatin, affecting gene expression. The distribution of estrogen-binding neurons (Stumpf, 1968, 1971; Pfaff, 1971; McEwen and Pfaff, 1973) and of corticosterone-binding neurons (Gerlach and McEwen, 1972) in the brain has been studied extensively. In order to understand the molecular mechanisms involved in functional changes of the neuroendocrine system, or changes in biological responses to hormones during aging, it is necessary to determine whether changes occur in hormone uptake and their receptors in the hypothalamus during aging. The methods used to study hormone uptake and receptors in target cells are well established.

2. Sex Steroid Uptake and Receptor Binding in the Hypothalamus during Aging

2.1. Estrogen Receptor Binding

Peng and Peng (1973), using homogenates of tissue, found decreased [^{3}H]estradiol uptake in the anterior hypothalamus and adenohypophysis of 2-year-old female rats, which show PVC and the ANE, 1 hr after i.p. injection of [^{3}H]estradiol, and 30 min after *in vitro* incubation of the tissues with [^{3}H]estradiol. The decreases in hypothalamic

[³H]estradiol uptake showed regional differences. The posterior hypothalamus of PVC and ANE rats did not show decreased uptake in an *in vivo* experiment. The results of the *in vivo* experiments are shown in Fig. 1.

Kanungo *et al.* (1975) reported that the cerebral hemispheres of 44-week-old and 108-week-old female rats had a lower cytosol–estradiol binding than 7-week-old rats. Jiang and Peng (1981) divided the brain of ovariectomized rats into the corticomedial amygdala (AMYG), preoptic area (POA), basomedial hypothalamus (BMH), and dorsomedial hypothalamus (DH), and measured specific [³H]estradiol binding (subtracting the nonspecific binding represented by the radioactivity in the tissue of the diethylstibestrol-pretreated rats injected with [³H]estradiol, from total binding represented by the radioactivity in the tissue of the rats injected with [³H]estradiol only) in the cytosol and nuclear fraction of the tissues. They found that [³H]estradiol binding in the nuclear fraction in the POA and BMH, 0.5 or 1 hr after i.v. injection, was lower in old noncyclic rats (including PVC rats and ANE rats averaging 29.5 months of age) than in young adult female rats (4-month-old). These

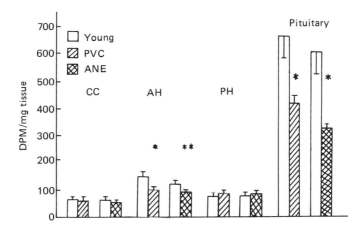

Fig. 1. Estradiol uptake in brain tissues and anterior pituitary of old constant estrous rats (22-month-old), anestrous rats (26-month-old), and young adult female rats (5-month-old) 1 hr after intraperitoneal injection of [³H]estradiol. Rats were ovariectomized one week before the experiment. Each column represents mean of four determinations and bar indicates SEM. * and ** indicate that difference between young adult rats are statistically significant at levels of 5% and 1%, respectively. CC indicates cerebral cortex, AH anterior hypothalamus, PH posterior hypothalamus, PVC prolonged vaginal cornification, and ANE anestrus. (From data published in *Fertil. Steril.* **24:**534–539, 1973, by permission of The American Fertility Society.)

results are shown in Fig. 2. In order to determine the relationship between cytosol receptors and nuclear receptors, the AMYG, POA, and BMH were pooled and designated as HPA. The brain of long-term ovariectomized rats was dissected 1 hr after s.c. injection of unlabeled estradiol (E_2) or physiological saline. Estradiol binding in the cytosol *in vitro* was assessed as described for cytosol E_2 receptor binding by Korach and Muldoon (1974), and the nuclear receptor E_2 complex was determined by the E_2 exchange assay of Anderson *et al.* (1973). One hour after E_2 injection, there was a significant increase in the nuclear E_2 receptor in the HPA and anterior pituitary of young adult female rats. On the other hand, no increase in the nuclear E_2 receptors was observed in the HPA and anterior pituitary of old PVC rats (average age, 20.8-month-old) 1 hr after E_2 injection (Fig. 3). The results indicate that there was an apparent decrease in translocation of E_2 from the cytosol to the nucleus by estrogen priming in old PVC rats. Moudgil and Kanungo (1973) reported decreased induction of acetylcholinesterase in the brain by estrogens in old rats.

Gosden (1976) reported that the uptake of tritiated 17β-estradiol in 14- to 17-month-old female mice was significantly lower than in young mice only in the pituitary, whereas uptake in the cerebrum and hypo-

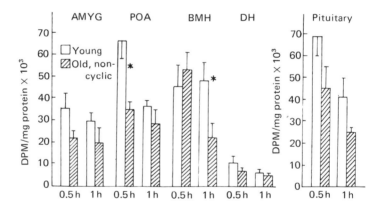

Fig. 2. Nuclear binding of estradiol in various regions of the brain and anterior pituitary of old non-cyclic female rats (30-month-old) and young adult female rats (4-month-old), 0.5 and 1 hr after intravenous injection of [^{3}H]estradiol. Rats were ovariectomized 48 hr prior to the injection. Each column represents mean of 5–6 determinations and bar indicates SEM. * indicates statistically significant at level of 5% as compared with young adult female rats. AMYG indicates amygdala, POA preoptic area, BMH basomedial hypothalamus, and DH dorsal hypothalamus. (Redrawn from data published in *Gerontology* **27:**51–57, 1981, by permission of S. Karger, Basel.)

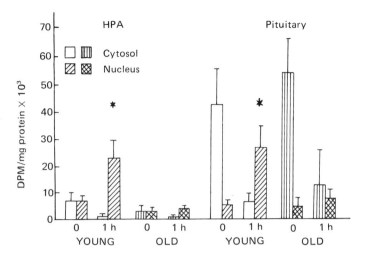

Fig. 3. Cytosol and nuclear estrogen receptors of the brain and anterior pituitary after *in vitro* incubation with [³H]estradiol, with or without cold estradiol priming 1 hr before dissection of the tissues. Rats were long-term ovariectomized. Each column represents mean of six determinations and bar indicates SEM. * indicates statistically significant at 5% level as compared with 0 in the same age group. 0 and 1 hr indicate treatments with and without cold estradiol priming, respectively. HPA indicates pooled brain tissues of amygdala, preoptic area, and basomedial hypothalamus. (Reproduced from *Gerontology* **27**:51–57, 1981, by permission of S. Karger, Basel.)

thalamus was similar in both age groups. Nelson *et al.* (1980) studied the relation between cytosol E_2 receptors and plasma E_2 levels in intact C57BL/ 6J mice. At proestrus, when plasma E_2 elevations were similar in 5- and 12-month-old mice, depletion of cytoplasmic receptors in the hypothalamus and pituitaries was similar in both age groups. However, during the different stages of the estrous cycle, when older mice showed decreased plasma E_2, a larger fraction of receptors remained in the cytoplasm. There is no evidence for age-related impairment in translocation of E_2 receptors. Possibly the delay of nuclear receptor occupancy associated with the slower preovulatory rise of E_2, is a factor in prolongation of estrous cycles. It seems that there is a species difference between rats and mice in respect to E_2 uptake and estrogen receptors in old age. However, a difference in age of the old animals used (mice = 12 and 14 months old, and rats = 20.8 and 29.5 months old) may have introduced a discrepancy. In contrast to old female rats, Peng *et al.* (1973) found no significant difference in E_2 uptake in the hypothalamus and adenohypophysis between old and young adult male rats.

2.2 Androgen Receptor Binding

Decreased testosterone binding in the hypothalamus of old male rats (Chouknyiska and Vassileva-Popova, 1977), and lower affinity of the hydrotestosterone-binding reaction in the hypothalamic, neocortical, and amygdaloid cytosols, have been reported in 18-month-old male rats (Greenstein, 1979).

2.3. Relation between Changes in Sex Steroid Uptake in the Hypothalamus and Changes in Feedback Response to Sex Steroids during Aging

In other chapters in this book, negative and positive feedback responses to E_2 were shown to be decreased in old female rats. The site of the negative feedback action of E_2 is believed to be in the BMH of female rats (Lisk, 1960; Chowers and McCann, 1961; Ramirez et al., 1964). The positive feedback action of E_2 has been localized in the POA, anterior hypothalamic area (Döcke and Dörner, 1965; Kalra and McCann, 1975; Goodman, 1978) and in the BMH (Palka et al., 1966).

In the rat, a relationship appears to exist between decreased E_2 binding and biological responses to estradiol. For example, negative and positive feedback responses to E_2 were decreased concomitantly with decreased nuclear [^{3}H]estradiol binding in the POA and BMH, 0.5 or 1 hr after injection of [^{3}H]estradiol (Jiang and Peng, 1981). In contrast, a progressive age-related reduction in the induced luteinizing hormone (LH) surge was found in old mice despite the ability of hypothalamic E_2 receptors to translocate normally at proestrus (Nelson et al., 1980), without decreased E_2 uptake in the hypothalamus (Gosden, 1976).

The negative feedback response to testosterone is increased in old male rats (Shaar et al., 1975; Pirke et al., 1978). The site of negative feedback action of testosterone is in the BMH in male rats (Lisk, 1962; Smith and Davidson, 1967). However, results showing decreased testosterone binding in the hypothalamus (Chouknyiska and Vassileva-Popova, 1977) and lower affinity of the hydrotestosterone-binding reaction in the hypothalamus (Greenstein, 1979), do not correlate well with the increased negative feedback response to testosterone in old male rats. Whether the increased negative feedback response to testosterone in old male rats relates to changes in extrahypothalamic influence (disinhibition) and/or to changes in catecholamine and serotonin metabolism, remains to be elucidated.

2.4. Relation between Changes in Sex Steroid Binding to Receptors in the Hypothalamus and Changes in Hypothalamic Neuronal Numbers during Aging

Hsü and Peng (1978) counted the number of neurons in the POA, supraoptic nucleus (SO), paraventricular nucleus (PVN), anterior hypothalamic area (AHA), arcuate nucleus (ARN), ventromedial nucleus (VMN), and dorsomedial nucleus (DMN). They found significant loss of neurons in the POA, AHA, and ARN, but no neuronal loss in the SO, PVN, and DMN in PVC rats and ANE rats (Fig. 4). Lin *et al.* (1976) measured neuronal nuclear volume (NNV) in these areas, and found that NNV of female rats was reduced in old age to different degrees in the measured areas. The percent decrease of neuronal numbers and NNV in old compared to young adult female rats is shown in Table 1. When these two measures are combined, we can see marked decreases in the POA, AHA, and ARN in PVC and ANE rats; and moderate decreases in the SO, PVN, DMN, and VMN in PVC and ANE rats. The SO and PVN do not have estrogen-responsive neurons. Thus, the de-

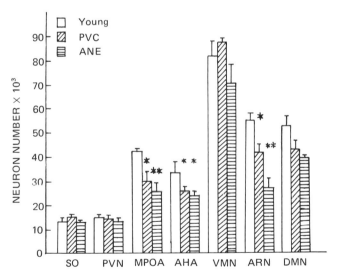

Fig. 4. Neuron number in hypothalamic nuclei of old female rats (24 months or older). Each column represents the mean of measurements from 3–5 PVC rats, 4–5 ANE rats, and 4–10 young adult rats. The bar indicates SEM. * and ** indicate statistically significant at 5% level.

Table 1. Percent of Neuron Numbers and Neuronal Nuclear Volume (NNV) in Different Hypothalamic Nuclei of Old as Compared to Young Adult Rats[a]

	POA	SO	PVN	AHA	ARN	VMN	DMN
PVC[b]							
Neuron no.	70	111	97	77	77	108	81
NNV	89	65	83	81	92	95	81
Overall	62	72	81	62	71	103	66
ANE[b]							
Neuron no.	61	99	86	72	50	86	74
NNV	82	69	81	75	93	78	87
Overall	50	68	70	54	47	67	64
Old males							
Neuron no.	88	97	101	114	98	103	96
NNV	99	89	96	99	95	95	103
Overall	87	86	97	113	93	98	99

[a] Recalculated from the data published in *Neuroendocrinology* **21**:247–254, 1976, and *Gerontology* **24**:434–440, 1978, by permission of S. Karger, Basel.
[b] PVC indicates prolonged vaginal cornification in old female rats; ANE indicates anestrus in old female rats.

creased E_2 binding in the POA and BMH in old noncyclic female rats correlates fairly well with the decrease in neuron number and NNV.

Contrary to old female rats, old male rats do not show changes in neuronal numbers and NNV when compared with young adult male rats (Lin *et al.*, 1976; Peng and Hsü, 1981; Table 1; Fig. 5).

Although decreased neuron number in the POA, AHA, and ARN can explain the decreased nuclear E_2 binding in noncyclic female rats, the remaining neurons show decreased NNV and the nuclear E_2 receptors do not increase after E_2 priming *in vivo*, indicating that the remaining neurons in the hypothalamus do not function normally. These results are consistent with the observations of Babichev (1973) that single unit electrical activity of neurons in the preoptic area, arcuate nucleus, and ventromedial nucleus becomes less sensitive to estrogen in old cyclic female rats.

3. Corticosteroid Uptake and Binding to Receptors in the Hypothalamus during Aging

Approximately a 35% reduction occurs in cerebral cortical corticosteroid receptors, which is progressive from 3–25 (or more) months

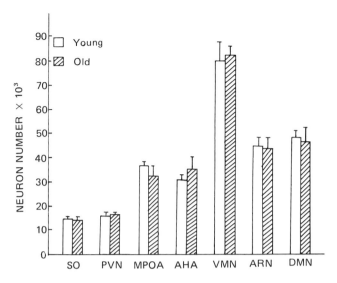

Fig. 5. Neuron number of hypothalamic nuclei of old male rats (24 or more months of age). Each column represents mean of measurements from 4–5 rats and bar SEM. SO: supraoptic nucleus, PVN: paraventricular nucleus, MPOA: medial preoptic area, AHA: anterior hypothalamic area, VMN: ventromedial nucleus, ARN: arcuate nucleus, DMN: dorsomedial nucleus. (Regraphed from the data published in *Gerontology*, 1981, by permission of S. Karger, Basel.)

of age in rats (Roth, 1974). When neuronal perikarya are extracted from the cerebrum of mature and old rats, the reduction in corticosteroid receptors with age is much greater, about 65% (Roth, 1976). In contrast, there are no age-related changes in the corticosterone-binding capacity of cytosol in the cerebral cortex, hippocampus or hypothalamus in C57BL/6J male mice at 28–32 months of age (Nelson *et al.*, 1976). Species differences between rats and mice in corticosterone-binding also have been shown for estrogen binding.

Both chronic and acute dexamethasone treatment produced greater adrenocortical inhibition in young than in aged rats (Riegle and Hess, 1972). Adrenocortical responses to restraint stress or to ether vapor stress were greater in young than in aged rats (Riegle, 1973). These observations indicate decreased sensitivity of the hypothalamic-pituitary-corticotropin control mechanism in aged rats. Corticosterone receptor levels in the hypothalamus and hippocampus of old rats need to be studied in order to correlate changes in hypothalamic and extrahypothalamic responses to corticosteroids during aging.

4. Summary

Decreased [^{3}H]estradiol uptake in the anterior hypothalamus and adenohypophysis of 2-year-old PVC and ANE female rats resulted in decreased specific [^{3}H]estradiol binding in the nuclear fraction of the POA and BMH. There also was no increase in the nuclear estradiol receptor complex in the HPA (including amygdala, POA, and BMH) and pituitary after estradiol priming. These results correlate fairly well with the decreased positive and negative feedback responses to estrogen, and with the loss of neurons and neuronal nuclear volume changes observed in the hypothalamus of PVC and ANE rats. In old mice, on the contrary, a progressive age-related reduction in the induced LH surge occurs without decreased E_2 uptake by the hypothalamus.

Species difference between rats and mice in corticosterone binding in the brain in old age also has been reported. There is decreased specific corticosterone binding in the cerebral cortex of old as compared to young rats, but no significant difference in cerebral cortical corticosteroid receptor content in cerebral cortex of old and young mice.

5. References

Anderson, J. N., Peck, E. J., Jr., and Clark, J. H., 1973, Nuclear receptor complex: accumulation, retention and localization in the hypothalamus and pituitary, *Endocrinology* **93:**711–717.

Aschheim, P., 1964, Resultants fournis par la greffe hétérochrone des ovaires dans l'étude regulation hypothalamo-hypophyso-ovarienne de la ratte senile, *Gerontologia* **10:**65–75.

Babichev, V. N., 1973, Characteristics of neurons in the areas of the hypothalamus regulating the gonadotropic function of the hypophysis in old female and male rats, *Bull. Exp. Biol. Med. USSR* **75:**3–5; cit. from *Hypothalamus Pituitary and Aging* (A. V. Everitt and J. A. Burgess, eds.), Charles C. Thomas, Springfield, Illinois, pp. 376–418.

Chouknyiska, R., and Vassileva-Popova, J. G., 1977, Effect of age on the binding of ^{3}H-testosterone with receptor protein from rat brain and testes, *C. R. Acad. Bulg. Sci.* **30:**133–135; cit. from G. S. Roth, 1979, Hormone receptor changes during adulthood and senescence: Significance for aging research, *Fed. Proc.* **38:**1910–1914.

Chowers, I., and McCann, S. M., 1961, Comparison of the effect of hypothalamic and pituitary implants of estrogen and testosterone on reproductive system and adrenal of female rats, *Proc. Soc. Exp. Biol. Med.* **124:**260–266.

Döcke, F., and Dörner, G., 1965, The mechanism of the induction of ovulation by oestrogens, *J. Endocrinol.* **33:**491–498.

Finch, C. E., Felicio, L. S., Flurkey, K., Gee, D. M., Mobbs, C., Nelson, J. F., and Osterburg, H. H., 1980, Studies on ovarian-hypothalamic-pituitary interactions during reproductive aging in C57BL/6J mice, *Peptides* (Suppl. 1)**1:**163–175.

Gerlach, J. L., and McEwen, B. S., 1972, Rat brain binds adrenal steroid hormone: Radioautography of hippocampus with corticosterone, *Science* **175:**1133–1136.

Goodman, R. L., 1978, The site of the positive feedback action of estradiol in the rat, *Endocrinology* **102**:151–159.

Gosden, R. G., 1976, Uptake and metabolism *in vivo* of tritiated estradiol-17-beta in tissues of aging female mice, *J. Endocrinol.* **68**:153–157.

Greenstein, B. D., 1979, Androgen receptors in the rat brain, anterior pituitary gland and ventral prostate gland: Effects of orchidectomy and aging, *J. Endocrinol* **81**:75–81.

Hsü, H. K., and Peng, M. T., 1978, Hypothalamic neuron number of old female rats, *Gerontology* **24**:434–440.

Huang, H. H., and Meites, J., 1975, Reproductive capacity of aging female rats, *Neuroendocrinology* **17**:289–295.

Jiang, M. J., and Peng, M. T., 1981, Cytoplasmic and nuclear binding of estradiol in the brain and pituitary of old female rats, *Gerontology* **27**:51–57.

Kalra, S. P., and McCann, S. M., 1975, The stimulatory effect on gonadotropin release of implants of estradiol or progesterone in certain sites in the central nervous system, *Neuroendocrinology* **19**:289–302.

Kanungo, M. S., Patnaik, S. E., and Koul, O., 1975, Decrease in 17β-estradiol receptor in brain of aging rats, *Nature (London)* **253**:366–367.

Korach, K. S., and Muldoon, T. G., 1974, Studies on the nature of the hypothalamic estradiol-concentrating mechanism in the male and female rats, *Endocrinology* **94**:785–793.

Krohn, P. L., 1955, Tissue transplantation technique applied to the problem of the aging of the organ of reproduction, in: *Ciba Foundation Colloquia on Aging, General Aspects*, Vol. 1 (G. E. W. Wolstenholme and M. P. Cameron, eds.), Little, Brown, Boston, pp. 141–161.

Lin, K. H., Peng, Y. M., Peng, M. T., and Tseng, T. M., 1976, Changes in the nuclear volume of rat hypothalamic neurons in old age, *Neuroendocrinology* **21**:247–254.

Lisk, R. D., 1960, Estrogen-sensitive centers in the hypothalamus of the rat, *J. Exp. Zool.* **145**:197–207.

Lisk, R. D., 1962, Testosterone-sensitive centers in the hypothalamus of the rat, *Acta Endocrinol. (Kbh.)* **41**:195–204.

Lu, K. H., Hopper, B. R., Vargo, T. M., and Yen, S. S. C., 1979, Chronological changes in sex steroid, gonadotropin and prolactin secretion in aging female rats displaying different reproductive states, *Biol. Reprod.* **21**:193–203.

McEwen, B. S., and Pfaff, D. W., 1973, Chemical and physiological approaches to neuroendocrine mechanisms: Attempts at integration, in: *Frontiers in Neuroendocrinology* (W. F. Ganong and L. Martini, eds.), Oxford University Press, New York, pp. 267–335.

Moudgil, V. K., and Kanungo, M. S., 1973, Effect of age of the rat on induction of acetylcholinesterase of the brain by 17β-estradiol, *Biochim. Biophys. Acta* **329**:211–220.

Nelson, J. F., Holinka, C. F., Latham, K. R., Allen, J. K., and Finch, C. E., 1976, Corticosterone binding in cytosol from brain regions of mature and senescent male C57BL/6J mice, *Brain Res.* **115**:345–351.

Nelson, J., Felicio, L., Sinha, Y. N., and Finch, C. E., 1980, Ovarian hormones and the etiology of reproductive aging in mice, in: *Aging—Its Chemistry* (A. A. Dietz, ed.), Am. Soc. Clin. Chemists, Washington, D. C., pp. 64–81.

Palka, Y., Ramirez, V. D., and Sawyer, C. H., 1966, Distribution and biological effects of tritiated estradiol implanted in the hypothalamo-hypophysial region of female rats, *Endocrinology* **78**:487–499.

Peng, M. T., and Hsü, H. K., 1982, No neuron loss from hypothalamic nuclei of male rats in old age, *Gerontology* **28**:19–22.

Peng, M. T., and Huang, H. H., 1972, Aging of hypothalamic-pituitary-ovarian function in the rat, *Fertil. Steril.* **23**:535–542.

Peng, M. T., and Peng, Y. M., 1973, Changes in the uptake of tritiated estradiol in the hypothalamus and adenohypophysis of old female rats, *Fertil. Steril.* **24:**534–539.

Peng, M. T., Pi, W. P., and Peng, Y. M., 1973, The hypothalamic-pituitary-testicular function of the old rat, *J. Formosan Med. Assoc.* **72:**495–502.

Pfaff, D. W., 1971, Steroid sex hormones in the rat brain: Specificity of uptake and physiological effects, in: *Steroid Hormones and Brain Function* (C. H. Sawyer and R. A. Gorski, eds.), University of California Press, Los Angeles, pp. 103–112.

Pirke, K. M., Geiss, M., and Sintermann, 1978, A quantitative study on feedback control of LH by testosterone in young adult and old male rats, *Acta Endocrinol. (Kbh)* **89:**789–795.

Ramirez, V. D., Abrams, R. M., and McCann, S. M., 1964, Effect of estradiol implants in the hypothalamo-hypophysial region of the rat on the secretion of luteinizing hormone, *Endocrinology* **75:**243–248.

Riegle, G. D., 1973, Chronic stress effects on adrenocortical responsiveness in young and aged rats, *Neuroendocrinology* **11:**1–10.

Riegle, G. D., and Hess, G. D., 1972, Chronic and acute dexamethasone suppression of stress activation of the adrenal cortex in young and aged rats, *Neuroendocrinology* **9:**175–187.

Roth, G. S., 1974, Age-related changes in specific glucocorticoid binding by steroid responsive tissues of rats, *Endocrinology* **94:**82–90.

Roth, G. S., 1976, Reduced glucocorticoid binding site concentration in cortical neuronal perikarya from senescent rats, *Brain Res.* **107:**345–354.

Shaar, C. J., Euker, J. S., Riegle, G. D., and Meites, J., 1975, Effects of castration and gonadal steroids on serum luteinizing hormone and prolactin in old and young rats, *J. Endocrinol.* **66:**45–51.

Smith, E. R., and Davidson, J. M., 1967, Differential responses to hypothalamic testosterone in relation to male puberty, *Am. J. Physiol.* **212:**1385–1390.

Stumpf, W. E., 1968, Estradiol-concentrating neurones: Topography in the hypothalamus by dry mount autoradiography, *Science* **162:**1001–1003.

Stumpf, W. E., 1971, Hypophysiotropic neurons in the periventricular brain: Topography of estradiol concentrating neurons, in: *Steroid Hormones and Brain Function* (C. H. Sawyer and R. A. Gorski, eds.), University of California Press, Los Angeles, pp. 215–226.

Zeilmaker, G. H., 1969, Effect of prolonged feeding on an ovulatory inhibitor (Lyndiol) on aging of the hypothalamic-ovarian axis and pituitary tumorigenesis in rats, *J. Endocrinol.* **43:**21–22.

CHAPTER 6

Relation of Neuroendocrine System to Reproductive Decline in Female Rats

PIERRE ASCHHEIM

1. Introduction

The reproductive decline in female mammals is universal. Age-related sterility in rats is complete at about 15–17 months (Miller *et al.*, 1979), when approximately 50–60% of the lifetime is spent. This type of sterility is multifactorial, the most important factor being senescence of the uterus. Oocyte alterations also occur. Disregarding these reproductive aspects, we will focus on aging of the hypothalamic-hypophysial-ovarian axis.

When this work was started 20 years ago, the contrast soon became apparent between (1) the modified, but persistent ovarian function in rats until the end of their lifespan, and termination of ovarian function in women at menopause, (2) the predominance of aging of the neuroendocrine regulatory mechanisms in the rat, and the predominance of intrinsic ovarian aging in women. Since menopause is restricted to humans and some infrahuman primates, the rat improperly appeared to be a model for other mammalian reproductive aging, a model characterized by hypersecretion of prolactin (PRL) during aging, implicating age-related alterations in hypothalamic-pituitary sensitivity to control input, and changes in neurotransmitter activity.

At present, it is known (Parkening *et al.*, 1980a) that reproductive aging in other rodents is different than in rats. There is no age-related

PIERRE ASCHHEIM • Unité de Recherches Gérontologiques, INSERM U.118, 75016 Paris, France.

increase in plasma PRL concentration in C57BL6 mice, Chinese hamsters or Mongolian gerbils. In Syrian hamsters, PRL concentration even decreases with age. Moreover, CBA mice represent the closest rodent model known at present for human ovarian aging! (Aschheim, 1982). But three reasons remain for justifying research in the rat model: (1) it is necessary to understand age-related changes in sexual neuroendocrinology in the rat, since it is the most widely used laboratory animal in this field; (2) it is necessary to establish reference data for age controls in studies on chronic drug administration, and, (3) the early aging of the neuroendocrine control system of ovarian function in the rat is an interesting model *per se,* and may explain the plasticity of ovarian aging and the facility of its experimental manipulation.

This chapter will attempt to disclose new trends in research in reproductive aging. During the last three years (from mid-1978 to mid-1981), there appeared nearly as many publications on this subject as in the preceding 15-year period. This resulted, at least in part, from (1) the increased use of hormone radioimmunoassays (RIAs), especially by collection of serial blood samples, and (2) the fully justified interest and use of middle-aged rats, during cyclicity or in the transition period from cyclicity to senile disruptions of the estrous cycle. In addition to accumulation of new data which are sometimes contradictory, two tendencies can be observed: (1) a greater awareness of difficulties in interpreting age-related hormonal blood concentrations in terms of secretion rate, when other possibly age-related changes in parameters of hormonal kinetics remain uncontrolled, and (2) a justified reserve in attributing hormonal changes to aging *per se* when they may result only from previous differences in the hormonal milieu. In this respect, the influence of ovarian steroids on central (hypothalamic-hypophysial) aging has recently been reevaluated.

The chapter begins with comments on the above points. It then describes aging of the ovary and its neuroendocrine regulation in old rats displaying senile deviations of the cycle (SDC), and in aging rats during the period of cyclicity and the transition period to acyclicity. Consideration is given next to experimental modifications of hypothalamic-hypophysial-ovarian aging. Finally, extrinsic and intrinsic aging and their physiological significance will be discussed.

2. Preliminary Comments on Hormonal Data in Old Rats

The numerous hormonal data reported for old rats in recent years are difficult to present in tabulated form. This results not only from the normal discrepancies found in animal husbandry, technical procedures, experimental designs, etc., but because aging itself is a complex and diverse process.

The activity of hormones is usually inferred from their concentrations in serum or plasma. In addition, age can modify hormone availability by altering vascular supply as well as the number and (or) quality of target cell receptors. But when hormone production rate is inferred from serum concentration alone, it is only justified if other parameters of hormonal kinetics are held constant. Table 1 presents some possible age-related changes which may alter the significance of blood hormone concentrations. A decrease in metabolic clearance rate (MCR) of luteinizing hormone (LH) is suggested by Fig. 1 (data from Riegle and Miller, 1978, by permission). By 75 min after injection of LH-releasing hormone (LHRH), its stimulatory effect disappears, but the residual LH level remains higher in old than in young rats, particularly after the second injection of LHRH. With a decrease of MCR, hormone concentration overestimates the production rate.

Both plasma volume and body weight increase with age. The expanded plasma volume in the larger body mass of old rats has been measured in males by Kaler and Neaves (1981), and in females by Aschheim and Fayein (unpublished). Whereas, in old recurrently pseudo-

Table 1. Parameters Whose Possible Age-Changes May Alter the Significance of Hormonal Blood Concentration in Terms of Secretion Rate in Old Rats

Metabolic clearance rate	Unknown. Decrease suggested for LH by Fig. 1[a]
Plasma volume	Increases with body weight which increases with age. Male rat,[b] female rat[c]
Hormonal transport	Unknown. No specific binding proteins for estrogen in adult rats.[d] Other binding proteins?
"Aged" hormones	Big LH molecule in male rats.[e] Discrepancy between LH concentration measured by RIA or RRA suggests also alteration of LH molecule in aged female mice[f]
Number and/or size of hormone producing cells	Increase in number of prolactin-producing pituitary cells.[g] Decrease in number and nuclear size of hypothalamic neurons[h,i]

[a] Riegle and Miller, 1978.
[b] Kaler and Neaves, 1981.
[c] Aschheim and Fayein (unpublished).
[d] Germain et al., 1978.
[e] Conn et al., 1980.
[f] Parkening et al., 1980b.
[g] Kawashima, 1974.
[h] Hsu and Peng, 1978.
[i] Lin et al., 1976.

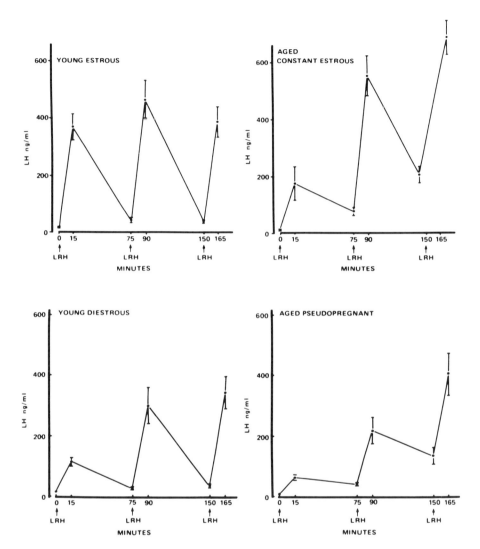

Fig. 1. Effect of three intravenous injections of 500 ng of LHRH on serum LH in young estrous and diestrous, and aged constant estrous and persistent diestrous, female rats. Serum LH is shown as the group mean with indicated SEM. Serial blood samples were taken before LHRH injection (0, 75 and 150 min) and 15 min after LHRH stimulation (15, 90, and 165 min). From G. D. Riegle and A. E. Miller, 1978, in: *The Aging Reproductive System* (E. L. Schneider, ed.), Raven Press, New York, with permission.

pregnant rats, progesterone concentration is elevated but significantly lower during the plateau period of luteal function than in young pseudo-pregnant controls (Fayein and Aschheim, 1980), the total amount of circulating progesterone is similar in both groups (which differ by 30% in their respective body weights). Due to this hormonal dilution in old rats, hormone concentrations in the blood underestimate secretion rate. This applies to progesterone hypoconcentration as well as to PRL-hy-perconcentration.

In female rats, little is known about age-related changes in binding proteins and free or bound hormonal fractions. But "aged hormones" deserve comment. Conn *et al.* (1980) described a large molecular size of LH in aged male rats. Castration of young rats resulted in similar alterations, reversed by steroid treatment, suggesting a relation not to aging *per se* but to changed testosterone milieu. Moreover, the MCR of the large LH form was decreased. Discrepancies between immunological and biological activities of LH in aged female mice, as reported by Parkening *et al.* (1980b), may also be due to such a qualitative change.

For the gerontologist, age-related changes in hormonal concentration reflecting production rate, must ultimately be ascribed to the number and/or quality of hormone producing cells. There is a proliferation with age (leading to tumors) of pituitary PRL producing cells (Kawashima, 1974). The concentration of serum PRL increases significantly. The increase in PRL production by the pituitary of acyclic rats is also seen *in vitro*. But when expressed as per mg of pituitary weight, accounting for cell proliferation in old age, the unitary activity of these newly formed cells decreases significantly (Aschheim and Rasolonjanahary, 1979).

Hormonal data must also be related to age changes in hormonal rhythmicity, pulsatile secretory pattern of LH, PRL surges, etc., as will be seen later. Hormonal concentration results from intricate, multidirectional processes, and therefore contradictory age-related changes in numerous parameters can occur. By itself, hormone concentration cannot clarify an endocrinological condition in the aged rat. It must be completed by stimulation and inhibition tests, by *in vitro* studies, and by examination of target structures. This is not intended to discredit measurements of hormonal concentrations, but to indicate that their critical evaluation may involve many interesting new gerontological aspects of homeostatic regulation.

The second comment concerns the gerontological validity of hormonal comparisons, a point which I emphasized many years ago and which is now taken into consideration by most investigators. Young cyclic and old acyclic rats differ not only by age, but also by their hormonal background, which in turn is "spontaneously" age related. Valid comparisons dealing only with age must also be made between young and middle-aged cyclic rats. Old, previously acyclic, but experimentally "recycled" rats can be usefully added to the study. Likewise, persistent estrous rats must be compared at different developmental stages of this condition, complemented by young rats made persistent-estrous, for example, by constant illumination. Stimulation and inhibition tests are frequently performed on ovariectomized or ovariectomized rats given hormone replacement. Here too, it is advisable to standardize the neuroendocrine status preceding ovariectomy and the time elapsed after ovariectomy, when hormonal changes due only to aging are investigated.

3. Relation of Neuroendocrine System to Ovarian Function after the End of Cyclicity

3.1. Senile Patterns of Ovarian Function

3.1.1. Senile Deviations of the Estrous Cycle

The incidence of regular 4- or 5-day estrous cycles decreases with age as indicated in Wistar rats by the first two lines in Table 2. At the end of the first year of life, estrous cycles are progressively replaced by two SDCs: persistent estrus (PE) and recurrent pseudopregnancies (RPP; Aschheim, 1961). PE predominates during the second and RPP during the third and last year of life. All PE rats were previously cyclic, as were most RPP rats. But some of the latter derive from PE, implicating resumption of ovulation. Another, rather unusual pattern, senile anestrus, has been described, but it could be pathological and will be disregarded here. Cyclic rats represent 5–10% of the population after the age of 18 months.

PE, characterized by a persistent cornified vaginal smear, is an anovulatory condition. The ovaries are devoid of corpora lutea and therefore are relatively small (weight = 40–60 mg). They contain numerous follicles of all sizes, healthy as well as atretic, and in addition cystic follicles, particularly in rats which aged during the PE condition. Estradiol levels are moderate, 18 pg/ml at 11–13 months, 30 pg/ml at 16 and 30 months of age (Lu *et al.*, 1979) and rather constant (Huang *et al.*, 1978). Low to medium levels were reported for estrone, testosterone, and androstenedione, and very low levels for progesterone and 20α-

Table 2. Evolution of Some Biological Parameters during Aging of Cyclic Rats.[a,b]

	Age in months								
	2–3	3–4	4–5	6–7	7–8	9–10	10–11	11–12	12–13
Cyclic rats	100	94	85	77		72	60	<60	>40
Regular Wistar cyclers at									
4 days	60	50	50	26		16			
5 days	20	30	40	60		70			
Persistence of cycles during the month following hemiovariectomy		100				65			40
Long-term persistence of ovulatory compensation after hemiovariectomy at 30 days of age		79				61	38		0
Persistence of the cycle after injection of 5 µg of estradiol benzoate at estrus		94	81		63	33			17
Increase of circulating FSH 1 mth after castration		510						380	
Increase of circulating LH 1 mth after castration		560						350	

[a] Values are given as percentages.
[b] From P. Aschheim (1979), with permission.

hydroxyprogesterone (Lu *et al.*, 1979). In PE rats, moderate amounts of estradiol are secreted continuously, unopposed by progestogens.

RPP are characterized by prolonged diestrous vaginal smears, lasting 15 days or more, interspaced by proestrus and/or estrus associated with ovulation of a normal number of oocytes, and then followed by a new diestrous period. The ovaries (weighing 80–110 mg) contain large corpora lutea and well-developed follicles. Traumatic deciduomata can readily be induced by irritation of the uterus at day (D) 4 of pseudopregnancy (Aschheim, 1961). As in young rats displaying RPP in the presence of vasectomized males, circulating progesterone concentration shows a rapid increase until D3, an elevated plateau level of 56 ng/ml until D9 (longer extension in old rats), and a decline afterwards (Fayein and Aschheim, 1980). As mentioned in Section 2, the plateau progesterone values are lower in old than in young rats, but the total amount of circulating progesterone is equal in the two groups. The 20α-hydroxyprogesterone values are also increased (Lu *et al.*, 1979). Estradiol levels are very low at diestrus (Lu *et al.*, 1979). In contrast to previous statements (Huang *et al.*, 1978), old RPP rats display a cyclic pattern in terms of luteal function.

3.1.2. Hormonal Data

Data on pituitary hormones in SDC can be summarized by an age-related hypersecretion of PRL associated with moderate or low levels of follicle-stimulating hormone (FSH) and LH, which clearly are not increased as after ovariectomy.

Pituitary PRL content is high in PE rats (Clemens and Meites, 1971), including nontumorous pituitary glands (Kawashima, 1974). Circulating PRL levels are also elevated in old PE rats. Kawashima (1974), Watkins *et al.* (1975a), Huang *et al.* (1976a), Lu *et al.* (1979) and Rasolonjanahary (1979) reported values of 160–400 and even 1200 ng/ml. But it is important to emphasize that this hormonal increase is age-related. Prolactin levels at the beginning of PE, in rats 11–16 months old (Lu *et al.*, 1979) or 8 months old (Rasolonjanahary, 1979), are significantly lower than at 18 months or afterwards, and are similar to basal PRL values of cycling rats of the same age. Damassa *et al.* (1980) studied the 24-hr pattern of PRL secretion in PE rats and demonstrated a diurnal surge at 1700 hr, whereas at 200 hr, a smaller nocturnal rise did not show statistical significance. Prolactin values were also elevated in RPP rats, but less than in PE, to 100–200 ng/ml (Watkins *et al.*, 1975a; Huang *et al.*, 1976a; Lu *et al.*, 1979; Rasolonjanahary, 1979). There is a moderate age-related increase in blood PRL values from 18 to 24 months (Fayein and Aschheim, 1980). The PRL surge is nocturnal in old spontaneous RPP rats (Damassa *et al.*, 1980), whereas in young rats with induced pseudopregnancy, daily diurnal and nocturnal surges are observed. The suppression of the former may be related to the low estradiol level in old RPP rats (Gilman *et al.*, 1981).

Pituitary content of FSH is high in PE (Clemens and Meites, 1971). LH content in PE is low, whereas in RPP it increases throughout the pseudopregnancy sequence to three-fold the PE level and then falls at ovulation (Aschheim, 1968). Variations in circulating FSH and LH concentrations in old PE and RPP rats do not differ markedly from those seen during the estrous cycle (excluding ovulatory surges) of adult rats (Huang *et al.*, 1978; Lu *et al.*, 1979). FSH and LH basal values are higher in PE than in RPP, as reported by Huang *et al.* (1978), although no major differences were noted by Lu *et al.* (1979). In these rats, there is no hypersecretion of FSH as after ovariectomy, and no significant hyposecretion of basal LH. But as discussed in Section 2, changes in plasma volume, MCR, pulsatile secretory pattern, or biological activity of gonadotropin molecules can alter the significance of assays of hormonal concentrations in the blood.

Hypothalamic LHRH content is not altered in aged rats (Steger *et al.*, 1979a). LHRH is present in sufficient amount to sustain basal LH secretion *in vitro* (Riegle and Miller, 1978). Meites *et al.* (1979) described a depressed catecholamine and an enhanced serotonin activity in old male rats as compared to young ones, and mentioned a similar difference between old and young females. Hypothalamic dopamine (DA) concentration was reduced in old RPP rats (Clemens, 1979). Walker (1981) reported the interesting finding that the circadian rhythm of hypothalamic serotonin turnover, seen in cyclic rats, is abolished in old PE (as well as in other conditions leading to PE). Reinitiation of cycling in old rats restored the rhythm of serotonin dynamics.

3.1.3. Structural Changes in the Ovary, Pituitary, and Hypothalamus

Ovary. No age-related regression of ovarian weight or of ovarian vascularization occurs in rats. As in all other mammals, there is an age-related decrease in the number of oocytes; but in rodents, except for the CBA mouse, a complete exhaustion of oocytes does not occur by the end of life. In mice, the proportion of oocytes lost per 100-day interval remains constant and is strain-specific. But in rats, it decreases contin uously with increasing age; between 100 and 200 days of age, the proportion lost is 0.281; between 500–600 days, it is only 0.082. During the first mentioned interval, a loss of 1140 oocytes results in 2924 residual oocytes, and during the second interval, a loss of 154 results in 1734 residual oocytes (Mandl and Zuckerman, 1951). An ultrastructural alteration in preovulatory oocyte morphology will be dealt with in Section 4.1, since it has been described in aging cyclic rats. Growing and mature follicles in acyclic old rats do not differ microscopically from those seen in young rats. Gonadotropin binding and aromatase activity in granulosa cells of mature Graafian follicles are similar in old PE and young proestrous rats (Erickson *et al.*, 1979). Corpora lutea of old RPP show the same binding capacity for LH and the same 3β-hydroxysteroid dehydrogenase (3β-IISD) activity as those of young rats (Steger *et al.*, 1976).

In about 25% of old acyclic rats, mostly in PE, 2–4 follicles per ovary can be observed which exhibit a striking densification of granulosa cells (Aschheim, unpublished). Follicles measure about 350 μm in diameter, and the external limits are regular (round or slightly waving). A small antrum is present, with or without an oocyte. Granulosa cells are numerous, small, densely packed, proliferating to the center, with few mitoses. In a few instances, I have observed a true intraovarian follicular rupture without any sign of luteinization, the oocyte lying in a nearby lymphatic space. All the granulosa cells show a very high 3β-HSD activity, which usually is seen only in the external layer of granulosa cells of preovulatory follicles. I could show experimentally that these follicles are not precursor structures of granulosa-cell tumors, but they may represent abortive steps to ovulation occurring during PE.

Other structural changes occur in old ovaries, including thickening of the basement membrane of small follicles, proliferation of the surface ("germinal") epithelium and of the rete ovarii, and accumulation of numerous phagocytes filled with lipofuscin granules in the interstitial compartment. Interstitial cells of thecal origin are transformed into "deficiency" or "wheel" cells which are considered to result from decreased biological activity of LH. Testis-like tubes, a particular form of follicular atresia, are present, and epithelial cellular cords appear, proliferate, and may become tumorous. In electron microscopy, epithelial cord and deficiency cells show a low steroidogenic activity, which can be normalized and notably increased by treatment with exogenous human chorionic gonadotropin (hCG) (Crumeyrolle-Arias et al., 1976). Few of these structural changes are due to intrinsic ovarian aging, as will be seen in Section 6, by comparison with ovarian aging in rats hypophysectomized when 26 days old.

Pituitary. The proportion of PRL-producing cells increases with age (Kawashima, 1974). Enlarged pituitaries, weighing more than 23 mg, are encountered in 12.5% of acyclic rats at 13–14 months of age; the proportion increases to almost 50% at 16–18 months (Aschheim, 1975). At 24 months, all rats show macroscopic adenomas or microscopic proliferation of PRL-producing cells (Aschheim and Pasteels, 1963). Their ultrastructure has been studied by Kawashima (1974) and by Kovacs et al. (1977), who also demonstrated by immunoperoxidase staining the presence of immunoreactive PRL and the absence of growth hormone (GH) and thyrotropin (TSH). Peng and Peng (1973) measured the uptake of tritiated estradiol in the pituitary of old rats in SDC, and reported that per mg of hypophysial tissue it was significantly lower than in young rats, but per pituitary it was the same.

Hypothalamus. Morphometric studies have been done in hypothalamic areas concerned with gonadotropin regulation (Lin et al., 1976; Hsu and Peng, 1978). The preoptic area implicated in cyclic release of these hormones in adults shows a large decrease of the total number of neurons and of individual nuclear volume in 24–30-month-old rats. In the areas implicated in tonic release, the situation differs; the arcuate nucleus shows a large decrease in neuron numbers and a moderate one in nuclear volume, whereas in the ventromedial nucleus there is no cellular loss and a variable reduction of nuclear volume. Uptake of tritiated estradiol is also significantly lower in the anterior hypothalamus of old rats compared with young rats (Peng and Peng, 1973). Analysis of its subcellular distribution reveals an impaired (decreased) translocation of estradiol from cytosol to nucleus in old PE rats (Jiang and Peng, 1981). Unfortunately, nothing is known about the evolution of these parameters between the ages of 4–24 months.

An interesting morphological change has been reported by Brawer (Brawer *et al.*, 1980; Schipper *et al.*, 1981). During aging of PE rats, an ovary-dependent degeneration occurs selectively in the arcuate nucleus. It is characterized by a significant increase in the numbers of astrocytic granules, starting during cyclicity, and principally in the numbers of reactive microglial cells, starting with PE. This "gliosis" within the arcuate nucleus is not related to neuronal degeneration of perikarya, but rather of axons, terminals, and sometimes dendrites connecting the medial preoptic area to the medial basal hypothalamus. This neurotoxic effect is absent in aging rats ovariectomized when young. At present, it is not known if morphological changes representing chemical deafferentation also occur in the hypothalamus of RPP rats.

Immunostaining demonstrated LHRH-positive perikarya in the medial preoptic and septal area (but not in the arcuate nucleus), of 16–20-month-old PE rats, in contrast to young rats. Staining intensity of LHRH-containing nerve elements, especially axon terminals in the median eminence, was also much higher in old than in young rats (Merchenthaler *et al.*, 1980). Age-related subneuronal distribution of LHRH has been studied by Barnea *et al.* (1980). With aging, an increase in the LHRH content of the hypothalamus occurs predominantly in subneuronal structures which give rise to fragile synaptosomes and free granules, suggesting alterations in the physicochemical properties of the plasma membranes of the neuronal terminals.

3.2. Aging of the Neuroendocrine Regulation of Ovarian Function

3.2.1. Physiological Aspects: Reinstatement of Cyclicity, Heterochronic Grafts of Ovary and Pituitary

SDC do not represent a fixed status. I have already mentioned the "spontaneous" transition from PE to RPP, indicating resumption of ovulation. RPP rats exposed to permanent light change to PE and resume RPP when returned to alternating photoperiods (Aschheim, 1961). Whereas these rats continue to show senile neuroendocrine regulation, they can secrete the ovarian hormones, progesterone and estrogen, previously lacking. Different agents have been used to reinstate ovarian cycles. In PE rats, this is achieved in order of decreasing efficiency by administration of progesterone, adrenocorticotropic hormone (ACTH), ether stress, L-dopa and other drugs, correcting a hypothalamic deficiency of catecholamines (Huang *et al.*, 1976b, Linnoila and Cooper, 1976). Luteinizing hormone (LH) surges have been observed on proestrous days of induced cycles in old PE rats by use of progesterone and ACTH (Huang *et al.*, 1976b). The incidence, amplitude, and timing of LH surges are more irregular than in young rats. Epinephrine treatment, injection of LHRH, and electrical stimulation of the preoptic area, can also induce ovulation (Meites, *et al.*, 1978). RPP rats resume cycles during treatment with lergotrile mesylate, a DA agonist (Clemens, 1979).

SDC are reversible, since cyclicity can be reinstated by a unique "trigger" mechanism. The resultant sequence of ovarian cycles is self-sustained. A single injection of hCG or LH in old PE rats first induces a pseudopregnancy, followed by a succession of about 11 autonomous ovarian cycles (Aschheim, 1965). Middle-aged PE rats generally resume short cycles directly after the induced ovulation, without pseudopregnancy, because of their lower PRL values (Everett, 1980; for age-related PRL concentration in PE, see Section 3.1.2). A single modification of environmental conditions can also restore cyclicity in a certain percentage of SDC, e.g., exposure of PE rats to constant darkness (Aschheim, 1965), isolation of previously grouped RPP, or chronic exposure to cold (+ 5°C) (Aschheim and Latouche, 1975).

Reinstatement of cyclicity is more or less easy to realize and is generally of limited duration. But an efficient treatment like a single injection of hCG in PE produces cycling in a large number of old rats and allows for comparison with young rats. Moreover, reversibility of the PE condition is an argument against an intrinsic cellular deficiency in hormone production or release at any one of the sites implicated in regulation of cyclicity, or in related neurotransmitter activity. It points more to a deficiency in the control mechanisms of cellular activity, and to changes in the sensitivity of regulatory structures (Aschheim, 1965).

Studies of heterochronic ovarian grafts demonstrate that the ovary is not primarily responsible for SDC. Adult cycling rats, ovariectomized and grafted with old ovaries originating from rats in SDC, resume cycles. Old PE or RPP rats, ovariectomized and grafted with prepubertal ovaries, resume PE or RPP, respectively (Aschheim, 1964/5). Grafting of an old pituitary under the median eminence of a young previously hypophysectomized rat results in resumption of ovarian cycles, but less frequently than grafts of young pituitaries (Peng and Huang, 1972). The grafted old gland seems to be more difficult to revascularize than the young pituitary and/or its functional performance is impaired.

3.2.2. Changes in Steroidal Feedback Regulation of the Hypothalamus, Neurotransmitter Activity, and Pituitary Response to LHRH

A significant increase of pituitary LH stores was found after ovariectomy of PE or RPP old rats, but was significantly lower than in ovariectomized young or old formerly cyclic rats. Prolactin was implicated, since in PE rats "recycled" during the month before ovariectomy, the postcastration rise of LH stores was enhanced (Aschheim, 1970). A complete study of circulating FSH, LH, and PRL levels after ovariectomy or ovariectomy and estrogen treatment has been reported by Huang *et al.* (1976a). Postovariectomy levels of FSH and LH in PE and RPP old rats were significantly greater than in intact control rats, but lower than in young ovariectomized rats. The rise was nullified by estrogen treatment. After ovariectomy, PRL values decreased significantly in young cyclic and old PE rats (but residual PRL concentration remained higher in PE), but did not change in RPP. Estrogen treatment increased PRL values in all categories. Is the smaller increase of gonadotropins after ovariectomy in old rats directly related to age or is it due, at least partly, to the higher residual levels of circulating PRL, a hormone known to inhibit the postcastration rise of LH? (Grandison *et al.*, 1977). Clemens (1979) reported that in ovariectomized, formerly RPP rats, lergotrile mesylate inhibited PRL secretion, but did not allow serum LH levels to rise.

The positive feedback of injected estradiol or progesterone on the LH surge in old acyclic rats, ovariectomized and pretreated with estrogen, is also diminished (Howland, 1976; Huang *et al.*, 1980) or abolished (Gosden and Bancroft, 1976; Peluso *et al.*, 1977), when compared to results in young, formerly cyclic rats. Can the observed differences be ascribed, not to age *per se,* but to differences in the gonadal steroid background? In acutely ovariectomized old rats, the positive feedback of estradiol and progesterone on LH secretion was observed only in formerly RPP, not in formerly PE animals (Lu *et al.*, 1980). But in PE, the positive feedback effect was seen five weeks after ovariectomy (Lu *et al.*, 1981) and was significantly smaller than in young, formerly cyclic, controls. After chronic implantation of these two long-term ovariectomized groups with estradiol, it was abolished in both age groups (Lu *et al.*, 1981). Thus, estrogen is the discriminating factor in the divergent responses of RPP and PE rats of the same age, and can induce a similar deficiency of response in rats of different ages, possibly through its neurotoxic action on the hypothalamus. The smaller positive steroidal feedback effect in old PE than in young cycling rats five weeks after ovariectomy is ascribed by Lu *et al.* (1981) to an insufficient recovery period after the operation. But proof of a later restoration of the full magnitude of the neuroendocrine response is presently lacking, particularly since a previous paper (Lu et al., 1977) observed an age-related difference that persisted for 55 days after ovariectomy. This is another example of a condition where direct age effects and those due to a modified steroidal milieu are not yet entirely delineated.

Since there are differential age-dependent responses of LH to ovariectomy, it is not surprising that catecholamine responses also differed in the anterior hypothalamus (Huang et al., 1979) and the median eminence (Wilkes and Yen, 1981). In the anterior hypothalamus, norepinephrine concentration and turnover were lower in old than in young ovariectomized rats, whereas DA concentration did not differ. In the median eminence, ovariectomy did not increase norepinephrine concentration in old rats and the increase in DA concentration was smaller than in young rats.

The amplitude of LH pulses is significantly reduced in old ovariectomized, formerly PE rats (Steger et al., 1979b; Estes et al., 1980). This difference between old and young rats could account for the smaller increase of LH after ovariectomy, possibly mediated by the deficiency of neurotransmitter activity after ovariectomy, or it could result from the higher basal levels of PRL.

In contrast to the above changes, contradictory results were reported on acute hypophysial stimulation by LHRH in old intact or ovariectomized rats, with or without steroidal pretreatment. LH release was similar in old and young ovariectomized rats pretreated with estrogen (Peluso et al., 1977), and in intact old and young rats (McPherson et al., 1977). The peak serum levels of LH were attained later in old rats. According to Lu et al. (1980), circulating LH increased similarly after a single LHRH pulse in old PE and RPP rats. In long-term ovariectomized old and young rats chronically implanted with estradiol, LHRH induced a similar rise in circulating LH (Lu et al., 1981). Therefore, hypophysial sensitivity to LHRH was not impaired with aging. However, Watkins et al. (1975b) reported smaller LH release in intact old acyclic rats than in young cycling rats, as did Howland (1976) in ovariectomized old vs. young animals. Riegle and Miller (1978), using a single injection of LHRH, confirmed the results of Watkins et al. (1975b). The response to LHRH was modified after multiple injections (Fig. 1); the increase in LH was greater after the second and third LHRH injections in old PE and RPP rats, and reached levels similar to those obtained in young controls. Comparison of pituitary sensitivity to LHRH between young and old rats, respectively, in induced (young) and spontaneous (old) PE or RPP may clarify these discrepancies (see Section 2). Interpretation of results on age-related negative and positive steroidal feedback regulation, pul-

satile LH secretion, and pituitary sensitivity to LHRH, remains controversial, and will be considered further in Section 5.1.

4. Relation of Neuroendocrine System to Ovarian Function during Cyclicity and Transition Period

4.1. Aging of Ovarian Function during Cyclicity: Physiological and Structural Changes

The problem is to detect, measure, understand, and if possible,
modify age-related changes in ovarian cycles which can be latent, but
finally result in qualitative changes such as the SDC. Table 2 illustrates
changes in some parameters observed in Wistar rats (Aschheim, 1979).
The decrease in the percentage of cyclic rats is accentuated between
10–13 months. During that period, cyclers become the minority of a
stable population whose mortality is insignificant. In this strain, there is
an important shift between 3–10 months from regular four-day cyclers
to regular five-day cyclers. Rats with longer cycles are rather unusual,
even in older animals.

In 12-month-old Holtzman rats, six-day cycles appear, characterized
by delayed ovulation (Fugo and Butcher, 1971). Preovulatory overripe-
ness of ova results in an increased incidence of developmental anomalies,
similar to those seen after experimentally delayed ovulation of young
rats. The important hormonal difference with normal cyclers is the earlier increase of plasma estradiol levels (Butcher and Page, 1981). These
authors showed that in experimental six-day cyclers, this particular pattern of estrogen secretion was responsible for the detrimental effects on
the ova and uterine environment.

In 1976, Van der Schoot described a delayed LH surge with a reduced steepness in 10-month-old–five-day cyclers as compared to 5-
month-old controls, but without any significant difference in the numbers of ruptured follicles. Gray *et al.* (1980) confirmed that in four-day
cyclers the preovulatory LH surge was significantly lower in rats aged
11 months than in controls aged three months. Cooper *et al.* (1980)
showed a relationship between the time of the LH surge and its amplitude. Later surges, as in 10.5-month-old rats, were consistently lower
than the normally timed LH surges, as in 4.5-month-old controls.

Other age-related neurohormonal changes have been described at
other times of the ovarian cycle. In a study of 13 such parameters at
proestrous morning, Wilkes *et al.* (1979) found three modifications: norepinephrine concentration in the median eminence, circulating FSH,

and androstenedione levels were increased in 12- as compared to 6-month-old rats. The significance of these apparently linked changes, which did not persist after transition to PE, is not entirely clear. In our laboratory, Rasolonjanahary (1979) found a three- to four-fold increase in circulating PRL concentration on diestrous morning in five-day cyclers 2–16 months of age, with a first significant rise between 2–3 months of age, a plateau level until after nine months, and another sharp rise around 12 months of age. Prolactin is the only hormone in rats displaying an age-related increase during cyclicity as well as in SDC. The increase of PRL in old cyclic rats may result from the slightly higher estradiol levels reported by Lu and Kledzik (1981), rising earlier and declining later than in young controls. Moreover, estradiol-binding activities in both the hypothalamus and pituitary are greater in old than in young females throughout their cycles (Lu and Kledzik, 1981). Peluso *et al.* (1979) reported that estradiol concentration within the ovary was higher in old irregular than in young regular cyclers during proestrus and estrus.

Changes of cycle length, of estradiol, and of LH secretion patterns and levels may be related to some structural modifications occurring in aging ovaries. Peluso and England-Charlesworth (1981) examined, at the ultrastructural level, the transformation of preovulatory follicles into ovarian cysts which often result from ovulatory delay in old irregularly cycling rats. Peluso *et al.* (1981) also described several interesting ultrastructural alterations which occurred in 50% of the preovulatory oocytes. The most striking anomaly was the deterioration of the stacking arrangements of the cytoplasmic rays, which are composed of RNA. These oocytes could not resume meiosis *in vitro* and showed a reduced incorporation of [^{3}H]uridine into RNA. Are these changes due entirely or partly to intrinsic oocyte aging and/or to the age-related changes in hormonal milieu? Intrinsic oocyte aging may be detected in similar studies on long-term hypophysectomized rats after gonadotropic stimulation. The transformation of interstitial cells into "wheel" cells, reported in Section 3.1.3, already occurs in 13-month-old cyclic rats (Aschheim, 1976) and may be related to the decreased LH surge.

A synthetic view on neurohormonal modifications during cycles in middle-aged rats is not yet possible. It is my belief that the decreased and delayed LH surge and the oocyte alterations are the best established facts, and it is important that they occur only in part of the middle-aged population. The progressive character of aging changes during cyclicity and the latent heterogeneity of apparently homogenous cyclic age groups are better illustrated after adaptation tests (Aschheim, 1979; Table 2). Hemiovariectomy performed at increasing ages initiates an increasing proportion of SDC (Table 2, third line, represents the inverse expression of the same condition, the persistence of cycles during the month following the operation). After hemiovariectomy performed at 30 days of age, the number of rats displaying ovulatory compensation of the remaining ovary decreases with age (Table 2, fourth line). This forms part of an advanced aging complex (see Section 5.3). The decreasing persistence with age of the estrous cycle after injection of estradiol benzoate at estrus (Table 2, fifth line) is the basis for a biological aging test of ovarian cyclicity (Aschheim, 1974), as seen in the next section. All these adaptation tests demonstrate an age-dependent decreasing stability of ovarian cycles. They raise problems about the individual selection which they induce.

4.2. Aging of the Neuroendocrine Regulation of Cyclic Ovarian Function

4.2.1. An Aging Test of Cyclic Ovarian Function: Mechanism, Applications

The aging test (Aschheim, 1974) is based on the fact that the ability to respond by becoming pseudopregnant due to estradiol benzoate injection at estrus increases with age in cyclic rats. The dose–response curves are homologous for a wide range of injected estrogen. This age-related facility to release PRL in response to estrogen results in an increasing percentage of induced pseudopregnancies (Table 2, fifth line, represents the inverse expression of this condition, the decreasing persistence of cycles after the injection of 5 μg of estradiol benzoate at estrus). A maintained cycle represents a "young" response to the injection, pseudopregnancy an "old" one. After the experimental sequence, normal cycles recur. The aging test measures (a) in the same age group, the latent heterogeneity (the "biological" age) of an apparently homogeneous cyclic population, and (b) a possible modification of biological age by comparison between an experimental and a control group of the same chronological age.

The increased sensitivity to estrogen may act through the increased ability of this hormone to inhibit the production and/or the activity of the hypothalamic PRL-inhibiting factor, by its direct stimulation of the pituitary, or through both mechanisms. The hypophysial response also was investigated *in vitro* (Aschheim and Rasolonjanahary, 1979). Prolactin release was measured by RIA after incubation with or without addition of estradiol to the medium from pituitaries from cycling rats aged 3–14 months. They all released similar amounts of PRL, whereas *in vivo,* injected estrogen induced 6% pseudopregnancy at 3–4 months and 83% at 12–13 months of age. The aging test thus appeared to act at the hypothalamic and not at the hypophysial level.

Applications of the Test. In addition to retarded aging induced by contraceptive steroids (Section 5.2) and advanced aging due to early hemiovarietomy (Section 5.3), the following experimental conditions have been tested (Aschheim, unpublished results). Four-month-old rats were exposed for 4 months to either constant light, which induced persistent estrus, or the presence of vasectomized males, which induced repetitive pseudopregnancies. After the end of treatment and reinstatement of cycles, the aging test did not show any significant difference in biological age when these 9- to 10-month-old rats were compared with controls. Thus when two experimental disruptions of the cycle, similar to (but perhaps not identical with) those seen in old age were induced for 4 months in adults, they were not followed by a persisting "aging" change of hypothalamic regulation of ovarian function. Sixteen-month-old rats in PE, induced to cycle by hCG, were "biologically old" when tested at the fourth or fifth estrus following the treatment. Reinstatement of cyclicity does not signify rejuvenation of the control mechanism. Multiparous cyclic rats aged 13 months, with a mean of eight previous pregnancies, the last one occurring at 11 months, provided a significantly older test response than nulliparous controls.

4.2.2. Changes in Feedback Regulation and Pituitary Response to LHRH

These changes are generally similar to those described in old acyclic rats (see Section 3.2.2). The post-ovariectomy rise of circulating LH was attenuated at about 12 months of age in regular or irregular cyclers and in recently initiated PE rats (Steger *et al.*, 1980; Gray *et al.*, 1980; Gray and Wexler, 1980; see also our unpublished results in Table 2, seventh line). The negative feedback action of estradiol on LH was maintained or reduced and the positive feedback of estrogen and/or progesterone on LH release was absent or reduced (Lu *et al.*, 1977; Steger *et al.*, 1980; Gray *et al.*, 1980; Gray and Wexler, 1980). As for the rise of FSH after ovariectomy or the positive steroidal feedback on FSH release, an age effect has not yet been detected in these animals (Steger *et al.*, 1980). The pituitary response to LHRH was decreased in ovariectomized, formerly irregularly cycling rats, but was partially restored after steroidal priming (Steger and Peluso, 1979). In intact middle-aged rats which had just become acyclic, the pituitary response to LHRH was not altered in PE, but was decreased in RPP rats (Wise and Ratner, 1980). Like the biological parameters shown in Table 2, some of the hormonal changes can already be detected at the age of 8–9 months. During aging of cyclic rats, decreasing hypothalamic sensitivity to estrogen feedback on LH release is not inconsistent with increasing hypothalamic sensitivity to estrogen feedback on PRL release, since they could result in a decreased output of LHRH or PRL-inhibiting factor, respectively.

5. Experimental Manipulations of Hypothalamic-Hypophysial-Ovarian Aging

In the past, various experimental approaches contributed widely to a better understanding of the aging problem, e.g., use of heterochronic grafts of ovaries and pituitary, reinstatement of cyclicity in PE rats, etc. As will be shown in this and the next section, such manipulations continue to provide interesting models for further analysis.

5.1. Suspended Aging

At 375 days after hypophysectomy of 40-day-old rats, resumption of ovarian cycles occurred after a successful graft of a young pituitary (Smith, 1963; Table 3). When ovariectomy at 6 or 12 months was followed at 24–27 months of age by graft of young or old ovaries, cycling was restored (Aschheim, 1964/5; Table 3). During the postovariectomy interval, aging of the neuroendocrine regulating system was suspended by lack of steroidal action. Hormonal characterization and testing of the biological age of the restored cycles were not yet feasible in those years. As emphasized in Section 3.1.3, early ovariectomy prevented the development of gliosis in the arcuate nucleus area normally found in old PE rats (Brawer *et al.*, 1980; Schipper *et al.*, 1981).

Very interesting results have been reported recently in an abstract by Elias *et al.* (1979). In old rats, ovariectomized at 2 months of age and studied 22 months later, circulating LH was not maintained at castration levels reached 2 months after ovariectomy, and was no longer secreted in a pulsatile fashion (Table 3). As pituitary stores of LH were not reported, it is possible that there was an age-related dissociation between LH synthesis and release. But it is more likely that the decrease in circulating LH was due to a deficiency of LHRH activity, for stimulation by exogenous LHRH resulted in a normal pituitary response as in young ovariectomized controls. The positive steroidal feedback on LH was also similar in the two groups. The putative deficiency of LHRH activity is

Table 3. Long-Term Effects of Early Hypophysectomy (Hx) or Ovariectomy (Ovx) in Aging Rats

Source	Age at operation	Time elapsed	Results	Interpretation
[a]	26 days + Hx	7–24 months	Proliferation of ovarian epithelial cords; thickening of basement membranes (epithelial cords, testis-like tubes, small follicles)	Intrinsic aging of these ovarian structures
[b]	26 days + Hx	> 11 months	Intramitochondrial inclusions in ovarian insterstitial cells after hCG stimulation	Intrinsic aging seen only after stimulation
[c]	40 days + Hx	12–13 months	+ young pituitary graft: resumption of cycles	Suspended aging during Hx
[d]	6 or 12 months + Ovx	21 or 12 months	+ old or young ovarian graft: resumption of cycles	Suspended aging during Ovx
[e]	60 days + Ovx	22 months	Castration levels and pulsatile fluctuations of LH: not maintained; LH responses to E,[f] E + P[g] and LHRH: maintained	See text, no aging of pituitary sensitivity
[h]	45 days + Ovx	→ 12 months	Decrease of prolactin secretion *in vitro*; stimulation by E, inhibition by dopamine added *in vitro*: maintained	Intrinsic pituitary aging? no aging of pituitary sensitivity

[a] Crumeyrolle-Arias and Aschheim, 1981.
[b] Crumeyrolle-Arias, 1979.
[c] Smith, 1963.
[d] Aschheim, 1964/5.
[e] Elias et al., 1979.
[f] E = estradiol.
[g] P = progesterone.
[h] Rasolonjanahary, 1979.

not necessarily age-dependent in a linear way, since data are available only for 4- and 24-month-old rats, and LH levels may decrease abruptly in middle age and remain constant thereafter.

Prolactin secretion *in vitro* by pituitaries originating from rats ovariectomized at 45 days of age and sacrificed at regular intervals for 11 months demonstrated a significant decrease with age and/or a post-ovariectomy interval (Rasolonjanahary, 1979; Table 3). Since PRL production *in vitro* is considered to be spontaneous, and since the number of secretory cells does not increase after early ovariectomy, the decreased secretion may denote intrinsic cellular aging. But when estradiol or DA was added to the incubation medium, pituitary sensitivity to stimulation or inhibition, respectively, was maintained in all groups. As a rule, endocrinological aging results on the contrary, in maintained basal levels of hormones and deficiencies are observed after adaptive tests.

5.2. Retarded Aging

By addition of L-tyrosine to the diet, starting at 7.5 months of age, Cooper and Walker (1979) reported a significant extension of the period of ovarian cyclicity in rats, which possibly resulted from achieving an appropriate catecholamine to serotonin balance within the central nervous system.

It is well-known that caloric restriction in rodents extends lifespan and retards growth and sexual maturity. Growth and reproduction are resumed after return to *ad libitum* feeding. Merry and Holehan (1979) reported that a particular pattern of chronic dietary resriction (continuous adjustment so that body weight was 50% of that of controls) resulted in enhanced longevity, retarded onset of puberty, and a longer duration of fertility during treatment. Their data demonstrated the persistence of cyclicity for more than 18 months, as compared to less than 12 months in controls. Unless the additional cycles are hormonally abnormal, these two examples do not favor the hypothesis of a strictly programmed cumulative effect of estrogen on the hypothalamus which self-limits cyclicity.

The third example even suggests that the hypothalamus can be desensitized to estrogen. Ethinyl-estradiol, mestranol (5–7 μg/day), or a progestogen (700 μg/day) estrogen mixture was administered orally to rats for 4 or 8 months, starting at the age of 4–5 months (Aschheim, 1975). After cessation of treatment, cyclicity resumed. As compared to controls, there was a high percentage of cyclic rats and a significant decrease of the biological age of these cycles. The delay of aging was maintained for at least 4 months. At autopsy at 16–18 months, experimental rats demonstrated significantly fewer tumorous or hypertrophied pituitaries than controls. When steroid treatments were begun at 10 months of age in cyclic rats, they lost most of their effectiveness. Progestogen given alone did not produce the age-retarding effects. Delayed aging may be explained by a central "desensitization" to estrogen during treatment, counteracting the normally occurring age-related increase in sensitivity to estrogen and subsequent secretion of PRL.

5.3. Advanced Aging

Early hemiovariectomy advances the biological age of the hypothalamic-hypophysial-ovarian axis (Aschheim, 1979). It does so in a very stereotyped way. For several months after hemiovariectomy at 30 days of age, the usual compensatory hypertrophy of the remaining ovary manifests itself through maintained cyclicity, a true ovulatory and luteal compensation (10–12 eggs and fresh corpora lutea), and a resulting increase in ovarian weight. But progressively functional compensation ceases in an increasing number of rats (Table 2, fourth line) and the nature of the persistent gain in ovarian weight changes. Cycles are maintained, but the ovary ovulates no more than 5–8 eggs and shows a similar number of fresh corpora lutea. The maintained ovarian weight increase is now due to an increased persistence of old corpora lutea. A very close correlation exists between results of the aging test and ovulatory compensation. Rats with a "young" test ovulate 10–12 eggs, whereas those ovulating only 5–8 eggs give an "old" test result. At 11 months of age, the experimental group is significantly "older," according to the aging test, than the control group of intact rats. At 12 months of age, an important shift from ovarian cycles to PE occurs in the hemiovariectomized rats which is advanced by 4 months as compared to intact rats. The mechanism of this interesting model for advancing reproductive aging is presently unknown.

6. Extrinsic and Intrinsic Aging

Hypophysectomy (Hx) in early life isolates the ovary from the hormonal imbalance normally induced by aging of the neuroendocrine regulatory centers. Hx may thus produce experimental conditions allowing primary aging of ovarian structures to emerge. Jones and Krohn (1961), for example, reported that Hx in mice clearly retarded but did not abolish oocyte loss with time. Crumeyrolle-Arias and Aschheim (1981) reported on post-Hx ovarian senescence compared to the structural ovarian changes observed in intact aged rats (see Section 3.1.3). Most of the ovarian changes in intact old rats were due to extraovarian aging. For example, in old rats Hx when young, proliferation of the surface epithelium or phagocytes filled with lipofuscin granules was lacking in the ovaries. Intrinsic aging was restricted (Table 3) to thickening of basement membranes and proliferation of epithelial cords (whereas their induction was of extraovarian origin). Ovarian interstitial cells remained in a deficient condition after Hx, without alterations due to aging, and they could be restored in old age by hCG treatment (Crumeyrolle-Arias, 1979). However, the morphological reactivation was submaximal compared to results obtained earlier in life, and at 12 months of age and later, hCG induced large unusual mitochondrial inclusions. The physiological significance of intrinsic aging changes in both Hx and intact animals, such as proliferation of epithelial cords observed at 12 and 22 months of age, respectively, is probably unimportant since these old ovaries can function in a cyclic manner when grafted into young ovariectomized rats.

The decreased secretion *in vitro* of PRL cells originating from old rats, ovariectomized when young, has already been discussed in Section 5.1. Provided that it expresses intrinsic hypophysial aging, it is completely masked in SDC of intact rats by proliferation of PRL cells and decreased hypothalamic PRL release-inhibiting factor (PIF) activity, resulting in increased PRL secretion.

Recently observed hypothalamic alterations (Section 3.1.3) are by no means necessarily intrinsic. In Chapter 5, Peng demonstrated that aged males do not display the neuronal loss observed in several hypothalamic nuclei of females. It would be interesting to investigate the neuronal loss in the hypothalamus of old females that are ovariectomized when young. On the other hand, the neurotoxic effect of estrogen on the hypothalamus, leading to a chemical deafferentation in PE, is lacking in old ovariectomized rats.

It is paradoxical that intrinsic aging changes are exhibited by proliferation of ovarian cellular cords which do not play any discernible role in aging of ovarian function or of its central regulation, whereas aging changes in steroid-sensitive hypothalamic neurons do not presently provide evidence for their intrinsic nature. Moreover, it is clear that such a system assuming a regulatory function, can express aging only when it is responsive to stimuli and thus is necessarily exposed to extrinsic influences. One may speculate whether investigation of intrinsic aging changes in such neurons is not meaningless despite their postmitotic condition, and whether intrinsic aging *in vivo* is not limited to cells (or subcellular compartments) with terminal activity, without any feedback.

7. Conclusions

Considering what is known of the relation of the neuroendocrine system to the reproductive decline in female rats today, I would propose the following conclusions:

(1) Aging of the hypothalamic-hypophysial-gonadal axis differs in female and male rats. Neuronal loss and functional impairment of residual neurons are obvious in some steroid-sensitive areas of the hypothalamus in females; no neuronal loss is observed in old males (see Chapter 5, by Peng). There is an age-related decrease of hypothalamic sensitivity to negative estrogen feedback in females, but an increase of sensitivity to testosterone in males (see Chapter 8 by Steger and Huang).

(2) The reproductive aging pattern of female rats is common to all investigated strains, but differs from those observed in other rodents, including mice (see Chapter 9 by Finch), particularly the CBA strain.

(3) Reproductive aging is characterized by a persistent, but modified ovarian function displaying senile deviations of the estrous cycle. A common factor of SDC is their age-related increase of circulating PRL. This implies alterations in hypothalamic sensitivity to control input (hormonal or environmental) and changes in neurotransmitter activity. There is no doubt that the predominant factor responsible for the reproductive decline of female rats is aging of the neuroendocrine regulatory mechanisms. Some of these hypothalamic aging changes have recently been described. Hormonal input, especially estrogen, modulates these changes, but this does not mean that the starting-point of aging is in the ovary. In this respect, the results of heterochronic ovarian transplantation experiments remain conclusive. The influence of estrogen on hypothalamic aging is varied, depending probably on the pattern of exposure to the hormone. Estrogen removal by ovariectomy suspends aging, whereas administration of ethinyl-estradiol can be desensitizing and is then followed by a delay of aging. However, estrogen can also become neurotoxic, hastening PE by selective hypothalamic deafferentation.

(4) The deficiency of hypothalamic control mechanisms awaits further analysis at a cellular and subcellular level. It accounts for the plasticity of reproductive aging in rats, the facility of its experimental manipulation, the reversibility of SDC, and the early changes already occurring during ovulatory cycles which can be detected by a biological aging test. There are critical periods for aging in adulthood, just as there are critical periods for development at about the time of birth or puberty. Neuroendocrine aging is a "historical" process, recording and/or integrating past events.

Therefore, longitudinal investigations are meaningful, and hormonal snapshots of old age are not.

(5) Oocyte depletion in rats displays a very unusual "aging" pattern. Instead of exhibiting an increasing level of vulnerability with age, or at least a constant one as in mice, the proportion of oocytes lost per unit time decreases with age! Verification of this puzzle is needed.

ACKNOWLEDGMENTS. I am grateful to N. Breugnot for help in typing this manuscript and to J. Meites for correction of deficient English. Experimental work in this laboratory was supported by grants from INSERM and Faculté de Medecine, Paris Ouest, Université René Descartes.

8. References

Aschheim, P., 1961, La pseudogestation à répétition chez les rattes séniles, *C. R. Acad. Sci.* **253:**1988–1990.

Aschheim, P., 1964/5, Résultats fournis par la greffe hétérochrone des ovaires dans l'étude de la régulation hypothalamo-hypophyso-ovarienne de la ratte sénile, *Gèrontologia* **10:**65–75.

Aschheim, P., 1965, La réactivation de l'ovaire des rattes séniles en oestrus permanent au moyen d'hormones gonadotropes ou de la mise à l'obscurité, *C. R. Acad. Sci.* **260:**5627–5630.

Aschheim, P., 1968, Contenu hypophysaire en hormone lutéinisante (LH) et réaction histophysiologique à la LH circulante du tissu interstitiel ovarien chez divers types de rattes séniles, *C. R. Acad. Sci.* **267:**1397–1400.

Aschheim, P., 1970, La rétroaction ovarienne dans la régulation hypothalamique de la fonction gonadotrope LH de la ratte sénile, in: *Colloques Nationaux du CNRS, n° 927: Neuroendocrinologie* (J. Benoit and C. Kordon, eds.), CNRS, Paris, pp. 363–376.

Aschheim, P., 1974, A biological aging test for the hypothalamo-hypophyseal regulation of the estrous cycle in the rat, in: *Endocrinology of Sex. Differentiation and Neuroendocrine Regulation in the Hypothalamo-Hypophyseal-Gonadal System* (G. Dörner, ed.), J. A. Barth, Leipzig, pp. 352–358.

Aschheim, P., 1975, Effets de l'administration chronique de stéroides anticonceptionnels sur l'âge biologique des cycles ovariens de la ratte après arrêt du traitement, *Ann. Biol. Anim.* **15:**775–783.

Aschheim, P., 1976, Aging in the hypothalamic-hypophyseal ovarian axis in the rat, in: *Hypothalamus, Pituitary and Aging* (A. V. Everitt and J. A. Burgess, eds.), Ch. C. Thomas, Springfield, pp. 376–418.

Aschheim, P., 1979, Function of the aging ovary: Comparative aspects, *Eur. J. Obstet. Gynecol. Reprod. Biol.* **9:**191–202.

Aschheim, P., 1982, Deux modèles opposés du vieillissement de l'ovaire et de sa commande hypothalamo-hypophysaire: la ratte et la souris CBA, *Sci. Techn. Anim. Lab.* **7:**99–108.

Aschheim, P., and Latouche, J., 1975, Les effets du séjour au froid sur le cycle ovarien de la ratte et son âge biologique, in: *Problèmes Actuels d'Endocrinologie* (H. P. Klotz, ed.), Exp. Sci. Fr., Paris, pp. 95–110.

Aschheim, P., and Pasteels, J. L., 1963, Etude histophysiologique de la sécrétion de prolactine chez les rattes séniles, *C. R. Acad. Sci.* **257**:1373–1375.

Aschheim, P., and Rasolonjanahary, R., 1979, Age-dependency of pituitary prolactin secretion *in vitro* and of its sensitivity to estrogen in rats, in: *Recent Advances in Gerontology* (H. Ozimo, K. Shimada, M. Iriki, and D. Maeda, eds.), Excerpta Medica, Amsterdam, pp. 481–484.

Barnea, A., Cho, G., and Porter, J. C., 1980, Effect of aging on the subneuronal distribution of luteinizing hormone-releasing hormone in the hypothalamus, *Endocrinology* **106**:1980–1988.

Brawer, J. R., Schipper, H., and Naftolin, F., 1980, Ovary-dependent degeneration in the hypothalamic arcuate nucleus, *Endocrinology* **107**:274–279.

Butcher, R. L., and Page, R. D., 1981, Role of the aging ovary in cessation of reproduction, in: *Dynamics of Ovarian Function* (N. B. Schwartz and M. Hunzicker-Dunn, eds.), Raven Press, New York, pp. 253–271.

Clemens, J. A., 1979, CNS as a pacemaker of endocrine dysfunction in aging and its pharmacological intervention by lergotrile mesylate, in: *Interdiscipl. Topics Gerontol.,* Vol. 15 (H. P. von Hahn, ed.), S. Karger, Basel, pp. 77–84.

Clemens, J. A., and Meites, J., 1971, Neuroendocrine status of old constant-estrous rats, *Neuroendocrinology* **7**:249–256.

Conn, P. M., Cooper, R., McNamara, C., Rogers, D. C., and Shoenhardt, L., 1980, Qualitative change in gonadotropin during normal aging in the male rat, *Endocrinology* **106**:1549–1553.

Cooper, R. L., and Walker, R. F., 1979, Potential therapeutic consequences of age-dependent changes in brain physiology, in: *Interdiscipl. Topics Gerontol.,* Vol. 15 (H. P. von Hahn, ed.), S. Karger, Basel, pp. 54–76.

Cooper, R. L., Conn, P. M., and Walker, R. F., 1980, Characterization of the LH surge in middle-aged female rats, *Biol. Reprod.* **23**:611–615.

Crumeyrolle-Arias, M., 1979, *In vivo* aging of rat's ovarian interstitial cells made nondividing through hypophysectomy, *Gerontology* **25**:162.

Crumeyrolle-Arias, M., and Aschheim, P., 1981, Post-hypophysectomy ovarian senescence and its relation to the spontaneous structural changes in the ovary of intact aged rats, *Gerontology* **27**:58–71.

Crumeyrolle-Arias, M., Scheib, D., and Aschheim, P., 1976, Light and electron microscopy of the ovarian interstitial tissue in the senile rat: Normal aspect and response to HCG of "Deficiency Cells" and "Epithelial Cords," *Gerontology* **22**:185–204.

Damassa, D. A., Gilman, D. P., Lu, K. H., Judd, H. L., and Sawyer, C. H., 1980, The twenty-four hour pattern of prolactin secretion in aging female rats, *Biol. Reprod.* **22**:571–575.

Elias, K. A., Huffman, L. J., and Blake, C. A., 1979, Age of ovariectomy affects subsequent plasma LH responses in old age rats, *Program of the 61st Annual Meeting of the Endocrine Society, Anaheim, California* (Abst. 133), p. 106.

Erickson, G. F., Hsueh, A. J. W., and Lu, K. H., 1979, Gonadotropin binding and aromatase activity in granulosa cells of young proestrous and old constant estrous rats, *Biol. Reprod.* **20**:182–190.

Estes, K. S., Simpkins, J. W., and Chen, C. L., 1980, Alteration in pulsatile release of LH in aging female rats, *Proc. Soc. Exp. Biol. Med.* **163**:384–387.

Everett, J. W., 1980, Reinstatement of estrous cycles in middle-aged spontaneously per-sistent estrous rats: Importance of circulating prolactin and the resulting facilitative action of progesterone, *Endocrinology* **106:**1691–1696.

Fayein, N. A., and Aschheim, P., 1980, Age-related temporal changes of levels of circulating progesterone in repeatedly pseudopregnant rats, *Biol. Reprod.* **23:**616–620.

Fugo, N. W., and Butcher, R. L., 1971, Effects of prolonged estrous cycles on reproduction in aged rats, *Fertil. Steril.* **22:**98–101.

Germain, B. J., Campbell, P. S., and Anderson, J. N., 1978, Role of the serum estrogen-binding protein in the control of tissue estradiol levels during postnatal development of the female rat, *Endocrinology* **103:**1401–1410.

Gilman, D. P., Lu, K. H., Whitmoyer, D. I., Judd, H. L., and Sawyer, C. H., 1981, Rela-tionship between progesterone and prolactin surges in aged and young pseudopreg-nant rats, *Biol. Reprod.* **24:**839–845.

Gosden, R. G., and Bancroft, L., 1976, Pituitary function in reproductively senescent female rats, *Exp. Gerontol.* **11:**157–160.

Grandison, L., Hodson, C., Chen, H. T., Advis, J., Simpkins, J., and Meites, J., 1977, Inhibition by prolactin of post-castration rise in LH, *Neuroendocrinology* **23:**312–322.

Gray, G. D., and Wexler, B. C., 1980, Estrogen and testosterone sensitivity of middle-aged female rats in the regulation of LH, *Exp. Gerontol.* **15:**201–207.

Gray, G. D., Tennent, B., Smith, E. R., and Davidson, J. M., 1980, Luteinizing hormone regulation and sexual behavior in middle-aged female rats, *Endocrinology* **107:**187–194.

Howland, B. E., 1976, Reduced gonadotropin release in response to progesterone or gonadotropin releasing hormone (GnRH) in old female rats, *Life Sci.* **19:**219–224.

Hsu, H. K., and Peng, M. T., 1978, Hypothalamic neuron number of old female rats, *Gerontology* **24:**434–440.

Huang, H. H., Marshall, S., and Meites, J., 1976a, Capacity of old versus young female rats to secrete LH, FSH and prolactin, *Biol. Reprod.* **14:**538–543.

Huang, H. H., Marshall, S., and Meites, J., 1976b, Induction of estrous cycles in old noncyclic rats by progesterone, ACTH, ether stress or L-Dopa, *Neuroendocrinology* **20:**21–34.

Huang, H. H., Steger, R. W., Bruni, J. F., and Meites, J., 1978, Patterns of sex steroid and gonadotropin secretion in aging female rats, *Endocrinology* **103:**1855–1859.

Huang, H. H., Simpkins, J., and Meites, J., 1979, Hypothalamic norepinephrine and dopamine turnover in ovariectomized old rats treated with gonadal steroids, *Physiol-ogist* (Abst.) **22:**71.

Huang, H. H., Steger, R. W., Sonntag, W. E., and Meites, J., 1980, Positive feedback by ovarian hormones on prolactin and LH in old versus young female rats, *Neurobiol. Aging* **1:**141–143.

Jiang, M. J., and Peng, M. T., 1981, Cytoplasmic and nuclear binding of estradiol in the brain and pituitary of old female rats, *Gerontology* **27:**51–57.

Jones, E. C., and Krohn, P. L., 1961, The effect of hypophysectomy on age changes in the ovaries of mice, *J. Endocrinol.* **27:**497–509.

Kaler, L. W., and Neaves, W. B., 1981, The androgen status of aging male rats, *Endocri-nology* **108:**712–719.

Kawashima, S., 1974, Morphology and function of prolactin cells in old female rats, *Gumma Symp. Endocrinol.* **11:**129–141.

Kovacs, K., Horvath, E., Ilse, R. G., Ezrin, C., and Ilse, D., 1977, Spontaneous pituitary adenomas in aging rats. A light microscopic, immunocytological and fine structural study, *Beitr. Pathol.* **161:**1–16.

Lin, K. H., Peng, Y. M., Peng, M. T., and Tseng, T. M., 1976, Changes in the nuclear volume of rat hypothalamic neurons in old age, *Neuroendocrinology* **21**:247–254.

Linnoila, M., and Cooper, R. L., 1976, Reinstatement of vaginal cycles in aged female rats, *J. Pharmacol. Exp. Ther.* **199**:477–482.

Lu, J. K. H., and Kledzik, G. S., 1981, Chronological changes in ovarian function and morphology in aging rats and their relation to neuroendocrine responses, in: *Dynamics of Ovarian Function* (N. B. Schwartz and M. Hunzicker-Dunn, eds.), Raven Press, New York, pp. 291–296.

Lu, K. H., Huang, H. H., Chen, H. T., Kurcz, M., Mioduszewski, R., and Meites, J., 1977, Positive feed-back by estrogen and progesterone on LH release in old and young rats, *Proc. Soc. Exp. Biol. Med.* **154**:82–85.

Lu, K. H., Hopper, B. R., Vargo, T. M., and Yen, S. S. C., 1979, Chronological changes in sex steroid, gonadotropin and prolactin secretion in aging female rats displaying different reproductive states, *Biol. Reprod.* **21**:193–203.

Lu, J. K. H., Damassa, D. A., Gilman, D. P., Judd, H. L., and Sawyer, C. H., 1980, Differential patterns of gonadotropin responses to ovarian steroids and to LH-releasing hormone between constant-estrous and pseudopregnant states in aging rats, *Biol. Reprod.* **23**:345–351.

Lu, J. K. H., Gilman, D. P., Meldrum, D. R., Judd, H. L., and Sawyer, C. H., 1981, Relationship between circulating estrogens and the central mechanisms by which ovarian steroids stimulate luteinizing hormone secretion in aged and young female rats, *Endocrinology* **108**:836–841.

Mandl, A. M., and Zuckerman, S., 1951, The relation of age to numbers of oocytes, *J. Endocrinol.* **7**:190–193.

McPherson, J. C., Costoff, A., and Mahesh, V. B., 1977, Effects of aging on the hypothalamic-hypophyseal-gonadal axis in female rats, *Fertil. Steril.* **28**:1365–1370.

Meites, J., Huang, H. H., and Simpkins, J. W., 1978, Recent studies on neuroendocrine control of reproductive senescence in rats, in: *The Aging Reproductive System* (E. L. Schneider, ed.), Raven Press, New York, pp. 213–235.

Meites, J., Simpkins, J. W., and Huang, H. H., 1979, The relation of hypothalamic biogenic amines to secretion of gonadotropins and prolactin in the aging rat, in: *Physiology and Cell Biology of Aging* (A. Cherkin *et al.,* eds.), Raven Press, New York, pp. 87–94.

Merchenthaler, I., Lengvári, I., Horváth, J., and Sétáló, G., 1980, Immunohistochemical study of the LHRH-synthesizing neuron system of aged female rats, *Cell Tissue Res.* **209**:499–503.

Merry, B. J., and Holehan, A. M., 1979, Onset of puberty and duration of fertility in rats fed a restricted diet, *J. Reprod. Fertil.* **57**:253–259.

Miller, A. E., Wood, S. M., and Riegle, G. D., 1979, The effect of age on reproduction in repeatedly mated female rats, *J. Gerontol.* **34**:15–20.

Parkening, T. A., Collins, T. J., and Smith, E. R., 1980a, A comparative study of prolactin levels in five species of aged female laboratory rodents, *Biol. Reprod.* **22**:513–518.

Parkening, T. A., Collins, T. J., and Smith, E. R., 1980b, Plasma and pituitary concentrations of LH, FSH and prolactin in aged female C57 BL/6 mice, *J. Reprod. Fertil.* **58**:377–386.

Peluso, J. J., and England-Charlesworth, C., 1981, Formation of ovarian cysts in aged irregularly cycling rats, *Biol. Reprod.* **24**:1183–1190.

Peluso, J. J., Steger, R. W., and Hafer, E. S. E., 1977, Regulation of LH secretion in aged female rats, *Biol. Reprod.* **16**:212–215.

Peluso, J. J., Steger, R. W., Huang, H. H., and Meites, J., 1979, Pattern of follicular growth and steroidogenesis in the ovary of aging cycling rats, *Exp. Aging Res.* **5**:319–333.

Peluso, J. J., Hutz, R., and England-Charlesworth, C., 1981, Age-related alterations in preovulatory oocytes, in: *Dynamics of Ovarian Function* (N. B. Schwartz and M. Hunzicker Dunn, eds.), Raven Press, New York, pp. 303–308.

Peng, M. T., and Huang, H. H., 1972, Aging of hypothalamic-pituitary-ovarian function in the rat, *Fertil. Steril.* **23:**535–542.

Peng, M. T., and Peng, Y. M., 1973, Changes in the uptake of tritiated estradiol in the hypothalamus and adenohypophysis of old female rats, *Fertil. Steril.* **24:**534–539.

Rasolonjanahary, R., 1979, Evolution, en fonction de l'âge, de la sécrétion de prolactine hypophysaire *in vitro* chez le rat. Effet de l'oestradiol et de la dopamine, Physiology of Reproduction, Sc.D. Dissertation, Université Pierre et Marie Curie, Paris 6.

Riegle, G. D., and Miller, A. E., 1978, Aging effects on the hypothalamic-hypophyseal-gonadal control system in the rat, in: *The Aging Reproductive System* (E. L. Schneider, ed.), Raven Press, New York, pp. 159–192.

Schipper, H., Brawer, J. R., Nelson, J. F., Felicio, L. S., and Finch, C. E., 1981, Role of the gonads in the histologic aging of the hypothalamic arcuate nucleus, *Biol. Reprod.* **25:**413–419.

Smith, P. E., 1963, Postponed pituitary homotransplants into the region of the hypophysial portal circulation in hypophysectomized female rats, *Endocrinology* **73:**793–806.

Steger, R. W., and Peluso, J. J., 1979, Hypothalamic-pituitary function in the older irregularly cycling rat, *Exp. Aging Res.* **5:**303–317.

Steger, R. W., Peluso, J. J., Huang, H. H., Hafez, E. S. E., and Meites, J., 1976, Gonadotrophin-binding sites in the ovary of aged rats, *J. Reprod. Fertil.* **48:**205–207.

Steger, R. W., Huang, H. H., and Meites, J., 1979a, Relation of aging to hypothalamic LHRH content and serum gonadal steroids in female rats, *Proc. Soc. Exp. Biol. Med.* **161:**251–254.

Steger, R. W., Huang, H. H., and Meites, J., 1979b, Pulsatile LH release in old and young ovariectomized rats, *Program of the 61st Annual Meeting of the Endocrine Society, Anaheim, California* (Abst. 135), p. 106.

Steger, R. W., Huang, H. H., Chamberlain, D. S., and Meites, J., 1980, Changes in control of gonadotropin secretion in the transition period between regular cycles and constant estrus in aging female rats, *Biol. Reprod.* **22:**595–603.

Van der Schoot, P., 1976, Changing pro-oestrous surges of luteinizing hormone in aging 5-day cyclic rats, *J. Endocrinol.* **69:**287–288.

Walker, R. F., 1981, Reproductive senescence and the dynamics of hypothalamic serotonin metabolism in the female rat, in: *Brain Neurotransmitters and Receptors in Aging and Age-Related Disorders* (S. J. Enna, T. Samorajski, and B. Beer, eds.), Raven Press, New York, pp. 95–105.

Watkins, B. E., McKay, D. W., Meites, J., and Riegle, G. D., 1975a, L-Dopa effects on serum LH and prolactin in old and young female rats, *Neuroendocrinology* **19:**331–338.

Watkins, B. E., Meites, J., and Riegle, G. D., 1975b, Age-related changes in pituitary responsiveness to LHRH in the female rat, *Endocrinology* **97:**543–548.

Wilkes, M. M., and Yen, S. S. C., 1981, Attenuation during aging in the postovariectomy rise in median eminence catecholamines, *Neuroendocrinology* **33:**144–147.

Wilkes, M. M., Lu, K. H., Hopper, B. R., and Yen, S. S. C., 1979, Altered neuroendocrine status of middle-aged rats prior to the onset of senescent anovulation, *Neuroendocrinology* **29:**255–261.

Wise, P. M., and Ratner, A., 1980, LHRH-induced LH and FSH responses in the aged female rat, *J. Gerontol.* **35:**506–511.

CHAPTER 7

Changes in Ovarian Function and Gonadotropin and Prolactin Secretion in Aging Female Rats

JOHN K. H. LU

1. Introduction

In the female rat, reproductive function is characterized by several interesting features, including (1) estrous cycles and the concomitant changes in neuroendocrine function are repeated at frequent intervals (4–5 days), and (2) reproductive life represents less than one-third of the entire lifespan. Under optimal laboratory conditions, the female rat may have a lifespan of about three years. Puberty occurs around 35–40 days after birth, and regular estrous cycles are usually seen in animals older than 2 months of age. Between the ages of 2–12 months, most adult females display regular estrous cycles of 4- or 5-day duration, and this cyclicity is interrupted by a persistent-diestrous phase when the rat is in gestation, postpartum lactation, or in a pseudopregnant condition.

Beginning about 10–12 months of age, the regular estrous cycles gradually become lengthened and irregular (Ingram, 1959; Mandl, 1961; Huang and Mcites, 1975), and are most frequently characterized by extended periods of vaginal cornification indicative of sustained estrogen secretion and delayed ovulation (Lu *et al.*, 1979; Peluso *et al.*, 1979). After a transitional phase of irregular cycling, aging females soon become chronically anovulatory. During this state, aging rats display vaginal cytology of persistent cornification, i.e., persistent estrus (PES; Fig. 1). After a prolonged period of PES, older females display persistent-

JOHN K. H. LU • Departments of Obstetrics/Gynecology and Anatomy, University of California at Los Angeles School of Medicine, Los Angeles, California 90024.

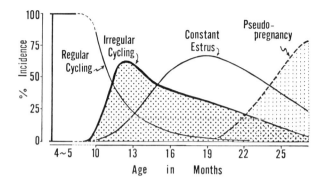

Fig. 1. Chronological changes in reproductive pattern in aging female rats (Long–Evans). Many females change from regular cycles to irregular cycles at about 10–12 months of age. Thereafter, aging rats become chronically anovulatory, and display persistent (or constant)-estrous vaginal smears. Older animals exhibit repetitive pseudopregnancies. (From Lu et al., 1979, with permission.)

diestrous vaginal cytology interrupted by 2–3 days of nucleated and cornified epithelial smears. These animals show intermittent ovulatory activity at irregular intervals, and become repetitively pseudopregnant (RPP; Aschheim, 1961). With further advancing age, the oldest rats become persistent-anestrous (Meites and Huang, 1976). Observations on multiparous rats of the Long–Evans strain indicate that 60–65% of the population change their reproductive patterns from regular cyclic to irregular cyclic around 10–12 months of age, and that 65–70% of females have become PES by 19 months (Lu *et al.,* 1979). Thus, most adult female rats display regular cyclicity between 2–12 months of age; thereafter, the animals experience a prolonged phase of postreproductive life. The question has been raised as to whether the reproductive decline that occurs in aging female rats is due primarily to changes in hypothalamic, pituitary, and/or ovarian function.

2. Changes in Ovarian Function

During the transition from regular to irregular cyclicity, many of the estrous cycles show extended periods of vaginal cornification or leukocytic smears. A few weeks later, estrous cyclicity ceases completely, and the aging rats become chronically anovulatory. During this state, ovarian follicular growth and, to some extent, maturation, persist, whereas the neuroendocrine signals essential for ovulation apparently disappear in the aging animals (Huang *et al.*, 1978; Lu *et al.*, 1979). Thus, the ovaries of PES rats contain small, medium, and even large follicles but no corpora lutea (Fig. 2; Lu *et al.*, 1979). In many of the large follicles, membrana granulosa are seen as thin layers of cells pushed against the follicular wall (Steger *et al.*, 1976). Substantial amounts of both estradiol and estrone are secreted by the ovaries of PES rats (Huang *et al.*, 1978; Lu *et al.*, 1979). Estradiol concentrations in PES rats are similar to values seen in cyclic females on diestrus day-2 evening, and estrone levels are within the highest values seen in cyclic animals (Fig. 3). The results from an *in vitro* experiment have shown that the granulosa cells taken from large antral follicles of PES rat ovaries exhibit a similar capacity for converting androstenedione to estrogens as cells from cyclic females on the day of proestrus (Erickson *et al.*, 1979). This may account for the persistent production of estrogens during the chronic anovulatory state. In the absence of corpora lutea, the adrenals but not the ovaries secrete small quantities of progesterone, while little progesterone is converted to 20α-OH-progesterone by ovarian enzymes (Lu *et al.*, 1979). The in-

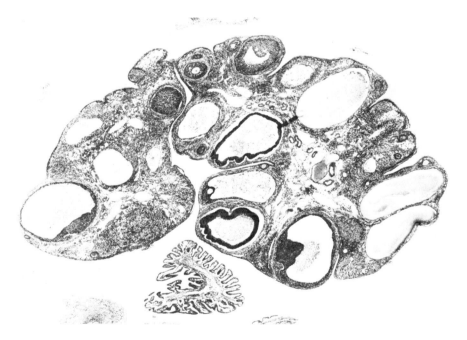

Fig. 2.   Cross-section of an ovary from a 13-month-old persistent-estrous rat showing several developing and large follicles but no corpora lutea, × 20. Reduced 28% for reproduction. (From Lu *et al.*, 1979, with permission.)

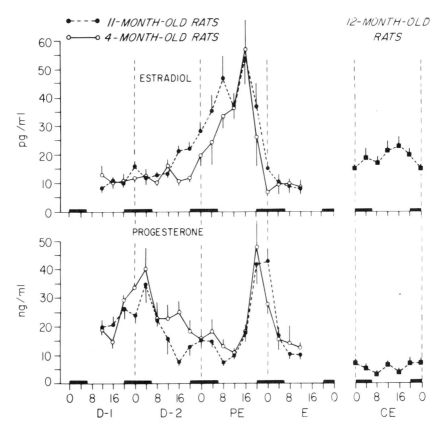

Fig. 3. Circulating concentrations of estradiol and progesterone in 4- and 11-month-old regularly cycling female rats and in 12-month-old constant-estrous (CE) females. D-1 = diestrus day-1; D-2 = diestrus day-2; PE = proestrus; E = estrus. The solid bars on the abscissa indicate the dark phases of the light-dark photoperiod, and the numbers are hours of the day. From D-2 afternoon until PE noon, estradiol values appear to be higher in old than in young cyclic animals, and estradiol levels in CE rats are similar to those of old cyclic animals on D-2 evening. By contrast, progesterone values in CE rats are persistently low.

terfollicular stromal tissue of PES rat ovaries contain small, "deficient" secondary interstitial cells (Crumeyrolle-Arias *et al.*, 1976; Erickson *et al.*, 1979), and this histological feature is associated with decreased androgen production (Fig. 4; Lu and Kledzik, 1981). Autoradiography studies show that LH-I[125] binds to granulosa cells and thecal cells in PES rat ovaries, but minimal binding is found in large cystic follicles (Steger *et al.*, 1976). Interestingly, a decreased production of androgens is accompanied by a significant increase in hCG-I^{125} binding capacity by PES rat ovaries (Lu and Kledzik, 1981), and the latter is probably due to chronic absence of a cyclic increase in LH secretion (Huang *et al.*, 1978; Lu *et al.*, 1979). The notion that the PES state is associated with a chronic deficiency of LH secretion is also consistent with the observation that ovulation can be induced in PES animals by administration of LH or LHRH (Aschheim, 1965; Meites *et al.*, 1978).

After a prolonged period of anovulation, older female rats resume spontaneous ovulatory activity, but ovulations occur at long and irregular intervals (Meites and Huang, 1976; Lu *et al.*, 1979). Following ovulation, corpora lutea are formed (Fig. 5) and their functions are maintained for 2–3 weeks or longer, presumably due to chronically elevated prolactin

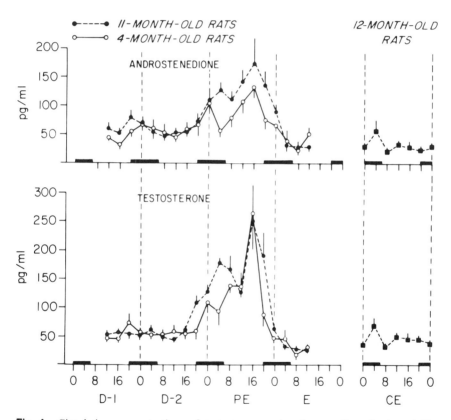

Fig. 4. Circulating concentrations of testosterone and androstenedione in 4- and 11-month-old regularly cyclic female rats and in 12-month-old CE females. Abbreviations are the same as in Fig. 3. The cyclic pattern of testosterone secretion is remarkably similar to that of estradiol. Persistent low levels of both androgens are found in CE females.

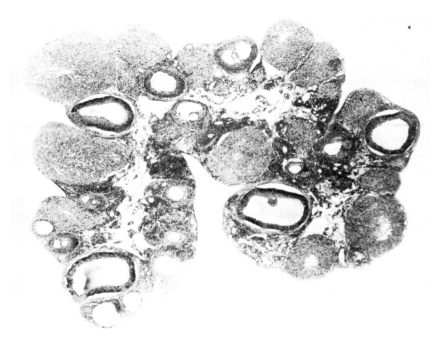

Fig. 5. Cross section of an ovary from a 27-month-old pseudopregnant rat showing follicles of various sizes and many prominent corpora lutea, × 20. Reduced 28% for reproduction. (From Lu *et al.*, 1979, with permission.)

in the circulation (Lu *et al.*, 1979). LH-I^{125} binds appreciably to the luteal cells, and high activity of 3β-hydroxysteroid dehydrogenase is found in the cells (Steger *et al.*, 1976). Histologically, the corpora lutea of old RPP rats consist of many enlarged luteal cells (Mandl, 1959) that secrete large amounts of progesterone (Huang *et al.*, 1978; Lu *et al.*, 1979, 1980; Fayein and Aschheim, 1980) and 20α-OH-progesterone (Lu *et al.*, 1979, 1980). It is known that prolactin inhibits 20α-hydroxysteroid dehydrogenase activity in granulosa and luteal cells of the rat ovary (Armstrong *et al.*, 1969; Wang *et al.*, 1979). In aged RPP rats, however, serum levels of both progesterone and 20α-hydroxyprogesterone are maintained at high values while prolactin secretion is also enhanced (Fig. 6).

Following the repetitive pseudopregnant state, the oldest females display constant anestrus characterized by persistent-diestrous vaginal cytology (Huang and Meites, 1975). This state is almost always associated with hemorrhage and/or tumors in the pituitary. The ovaries of anestrous rats contain little follicular and luteal tissues (Meites and Huang, 1976), and produce minimum quantities of steroids (Huang *et al.*, 1978).

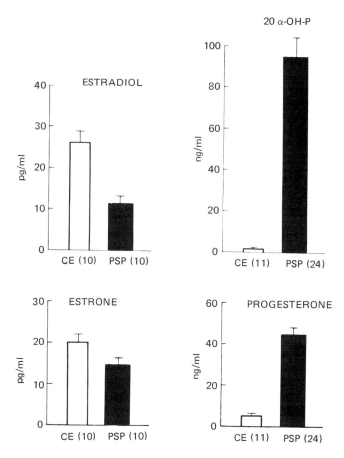

Fig. 6.   Serum concentrations of estradiol, estrone, progesterone, and 20α-OH-P in intact old constant-estrous (CE) and repetitive-pseudopregnant (PSP) rats. The CE and PSP states are characterized by high circulating levels of estrogen and progestin, respectively. (From Lu *et al.*, 1980, with permission.)

It is likely that anestrus in old female rats represents a pathological rather than a physiological state (Aschheim, 1979).

3.   Changes in Gonadotropin Secretion

It has been shown that lower luteinizing hormone (LH) but higher follicle-stimulating hormone (FSH) content is found in the pituitaries of old PES rats than in young females (Clemens and Meites, 1971), suggesting differential effects of aging on gonadotropin secretion. Several reports have shown changes in basal levels of serum gonadotropins associated with aging, but discrepancies exist among these findings (Shaar *et al.*, 1975; Huang *et al.*, 1976; Lu *et al.*, 1979). These differences are largely due to comparison of single assays randomly sampled during the day. Since pituitary hormones including gonadotropins may exhibit pulsatile secretion, a comparison based on a single blood sample may not be physiologically significant. In general, it has been found that the chronic anovulatory state in aging PES rats is associated with persistently low circulating levels of LH (Lu and Kledzik, 1981) and a lack of cyclic increases in LH and FSH secretion (Huang *et al.*, 1978; Lu *et al.*, 1979). However, basal levels of serum FSH are increased in PES females (Fig. 7). Adequate amounts of FSH secretion in the aging animals may account for the normal aromatase activity found in the granulosa cells of large ovarian follicles (Erikson *et al.*, 1979). The mechanism whereby the anovulatory state is associated with an increased FSH secretion is not known at present. Basal values of serum gonadotropins appear to be similar between aged RPP and PES females (Lu *et al.*, 1979). Since the RPP animals show follicular development and ovulatory activity, changes in gonadotropin secretion may occur at different phases of the pseudopregnancy.

Hypothalamic content of LHRH was shown to be similar between aging PES and young cyclic female rats (Steger *et al.*, 1979), although the increase in LHRH concentration that occurs in young proestrous females is not seen in the anovulatory animals. Administration of LHRH elicits an increase in LH release in PES rats, and the magnitude of LH rise is the same or lower than in young females (Watkins *et al.*, 1975; Meites *et al.*, 1978). Similarly, LHRH administration induces the same magnitude of increase in LH release in aged PES and RPP rats (Lu *et al.*, 1980). However, the LH response to LHRH is enhanced by estradiol treatment in RPP but not PES females, indicating differences in the central nervous response to estrogen modulation (Lu *et al.*, 1980).

Ovariectomy results in an increase in LH secretion in young and aged female rats, but the magnitude of the rise is less in aged than in young animals (Fig. 8; Steger *et al.*, 1980). Among aged females, the increase in LH secretion after ovariectomy is greater in RPP than in PES rats (Huang *et al.*, 1976). These observations suggest that chronic elevation of circulating estrogen during the anovulatory state in PES females may suppress the central nervous mechanism which mediates the steroid feedback on LH secretion (Lu *et al.*, 1980, 1981), and that progesterone appears to alleviate such a suppressive effect. Reports have shown that the postovariectomy increase in FSH secretion is unchanged

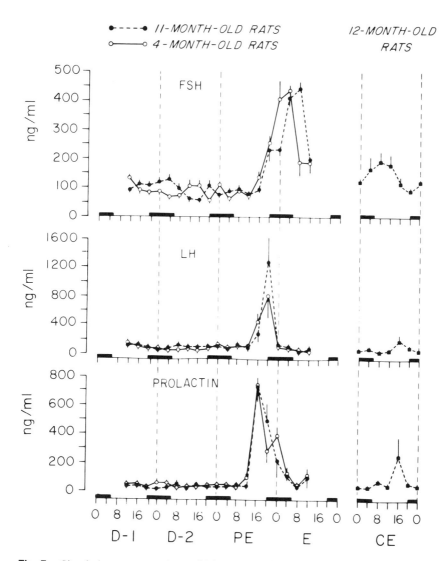

Fig. 7. Circulating concentrations of FSH, LH, and prolactin in 4- and 11-month-old regularly cycling female rats and in 12-month-old CE females. Abbreviations are the same as in Fig. 3. During the chronic anovulatory state in CE rats, morning basal values of serum FSH are elevated, whereas LH concentrations are maintained at low basal levels. Patterns of prolactin secretion in CE females show a diurnal surge.

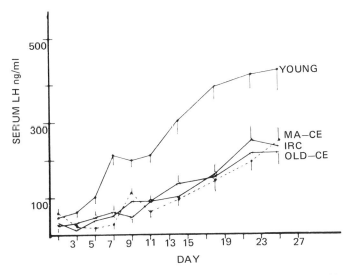

Fig. 8. Postovariectomy increases in serum LH levels in young (4 months old) regularly cycling and 14-month-old irregularly cycling (IRC) rats, and in constant-estrous females 14 months (MA-CE) and 20 months old (old-CE). (From Steger *et al.*, 1980, with permission.)

(Steger *et al.*, 1980) or markedly decreased in aged rats (Huang *et al.*, 1976). Under various conditions, there is a dissociation of FSH and LH secretion (Lu *et al.*, 1980; Steger *et al.*, 1980; Nass *et al.*, 1982).

In aging PES rats, there is a lack of cyclic increases in LH and FSH secretion and the absence of gonadotropin surges may be the immediate cause for anovulation (Meites *et al.*, 1978). Thus, in intact and acutely ovariectomized PES animals, ovarian steroids are less effective in producing an LH surge (Fig. 9; Lu *et al.*, 1980, 1981). However, estradiol or estradiol-progesterone elicits an increase in LH release in long-term ovariectomized PES rats (Fig. 10; Lu *et al.*, 1977, 1981; Steger *et al.*, 1980). In contrast, the stimulatory feedback of steroids on LH secretion is effective in intact and acutely ovariectomized RPP females (Fig. 9; Lu *et al.*, 1980). RPP animals are usually older than PES females (Lu *et al.*, 1979). As indicated earlier, the PES state in aging rats is characterized by a steroid environment of high estrogen and low progesterone, whereas the RPP animals secrete large amounts of progesterone and some estrogens (Fig. 6; Lu *et al.*, 1980). These observations suggest that alterations in ovarian steroid secretion during the PES state may influence the central nervous system functions regulating pituitary LH secretion. Furthermore, chronic placement of estradiol implants into long-term

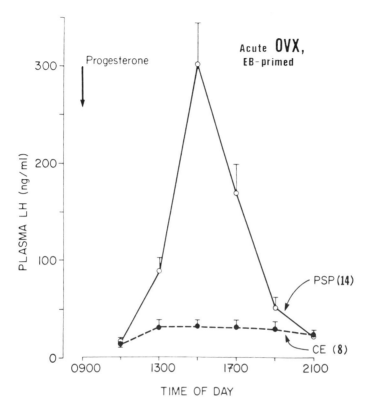

Fig. 9. Effects of progesterone injection (day-4) on plasma LH levels in acutely ovariec-tomized, estradiol benzoate-primed (day-1) old constant-estrous (CE) and repetitive pseu-dopregnant (PSP) rats. Progesterone administration elicits an LH surge in old PSP but not CE rats. (From Lu *et al.*, 1980, with permission.)

ovariectomized old and young rats abolishes the ability of steroids to elicit an LH surge (Fig. 10; Lu *et al.*, 1981). These results indicate that although the positive feedback mechanism of steroids on LH secretion is present in aging PES rats, a chronic elevation of circulating estrogen (Fig. 3) prevents the central nervous system (CNS) from responding normally to steroid stimulation by increasing LH secretion (Lu *et al.*, 1981). Since the stimulatory feedback of ovarian steroids on LH secretion is functioning in aged RPP but not PES females (Fig. 9), the differential absence of such neuroendocrine function in the PES animals appears to be due to hyperestrogenic conditions rather than to aging *per se*. It should be noted, however, that not all aged PES rats respond normally to es-tradiol or estradiol-progesterone administration by increasing LH se-

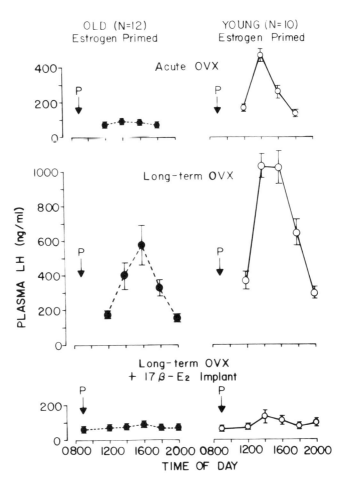

Fig. 10. Effects of progesterone injection (day-4) on plasma LH levels in estradiol benzoate-primed (day-1), acutely ovariectomized (OVX), and long-term OVX (5 weeks), old persistent-estrous rats (left panels), young females (cyclic at the time of OVX, right panels), and long-term OVX old and young rats implanted with 17β-estradiol (7 weeks old). (From Lu *et al.*, 1981, with permission.)

cretion after long-term ovariectomy (Steger *et al.*, 1980). Some animals show a consistent lack of response during a 60-day period of postovariectomy, and this is likely due to a prolonged inhibition of CNS function under hyperestrogenic conditions rather than to old age.

   The results of these studies indicate that a chronic increase in circulating estrogen associated with anovulatory function in aging female rats exerts a profound inhibition on both positive and negative feedback control of LH secretion, and that elimination of circulating estrogen after long-term ovariectomy reinstates the stimulatory feedback response in some but not all aging animals. The magnitude of the ovarian steroid-induced LH surge is always less in aged PES than in young rats under long-term ovariectomy conditions (Fig. 10; Lu *et al.*, 1981), as is the post-ovariectomy increase in basal LH secretion (Fig. 8; Steger *et al.*, 1980). Recent reports have shown that a chronic elevation of circulating estrogen in female rats causes histological degeneration in the hypothalamic arcuate nucleus (Brawer *et al.*, 1980), and a defect in tubero-infundibular dopamine neurotransmission (Casanueva *et al.*, 1982). The estrogen-induced defective dopamine function is associated with enhanced prolactin secretion (Casanueva *et al.*, 1982), and the degenerating synaptic structures may represent a selective disruption of neural connections between the medial preoptic area and the medial basal hypothalamus (Brawer *et al.*, 1980). It remains to be determined whether such functional and histological alterations in the arcuate nucleus are present in aging PES animals that demonstrate an impaired steroid feedback regulation on LH secretion. In contrast to the marked inhibition of LH secretion under the PES state, a chronic elevation of circulating estrogen appears to have little or no influence on the steroid feedback regulation of FSH secretion (Lu *et al.*, 1980; Steger *et al.*, 1980).

4. Changes in Prolactin Secretion

As discussed above, altered ovarian function and steroid production associated with aging undoubtedly influence hypothalamic-pituitary functions, including prolactin secretion. Reports have shown that higher pituitary and serum levels of prolactin are found in old PES than in young female rats (Clemens and Meites, 1971), and that hemorrhagic pituitaries and/or pituitary tumors are frequently found in old animals (Meites and Huang, 1976; Lu *et al.*, 1979). Ovariectomy at a young age tends to reduce the incidence of pituitary pathology and prevents the marked increase in prolactin secretion found in old females (Lu *et al.*, 1979), suggesting a causal relationship between ovarian steroids and abnormal prolactin secretion during aging. The results from a systematic study have revealed that, in aging PES rats, serum levels of prolactin are maintained at low basal values until they are increased at the age of 16 months and later (Fig. 11), suggesting the aging-related increase in pituitary prolactin secretion is probably a consequence of steroid hormonal changes due to chronic anovulation (Lu *et al.*, 1979). Basal values

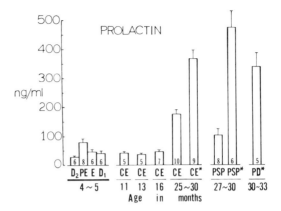

Fig. 11. Circulating concentrations of prolactin in young cycling rats and in old females in constant-estrus (CE), repetitive-pseudopregnant (PSP), or persistent-diestrous (PD) states. Abbreviations are the same as in Fig. 3. * = rats with pituitary tumors or lesions. Serum prolactin levels are markedly increased in old (25–30 months old) but not in young (11–16 months old) rats during the CE state. The values are much greater in animals with evidence of pituitary lesions. (From Lu *et al.*, 1979, with permission.)

of serum prolactin are lower in old RPP than in PES females (Fig. 11), presumably due to increased progesterone and decreased estrogen secretion during the repetitive pseudopregnant state (Lu *et al.*, 1979). Hemorrhagic pituitaries are commonly seen in both PES and RPP females beyond the age of 25 months, and serum prolactin values are 2–3-fold greater in animals with hemorrhagic pituitaries than in those with normal pituitaries (Fig. 11; Lu *et al.*, 1979). As indicated earlier, intact or acutely ovariectomized PES rats do not respond normally to estradiol-progesterone administration by increasing LH release (Lu *et al.*, 1980, 1981). Similar to this, estradiol-progesterone administration is ineffective in eliciting a prolactin surge in old PES animals, even when animals are tested at two weeks postovariectomy (Huang *et al.*, 1980). Thus, in aging PES rats administration of ovarian steroids elicits an FSH but not LH or prolactin surges (Steger *et al.*, 1980).

The 24-hr pattern of prolactin secretion reveals that 20- to 26-month-old PES and RPP rats exhibit predominantly diurnal and nocturnal surges of secretion, respectively (Damassa *et al.*, 1980), presumably due in part to differential patterns of ovarian estrogen and progesterone secretion in these two reproductive states (Fig. 6; Lu *et al.*, 1980). In ovariectomized young rats, estrogen administration is known to elicit a late afternoon prolactin surge (Neill, 1972). Perhaps the daily diurnal prolactin surge found in aging PES rats is due to chronically elevated circulating estrogen (Fig. 3; Lu *et al.*, 1981). It is interesting to note that, in ovariectomized, estradiol-progesterone treated rats formerly in PES, serum prolactin values are maintained at static high levels between 0900–2100 hr (Huang *et al.*, 1980). The results from another study also revealed that both PES and RPP rats that show evidence of pituitary tumors and/or lesions exhibit static high levels of circulating prolactin but no obvious surges of prolactin secretion (Damassa *et al.*, 1980). In RPP females, the daily nocturnal surges of prolactin release appear to be dependent on intact ovarian function and high circulating progesterone (Gilman *et al.*, 1981). These observations clearly indicate that ovarian secretion of estrogen and progesterone in aging rats during the prolonged PES and RPP states exert a profound influence on prolactin secretion, and that chronically increased circulating estrogen and decreased progesterone (Fig. 3) may be the important factors influencing prolactin secretion. It is possible that the estrogen-induced pituitary tumor or hyperprolactinemia observed in aging female rats may be due to a degeneration in the hypothalamic arcuate nucleus (Brawer *et al.*, 1980) and/or a defect in the tubero-infundibular dopamine neurotransmission (Casanueva *et al.*, 1982). It should be pointed out, however, that aging *per se* may be associated with functional and histological changes in the hypothalamus, and that a substantially increased estrogen exposure during the chronic anovulatory state may cause the hypothalamic aging observed in PES animals. Thus, alterations in gonadotropin and prolactin secretion in aging PES and RPP animals may be the combined result of ovarian steroid influence and developmental changes in organ function.

5. Alterations in Ovarian Steroid and Periovulatory Gonadotropin Secretion Preceding the Cessation of Regular Estrous Cycles

The foregoing discussions have dealt with changes in ovarian function and pituitary hormone secretion, and their relation to neuroendocrine response in aging females after complete cessation of estrous cycles. Reproductive aging in the female rat, however, is characterized initially by a gradual cessation of regular cyclicity beginning about 10–12 months of age (Lu and Kledzik, 1981). During this transition period, aging females display irregular instead of regular patterns of estrous cycles. Most of the irregular cycles are characterized by prolonged phases of vaginal cornification, indicative of sustained estrogen secretion and delayed ovulation (Lu *et al.*, 1979; Peluso *et al.*, 1979). These changes in reproductive function occur relatively early in the female rat. The question has been raised, therefore, whether any functional alterations in the hypothalamic-pituitary-ovarian axis precede the disruption of regular cyclicity in aging females.

We performed experiments to determine the patterns of LH, FSH, and ovarian steroid secretion in middle-aged (10–12 months old) female rats in proestrus and estrus of the regular cycle, as compared to patterns in young females (4 months old). Consecutive blood samples were taken through a jugular catheter at 90-min intervals from the afternoon of proestrus until noon of the next day. After the experiments, patterns of estrous cyclicity were followed in each animal for about 60–70 days. During that period, some middle-aged rats continued to show regular cyclicity (RC), whereas others became irregular cyclers or persistent-estrous (N-RC). Hormonal data revealed that during the 4-day regular estrous cycles, the magnitude of proestrous LH but not FSH surges was significantly decreased in aging rats that subsequently became N-RC, whereas the patterns of both LH and FSH surges in the middle-aged RC females were the same as in the young controls (Nass *et al.*, 1982). These results indicate that reproductive aging is characterized by a differential change in the steroid feedback on gonadotropin secretion, and such alteration in the neuroendocrine system occurs during aging but is not a direct consequence of chronological age *per se*. Other reports, however, showed that a reduction of the proestrous LH surge was seen in *all* middle-aged rats, regardless of subsequent changes in their estrous cyclicity (Cooper *et al.*, 1980; Gray *et al.*, 1980; Wise, 1982). Our data also demonstrated that the second increase in FSH secretion beginning about midnight of proestrus (Smith *et al.*, 1975) was greater in middle-aged regular cyclic rats than in young females. Thus, aging exerts differential effects on LH and FSH secretion prior to the disruption of regular estrous cyclicity. The sustained increase in FSH secretion seen in middle-aged female rats on the day of estrus may be associated with higher circulating estradiol levels on diestrus day-2 and on proestrus (Fig. 3). The greater amounts of circulating FSH and estradiol found in middle-aged rats during the regular cycles may be responsible for a slower rate of follicular atresia (Peluso *et al.*, 1979). Repeated exposure to higher circulating estrogen during recurrent estrous cycles at middle age may cause a progressive decrease in the sensitivity of the central nervous mechanism which mediates the positive feedback of steroids on LH secretion (Lu *et al.*, 1981). Histologically, such functional lesions may involve a degeneration of the hypothalamic arcuate nucleus (Brawer *et al.*, 1980).

In consonance with our findings on middle-aged regularly cycling rats, other reports have shown that the magnitude of the LH but not the FSH surge elicited by estradiol or estradiol-progesterone also is reduced in aging females (Steger *et al.*, 1980; Gray *et al.*, 1980). Furthermore, the postovariectomy increase in LH but not FSH secretion also is less in these middle-aged animals (Steger *et al.*, 1980). As expected, these attenuations of the steroid feedback regulation of LH secretion also are found in middle-aged rats displaying irregular estrous cycles (Steger *et al.*, 1980). These observations support the view that reproductive aging is associated with a progressive loss of steroid feedback on gonadotropin secretion, particularly LH secretion and enhanced FSH secretion. These functional changes in the neuroendocrine regulation of gonadotropin secretion presage the disruption of regular estrous cyclicity, and are related to an altered estrogen secretion pattern. In aging female rats, the functional relationship between ovarian physiology and changing neuroendocrine responses remains to be identified and vigorously examined.

6. Conclusions

In the female rat, aging is characterized by a progressive cessation of regular estrous cycles, and is preceded by specific alterations in both pituitary and ovarian secretion. During regular estrous cycles in middle-aged females, enhanced FSH secretion may result in advanced follicular growth and increased ovarian estrogen production. These, in turn, may cause a decrease of follicular atresia in the face of a smaller pool of ovarian follicles. At middle age, these subtle changes in hormone secretion and in ovarian function are probably repeated during successive regular cycles. As a result, repeated exposure to higher levels of circulating estrogen may eventually reduce the hypothalamic responsiveness to ovarian steroid feedback, and result in a progressive decrease in the magnitude of estrogen-elicited LH surges and/or a delayed onset of the LH surge. Either or both of these may affect the final process of follicular maturation and ovulation during the estrous cycle. With these alterations in ovarian and neuroendocrine functions, a gradual shift from regular cyclic to irregular cyclic patterns can be anticipated in middle-aged females. Once the estrogen-elicited LH surge is less than optimal in terms of either magnitude or timing, anovulation is seen in aging animals in the face of continued follicular growth. Much remains to be clarified as to why FSH secretion is enhanced in middle-aged female rats, and how the stimulatory feedback response to LH secretion is gradually attenuated.

After complete cessation of ovulatory cycles, continued follicular growth in the ovaries produces substantial amounts of circulating estrogen and decreased progesterone during the persistent estrous state. These may further suppress the central nervous mechanism which mediates the positive feedback of ovarian steroids on LH secretion. Under these conditions, ovarian steroid administration is ineffective in eliciting an LH or prolactin surge in persistent-estrous females. Elimination of circulating estrogen after long-term ovariectomy reinstates the stimulatory feedback actions of steroids on LH secretion. Following a prolonged period of anovulation, older females resume ovulatory activity at irregular and long intervals, and the mechanism(s) underlying this functional resumption is totally unknown at present. An extended period of pseudopregnancy follows ovulation in aged females, with prominent corpora lutea secreting large amounts of progesterone and 20α-OH-progesterone. Thus, in aged pseudopregnant rats, there is an increased circulating progestin and decreased estrogen, and positive feedback by steroids on LH secretion becomes functional. These and other findings from our recent studies provide evidence that chronic elevation of circulating estrogen prevents the central nervous system from responding normally to ovarian steroids by eliciting an LH surge essential for ovulation, and progesterone appears to alleviate the suppression by estrogen. Associated with these differential patterns of estrogen and progesterone secretion, aged persistent-estrous and pseudopregnant females exhibit predominantly daily diurnal and nocturnal surges of prolactin release, respectively.

ACKNOWLEDGMENTS. The author wishes to acknowledge the courtesy of *Endocrinology* and *Biology of Reproduction* for permission to reproduce illustrations. This work was supported by NIH research grant AG-01512 from the National Institute on Aging, and a Basic Science Grant (OB-40) from the UCLA School of Medicine.

7. References

Armstrong, D. T., Miller, L. S., and Knudsen, K. A., 1969, Regulation of lipid metabolism and progesterone production in rat corpora lutea and ovarian interstitial elements by prolactin and luteinizing hormone, *Endocrinology* **85**:393–401.
Aschheim, P., 1961, La pseudogestation a repetition chez les rattes seniles, *C. R. Acad. Sci.* **253**:1988–1990.
Aschheim, P., 1965, La reactivation de l'ovarie des rattes seniles en oestrus permanent au moyen d'hormones gonadotropes de la mise a l'obscurite, *C. R. Acad. Sci.* **260**:5627–5630.

Aschheim, P., 1979, Function of the aging ovary: Comparative aspects, *Eur. J. Obstet. Gynecol. Reprod. Biol.* **9**:191–202.

Brawer, J. R., Schipper, H., and Naftolin, F., 1980, Ovary-dependent degeneration in the hypothalamic arcuate nucleus, *Endocrinology* **107**:274–279.

Casanueva, F., Cocchi, D., Locatelli, V., Flavto, C., Zambotti, F., Bestetti, G., Rossi, G. L., and Müller, E., 1982, Defective central nervous system dopaminergic function in rats with estrogen-induced pituitary tumors, as assessed by plasma prolactin concentrations, *Endocrinology* **110**:590–599.

Clemens, J. A., and Meites, J., 1971, Neuroendocrine status of old constant estrous rats, *Neuroendocrinology* **7**:249–256.

Cooper, R. L., Conn, P. M., and Walker, R. F., 1980, Characterization of the LH surge in middle-aged female rats, *Biol. Reprod.* **23**:611–615.

Crumeyrolle-Arias, M., Scheib, D., and Aschheim, P., 1976, Light and electron microscopy of the ovarian interstitial tissue in the senile rat: Normal aspect and response to HCG of "Deficiency Cells" and "Epithelial Cords," *Gerontology* **22**:185–204.

Damassa, D. A., Gilman, D. P., Lu, K. H., Judd, H. L., and Sawyer, C. H., 1980, The twenty-four hour pattern of prolactin secretion in aging female rats, *Biol. Reprod.* **22**:571–575.

Erickson, G. F., Hsueh, A. J. W., and Lu, K. H., 1979, Gonadotropin binding and aromastase activity in granulosa cells of young proestrous and old constant estrous rats, *Biol. Reprod.* **20**:182–190.

Fayein, N. A., and Aschheim, P., 1980, Age-related temporal changes of levels of circulating progesterone in repeatedly pseudopregnant rats, *Biol. Reprod.* **23**:616–620.

Gilman, D. P., Lu, J. K. H., Whitmoyer, D. I., Judd, H. L., and Sawyer, C. H., 1981, Relationship between progesterone and prolactin surges in aged and young pseudopregnant rats, *Biol. Reprod.* **24**:839–845.

Gray, G. D., Tennent, B., Smith, E. R., and Davidson, J. M., 1980, Luteinizing hormone regulation and sexual behavior in middle-aged female rats, *Endocrinology* **107**:187–194.

Huang, H. H., and Meites, J., 1975, Reproductive capacity of aging female rats, *Neuroendocrinology* **17**:289–295.

Huang, H. H., Marshall, S., and Meites, J., 1976, Capacity of old versus young female rats to secrete LH, FSH and prolactin, *Biol. Reprod.* **14**:538–543.

Huang, H. H., Steger, R. W., Bruni, J. F., and Meites, J., 1978, Patterns of sex steroid and gonadotropin secretion in aging female rats, *Endocrinology* **103**:1855–1859.

Huang, H. H., Steger, R. W., Sonntag, W. E., and Meites, J., 1980, Positive feedback by ovarian hormones on prolactin and LH in old versus young female rats, *Neurobiol. Aging* **1**:141–143.

Ingram, D. K., 1959, The vaginal smear of senile laboratory rats, *J. Endocrinol.* **19**:182–188.

Lu, J. K. H., and Kledzik, G. S., 1981, Chronological changes in ovarian function and morphology in aging rats and their relation to neuroendocrine responses, in: *Dynamics of Ovarian Function* (N. B. Schwartz and M. Hunzicker-Dunn, eds.), Raven Press, New York, pp. 291–296.

Lu, K. H., Huang, H. H., Chen, H. T., Kurcz, M., Mioduszewski, R., and Meites, J., 1977, Positive feedback by estrogen and progesterone on LH release in old and young rats, *Proc. Soc. Exp. Biol. Med.* **154**:82–85.

Lu, K. H., Hooper, B. R., Vargo, T. M., and Yen, S. S. C., 1979, Chronological changes in sex steroid, gonadotropin and prolactin secretion in aging female rats displaying different reproductive states, *Biol. Reprod.* **21**:193–203.

Lu, J. K. H., Damassa, D. A., Gilman, D. P., Judd, H. L., and Sawyer, C. H., 1980, Differential patterns of gonadotropin responses to ovarian steroids and to LH-releasing hormone between constant-estrous and pseudopregnant states in aging rats, *Biol. Reprod.* **23:**345–351.

Lu, J. K. H., Gilman, D. P., Meldrum, D. R., Judd, H. L., and Sawyer, C. H., 1981, Relationship between circulating estrogens and the central mechanisms by which ovarian steroids stimulate luteinizing hormone secretion in aged and young female rats, *Endocrinology* **108:**836–841.

Mandl, A. M., 1959, Corpora lutea in senile virgin laboratory rats, *J. Endocrinol.* **18:**438–443.

Mandl, A. M., 1961, Cyclic changes in the vaginal smears of senile nulliparous and multiparous rats, *J. Endocrinol.* **22:**257–268.

Meites, J., and Huang, H. H., 1976, Relation of neuroendocrine system to loss of reproductive functions in aging rats, in: *Neuroendocrine Regulation of Fertility* (A. Kumar, ed.), Karger, Basel, pp. 246–258.

Meites, J., Huang, H. H., and Simpkins, J. W., 1978, Recent studies on neuroendocrine control of reproductive senescence in rats, in: *The Aging Reproductive System* (E. L. Schneider, ed.), Raven Press, New York, pp. 213–235.

Nass, T. E., LaPolt, P. S., and Lu, J. K. H., 1982, Alterations in ovarian steroid and preovulatory gonadotropin secretion preceding the loss of regular estrous cyclicity in aging female rats, *Program of the 64th Annual Meeting of The Endocrine Society*, Abst. No. 137.

Neill, J. D., 1972, Sexual differences in the hypothalamic regulation of prolactin secretion, *Endocrinology* **90:**1154–1159.

Peluso, J. J., Steger, R. W., Huang, H. H., and Meites, J., 1979, Pattern of follicular growth and steroidogenesis in the ovary of aging cyclic rats, *Exp. Aging Res.* **5:**319–333.

Shaar, C. J., Euker, J. S., Riegle, G. D., and Meites, J., 1975, Effects of castration and gonadal steroids on serum luteinizing hormone and prolactin in old and young rats, *J. Endocrinol.* **66:**45–51.

Smith, M. S., Freeman, M. E., and Neill, J. D., 1975, The control of progesterone secretion during the estrous cycle and early pseudopregnancy in the rat: Prolactin, gonadotropin and steroid levels associated with rescue of the corpus luteum of pseudopregnancy, *Endocrinology* **96:**219–226.

Steger, R. W., Peluso, J. J., Huang, H. H., Hafez, E. S., and Meites, J., 1976, Gonadotropin binding sites in the ovary of aged rats, *J. Reprod. Fertil.* **48:**205–207.

Steger, R. W., Huang, H. H., and Meites, J., 1979, Relation of aging to hypothalamic LHRH content and serum gonadal steroids in female rats, *Proc. Soc. Exp. Biol. Med.* **161:**251–254.

Steger, R. W., Huang, H. H., Chamberlain, D. S., and Meites, J., 1980, Changes in control of gonadotropin secretion in the transition period between regular cycles and constant estrus in aging female rats, *Biol. Reprod.* **22:**595–603.

Wang, C., Hsueh, A. J. W., and Erickson, G. F., 1979, Induction of functional prolactin receptors by follicle-stimulating hormone in rat granulosa cells *in vivo* and *in vitro*, *J. Biol. Chem.* **254:**11330–11336.

Watkins, B. E., Meites, J., and Riegle, G. D., 1975, Age-related changes in pituitary responsiveness to LHRH in the female rat, *Endocrinology* **97:**543–548.

Wise, P. M., 1982, Alterations in proestrous LH, FSH, and prolactin surges in middle-aged rats, *Proc. Soc. Exp. Biol. Med.* **169:**348–354.

CHAPTER 8

The Reproductive Decline in Male Rats

RICHARD W. STEGER and HENRY H. H. HUANG

1. Introduction

The aging male rat exhibits a gradual decline in reproductive function, but fertility is usually maintained throughout the normal lifespan (Meites et al., 1980; Steger et al., 1981). Only when the endocrine system is challenged by experimental manipulations or when the various components of the reproductive axis are closely examined, do age-related defects become apparent. This review will attempt to point out the "normal" aging events affecting the reproductive processes in the male rat, as well as the more common pathological findings seen in certain rat strains. Changes in hypothalamic neurotransmitter function and gonadotropin-releasing factor levels in relationship to male endocrine function have already been discussed in the chapter by Simpkins and will not be covered in this review.

2. Testicular Structure and Function

Although the testes maintain gametogenic and steroidogenic function throughout the lifespan of the male rat, there are several apparent defects that make these processes less efficient with aging.

RICHARD W. STEGER • Department of Obstetrics and Gynecology, University of Texas Health Science Center at San Antonio, San Antonio, Texas 78284.   HENRY H. H. HUANG • Research Laboratory, Mercy Hospital and Medical Center, Chicago, Illinois 60616.

2.1. Testicular Histology

Data from several strains of rats indicate that testes weights, on either an absolute or on a body weight basis, do not change significantly with age, although there is a trend toward an absolute increase in weight with advancing age (Leathem and Albrecht, 1974; Saksena *et al.*, 1979; Turek and Desjardins, 1979; Pirke *et al.*, 1979a; Prisco and Dessi-Fulgheri, 1980). However, data from other studies demonstrate that absolute testicular weight plateaus between 3–5 months of age and declines significantly thereafter (Peng *et al.*, 1974; Kaler and Neaves, 1981a). In the latter study, testicular volume also was shown to decline significantly between 12–24 months of age.

Histological analysis of the rat testes varies somewhat with the species, but, in general, basement membrane thickening and tubular fibrosis is commonly observed after 16–18 months of age (Peng *et al.*, 1974; Humphreys, 1977; Steger *et al.*, 1979). Despite the existence of fibrotic changes in the tubules of old rats, an analysis of the spermatogenic cycle (Table 1) showed no differences between young (3–4 months) and old (22 months) Wistar rats (Steger *et al.*, 1979). Similarly, a comparison of 5- and 17-month-old Sheffield–Wistar rats showed similar tubular pat-

Table 1. A Comparison of the Frequency of Observation of the Stages of the Spermatogenic Cycle in Aged vs. Young Adult Rats[a]

Stage of spermatogenic cycle	Frequency of observation	
	Young	Aged
I	10 ± 1.2	9 ± 1.7
II–III	12 ± 2.2	13 ± 2.6
IV–V	10 ± 2.4	13 ± 2.4
VI	8 ± 1.0	7 ± 0.93
VII	25 ± 3.4	25 ± 3.7
VIII	5 ± 1.8	4 ± 1.4
IX	3 ± 1.1	3 ± 1.2
X	4 ± 1.4	3 ± 1.7
XI	3 ± 0.94	4 ± 1.2
XII	11 ± 1.3	9 ± 2.0
XIII	4 ± 0.85	6 ± 1.1
XIV	5 ± 1.5	4 ± 1.8

[a] Counts were done in testicular sections from seven old animals and five young animals. The number of tubular cross sections scored per animal was 250. (From Steger *et al.*, 1979.)

terns, with the exception of the observation that 2% of the transverse tubular secretions in the older rats contained only basal cells and there was an increase in the number of undifferentiated spermatids in the tubules. By 24 months, only 20% of the tubules were normal in appearance, but every section had some tubules in which spermatogenesis was proceeding normally. Large numbers of undifferentiated spermatids were seen and it appeared that spermatogenesis was occurring to the early spermatid stage, but elongation was impaired (Humphreys, 1977).

An electron microscopic study of the aged testes showed changes in the Sertoli cell itself and in its relationship to the maturing spermatid (Humphreys, 1977). Cell division of spermatogonia and spermatocytes appeared to be similar in young and old animals, despite a reduction in age in the number of spermatocytes. Some, but not all old rats, show scattered areas of interstitial hyperplasia.

In F344 male rats, which frequently develop Leydig cell tumors, nodular interstitial cell hyperplasia is much more common and is seen as early as 10 months of age (Coleman *et al.*, 1977). In the F344 rat, during the advanced stages of interstitial cell proliferation, all germ and Sertoli cells are lost and eventually tubular elements become indistinguishable from interstitial tissue stroma (Turek and Desjardins, 1979).

A recent histometric analysis of the testes in 3-, 5-, 12-, and 24-month-old Sprague–Dawley rats demonstrated a significant age-related increase in the total number of Leydig cells per testis (Kaler and Neaves, 1981a). In the same study, the average volume of a single Leydig cell decreased with age, although not significantly. Thus, the total Leydig cell volume per testis remained constant with age as did the volume of interstitial tissue.

2.2. Sperm Count and Fertility

Total sperm population in the epididymis and vas deferens of male rats rises to a plateau at about 100 days of age (Fig. 1) and is maintained at this level to at least 15 months of age (Saksena *et al.*, 1979). Unfortunately, we are not aware of any similar studies investigating older rats. In the same study, 16- and 17-month-old rats were still fertile but, when mated to young proestrous females, the mean number of pups per mother decreased with age (Table 2). In our own colony, male rats as old as 24 months have still been able to successfully sire litters of only slightly reduced sizes (Steger, unpublished observations).

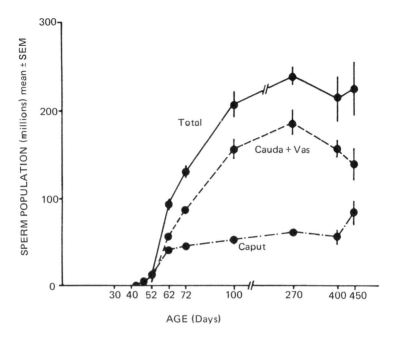

Fig. 1. Total sperm population in the epididymis and vas deferens of male rats from days 30–450 of age. Each point represents the mean of 5–7 animals and the vertical lines indicate the standard error of the mean. (From Saksena *et al.*, 1979.)

2.3. Serum Steroid Levels

In contrast to data from aging men and mice, there is almost universal agreement that testosterone levels in the male rat decrease significantly with age (Ghanadian *et al.*, 1975; Bruni *et al.*, 1977; Gray, 1978; Pirke *et al.*, 1979b; Saksena and Lau, 1979; Steger *et al.*, 1979; Kaler and Neaves, 1981a; Simpkins *et al.*, 1981; Frankel and Mock, 1982). Serum 5α-dihydrotestosterone, however, does not change with old age (24 months) and androstenedione shows only a slight decline with age (15 months); Ghanadian *et al.*, 1975; Saksena and Lau, 1979; Simpkins *et al.*, 1981). Simpkins and co-workers (1981) also have shown that the diurnal variations in plasma testosterone levels seen in young (3–4 months) male rats are absent in old (19–20 months) male rats.

Dehydroepiandrosterone decreases significantly between 9–12 months, while, at the same time, serum pregnenolone levels increase significantly (Saksena and Lau, 1979). Plasma progesterone levels also are elevated in old male rats, probably due to a significantly larger and

Table 2. Age-Related Changes in the Fertility of the Male Rat[a,e]

Male rat number	Number of young born[b] when mated on day						
	62	72	100	200	300	400	500
1	NM[c]	12	14	14	13	12	8
2	8	10	13	15	14	10	8
3	9	11	14	16	15	10	8
4	5	10	10	11	16	9	8
5	7	9	12	15	14	8	9
6	6	8	9	11	15	13	11
7	10	11	10	15	13	11	6
8	7	6	9	13	12	10	7
Mean ± SEM	6.40 ± 0.6[1]	9.6 ± 0.7[2,3,4]	11.4 ± 0.8[4,5]	13.8 ± 0.7[6]	14.0 ± 0.5	10.4 ± 0.6[3,5]	8.1 ± 5[1,2,d]

[a] Males were regularly used at least once in 10 days.
[b] Mated to virgin females of 200–250 g.
[c] NM = Not mated on two consecutive days.
[d] Figures with different superscripts (1,2,3 . . .) differ significantly at $p < .05$ (Duncan's test).
[e] From Saksena et al., (1979).

sustained diurnal elevation of progesterone in old, as compared to young male rats (Saksena and Lau, 1979; Simpkins *et al.*, 1981). The elevated progesterone levels were possibly due to increased adrenal cortical secretion, as demonstrated in the aging female rat (Steger and Peluso, unpublished observations). Estrone and estradiol levels were unchanged in Sprague–Dawley derived rats from 2–15 months of age (Saksena and Lau, 1979), in contrast to elevated levels seen in aging men. In the aging F344 rat, estradiol levels increase dramatically, possibly in association with the development of Leydig cell tumors (Turek and Desjardins, 1979).

2.4. Gonadotropin Response of the Old Testes

The aging testis appears to be less responsive to gonadotropin stimulation despite unimpaired LH binding (Steger *et al.*, 1979). The age-related decrease in endogenous LH is much less than the decrease in circulating testosterone levels, suggesting decreased testicular response in addition to decreased gonadotropin levels as a causative factor of reduced testosterone levels in old vs. young rats (Gray, 1978; Pirke *et al.*, 1978a). However, as will be discussed subsequently, decreased gonadotropin stimulation could lead to decreased gonadotropin responsiveness.

The data on the *in vivo* responsiveness of the aged testis to exogenous gonadotropin stimulation is somewhat contradictory, probably due to utilization of different age and animal strains, different regimens and doses of hormone administration, and differences in the expression of data. Riegle and Miller (1978) showed a decreased response with age to 1, 5, and 20 IU of human chorionic gonadotropin (hCG), but the relative responses, although not reported, appeared approximately equal in young and old rats (Fig. 2). The time course of testosterone release was similar in both age groups. Lin *et al.* (1980) also showed that plasma testosterone levels were significantly lower in old than in young males after a single injection of hCG. Kaler and Neaves (1981a) likewise showed a reduced plasma testosterone response to hCG with age, but an unchanged total circulating quantity of testosterone when differences in plasma volumes were considered.

Harman and co-workers (1978) showed that old (24 months) rats were initially less responsive to a single injection of 1 IU hCG, but within 2 hr of injection, testosterone levels were indistinguishable from younger (12 months) rats. However, it must be realized that defects in testosterone secretion appear as early as 7 or 8 months of age (Saksena and Lau, 1979; Frankel and Mock, 1982). Multiple injections of hCG over a 3-

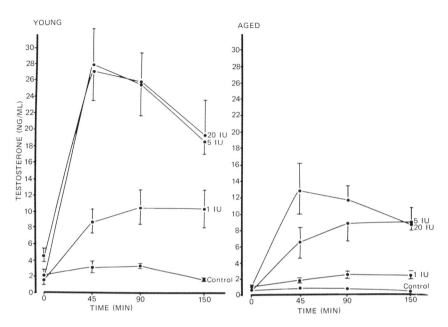

Fig. 2.   Effect of intravenous injection of 1, 5, and 20 IU of hCG on serum testosterone in young (4 months) and aged (22–30 months) male Long–Evans rats. Testosterone levels are shown as the group mean ± SEM. Blood samples were taken under light ether anesthesia before and at 45, 90, and 150 minutes after hCG or control (saline) injections. (From Riegle and Miller, 1978.)

day period (Harman *et al.*, 1978) or a 7-day period (Riegle and Miller, 1978) led to equal testosterone levels in young (3–4 months), middle-aged (12 months), and old (24–28 months) male rats (Fig. 3). Five daily injections of hCG likewise restored normal levels of testicular Δ^5-3β-hydroxysteroid dehydrogenase levels in old rats (Leathem and Albrecht, 1974), suggesting that chronic gonadotropin hypostimulation rather than changes in testicular gonadotropin response is the cause of age-related decreases in plasma testosterone levels. Lin *et al.* (1980), using 3 weeks of hCG administration, could not, however, restore circulating testosterone levels of old rats to basal levels seen in young rats.

Leydig cell function also may be impaired in old rats due to a decrease in testicular blood flow with age (Pirke *et al.*, 1979a). Multiple hCG injections reverse this age effect, offering another explanation for the ability of chronic hCG replacement to overcome the age-dependent decrease in testosterone secretion.

In vitro studies of basal and gonadotropin-stimulated testosterone

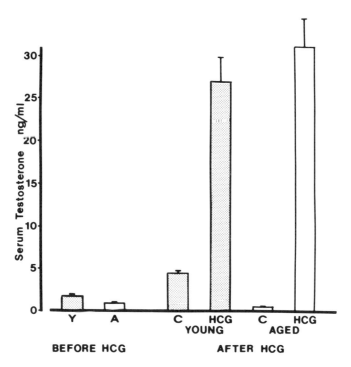

Fig. 3. Effect of daily subcutaneous injection of hCG (5 IU/100 g body weight for 7 days) on serum testosterone levels in young (shaded bars) and aged (open bars) male rats. Blood samples were taken before hCG treatment was started and at 24 hr after the final hCG injection. Control groups (C) received seven daily injections of the control vehicle. Values are shown as the mean ± SEM. (From Riegle and Miller, 1978.)

secretion show no age-related changes in testosterone secretion into the media (Pirke *et al.*, 1978b; Kaler and Neaves, 1981a,b). However, the testosterone production of Leydig cells isolated from testes of old rats was significantly less than that from young adult animals (Pirke *et al.*, 1979b; Chen *et al.*, 1981). The fact that the Leydig cell number increases with age in the rat (Pirke *et al.*, 1978; Kaler and Neaves, 1981a,b), accounts for the ability of the old testes to maintain *in vitro* testosterone secretion despite the age-related defect in Leydig cell function.

Several studies have shown that [125I]-LH binds equally to homogenates of old and young testes and [125I]-hCG uptake by the testes does not differ with age (Steger *et al.*, 1979; Pirke *et al.*, 1979b). A more recent study has shown that the number or affinity of binding sites for [125I]-hCG does not change with age (Kaler and Neaves, 1981b). However, these results were obtained in studies using testicular homogenates and did not take into account the increased number of Leydig cells in the old rat testis. Thus, gonadotropin binding expressed on a per Leydig cell basis might actually decline with age.

It has been suggested that the impairment in testosterone synthesis in old Leydig cells is beyond the gonadotropin receptor and cyclic AMP formation, since testosterone secretion is attenuated with age in isolated Leydig cells stimulated with either LH or 8-bromo-cyclic AMP (Lin *et al.*, 1980). Furthermore, the ability of old testes to convert pregnenolone and progesterone to testosterone is not impaired, suggesting that either cholesterol conversion to pregnenolone or cholesterol transport to the side chain cleavage enzyme is impaired in old rats (Chen *et al.*, 1981). The conversion of pregnenolone and progesterone to testosterone, which takes place on the smooth endoplasmic reticulum, was intact in the old Sprague–Dawley rat (Chen *et al.*, 1981). Kaler and Neaves (1981b) reported that the ability of the aging testis to synthesize cholesterol from octanoate and the conversion of cholesterol to pregnenolone were unchanged with age. Furthermore, the ability of the old testis to convert pregnenolone to testosterone was increased approximately 25% in the old, as compared to the young rat testis, in agreement with the findings of Chen *et al.* (1981). The studies of Kaler and Neaves (1981b) were based on testicular homogenates, which could explain the failure to note the impairment of testosterone synthesis with age as documented by Chen *et al.* (1981) using isolated Leydig cells.

2.5. Steroid Clearance

The age-related decrease in serum testosterone levels does not appear to be due to changes in metabolic clearance rate (MCR), since the MCR of testosterone has been demonstrated to be 2.5 times lower in old male rats (20–24 months) then in young (6–8 months) controls (Table 3; Huang *et al.*, 1979). Kaler and Neaves have argued that increases in plasma volume with age, as demonstrated by an isotope dilution method, are at least partially responsible for observed changes in testosterone levels due to a dilution effect. However, Frankel and Mock (1982) have refuted this "dilution" hypothesis based on comparisons of testosterone concentrations in testicular venous blood with testosterone levels in the systemic circulation. Since the ratio of mean peripheral to testicular venous testosterone did not change significantly with age in this latter study, the authors concluded that testosterone reductions with age were due to decreased testosterone secretion and not to increased plasma volume.

Table 3. Mean Serum Testosterone Levels of Old and Young Mature Rats after Bilateral Orchidectomy[a]

Groups and no. of rats		Intact	Time after castration						
			15 min	30 min	1 hr	3 hr	6 hr	12 hr	24 hr
Young	(8)	605 ± 121	212 ± 31	155 ± 14	73 ± 8	22 ± 4	10 ± 1	5 ± 1	4 + 0.3
Old	(8)	182 ± 43	64 ± 6	52 ± 9	57 ± 5	23 ± 9	16 ± 1	16 ± 0.7	10 ± 2

[a] From Huang et al. (1979).

It could also be argued that the dilution hypothesis does not hold, since age-related decreases in testosterone levels are comparable in Long–Evans, Wistar, F344, and Sprague–Dawley rats despite significant differences in growth curves.

3. Pituitary Structure and Function

In the aging female rat, several lines of evidence point to the normality of pituitary function with age and ascribe age-related changes in reproductive function to hypothalamic mechanisms. It appears likely that the conditions in the male rat are similar, but the evidence on pituitary function is not as strong.

3.1. Morphology

The pituitaries of old female rats show certain age-related changes, including vacuolation of basophils, increased colloid, and the frequent presence of adenomalike lesions (Steger et al., 1981). A careful histological study of the old male rat pituitary has not been undertaken.

3.2. Basal Gonadotropin Levels

In aging male rats, both serum LH and FSH are lower than in young controls (Shaar et al., 1975; Riegle and Meites, 1976; Bruni et al., 1977; Pirke et al., 1978a). These decreases occur despite a reduction in serum testosterone levels which could be expected to cause increased gonadotropin release if the hypothalamic pituitary axis were functioning normally. The pituitary content of LH in old male rats is reduced to 25%

of levels seen in young controls (Riegle *et al.*, 1977), possibly due to reduced hypothalamic stimulation.

The circulating form of LH may also change in the rat with age, as indicated by gel filtration studies (Conn *et al.*, 1980). From these studies, it appears that molecular weight of LH increases in old rats, possibly due to increased sialic acid content, as seen in young castrate rats.

Basal prolactin levels have been reported to be similar (Shaar *et al.*, 1975) or elevated (Riegle and Meites, 1976; Forman *et al.*, 1981) in old, as compared to young male rats. The age-related increase in prolactin or in the incidence of pituitary tumors, however, is much less in the old male than in the old female rat (Steger *et al.*, 1981). Pituitaries of old and young female rats are equally responsive to dopaminergic inhibition of prolactin release (Steger, 1981). Similar experiments have not been carried out in the male, although most evidence points to hypothalamic causes for increased prolactin levels (Forman *et al.*, 1981; Steger *et al.*, 1981; Steger, 1982; Simpkins *et al.*, 1977, this volume).

3.3. Steroid Negative Feedback

The postcastration rise of both LH and FSH is significantly attenuated in middle-aged (13 months) and old (23–30 months) rats as compared to young (3–6 months) controls (Table 4; Shaar *et al.*, 1975; Pirke *et al.*, 1978b; Huang *et al.*, 1979; Gray *et al.*, 1980). These changes have been related to alterations in hypothalamic monoamine turnover, as discussed in a previous chapter in this book.

Both old and middle-aged rats show a substantial increase in sensitivity to testosterone negative feedback (Table 5; Shaar *et al.*, 1975; Pirke *et al.*, 1978a; Gray *et al.*, 1980) in contrast to the decreased sensitivity to steroid feedback seen in aging female rats (Gray and Wexler, 1980). This change in testosterone response could be due to decreased testos-

Table 4. Mean Serum LH Levels of Old and Young Mature Rats after Bilateral Orchidectomy[a]

Groups and no. of rats		Intact	Time after castration						
			15 min	30 min	1 hr	3 hr	6 hr	12 hr	24 hr
Young	(8)	28 ± 4	35 ± 6	35 ± 9	22 ± 3	15 ± 3	51 ± 7	62 ± 9	248 ± 48
Old	(8)	12 ± 1	15 ± 0.5	13 ± 1	16 ± 2	19 ± 5	26 ± 10	30 ± 4	47 ± 13

[a] From Huang *et al.*, 1979.

Table 5. Mean Serum LH (ng/ml) Levels of Old and Young Mature Male Rats after Bilateral Orchidectomy and Testosterone Propionate (TP) Treatment[a,e]

Age	n	Intact[b]	Orchidectomy alone			TP (µg/100 g body wt)	Orchidectomy + TP treatment — Time after orchidectomy (days)				Recovery period after TP or vehicle treatment (weeks)	
			18 hr[b]	7 days[b]	12 days[b]		13	16[b,c,d]	20[b,c,d]	24[b,c,d]	2[b]	6[b]
Young	32	26.0	102.0	219.2	195.4							
Old	29	6.0	19.3	199.0	165.9							
Young	8					Vehicle	251.9	282.7	313.5	319.3	375.2	454.2
Old	7					Vehicle	191.5	198.1	224.5	214.5	209.8	224.2
Young	8					1.0	255.7	250.4	327.0	317.3	244.1	387.0
Old	8					1.0	242.7	220.3	192.6	222.0	217.9	231.0
Young	8					10.0	267.3	311.0	331.0	395.2	425.0	412.0
Old	7					10.0	182.8	51.0	45.8	36.7	299.1	264.4
Young	8					50.0	169.5	31.3	12.1	3.4	402.0	429.3
Old	7					50.0	198.9	9.2	10.1	7.0	181.0	199.7

[a] Blood samples were taken between 11:00 and 12:00 hr, 3 hr after treatment on days 13, 16, 20 and 24. Testosterone propionate was injected s.c. for 12 days, beginning on day 13 after orchidectomy.

[b] $p < 0.05$; young vs. appropriate old values.

[c] $p < 0.05$; TP-treated vs. vehicle-treated.

[d] $p < 0.05$; significant interaction between age and treatment.

[e] From Shaar et al., 1975.

terone clearance as demonstrated directly by Huang *et al.,* or indirectly by Pirke *et al.,* (1978a).

3.4. Pituitary LHRH Response

Riegle and Meites (1976) reported that the LH response to LHRH (500 ng/rat; body weights averaged 432 g in young and 468 g in old rats) was reduced 50% in old (22–30 months) as compared to young (4–6 months) Long-Evans rats. However, Bruni *et al.* (1977) showed that a larger dose of LHRH (450 ng/100 g body weight; young = 352 g; old = 887 g) was equally effective in old (21 months) and young (4 months) male Wistar rats in raising serum LH and FSH levels on a relative basis (Fig. 4). In the latter study, nine consecutive LHRH injections (50 ng/ 100 g) given at 26 min intervals resulted in significantly smaller increases in serum LH and FSH in the old than in the young male rats (Fig. 5).

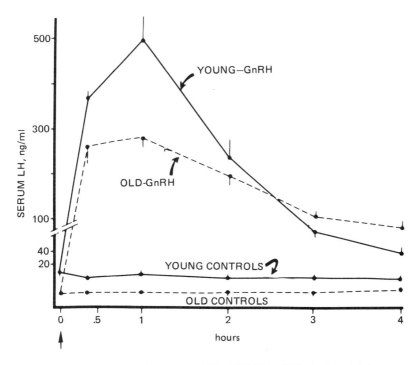

Fig. 4. Effect of a single injection (arrow) of GnRH (450 ng/100 g body weight) on serum LH in young (4 months) and old (21 months) male Wistar rats. Values are expressed as mean ± SEM. (From Bruni *et al.,* 1977.)

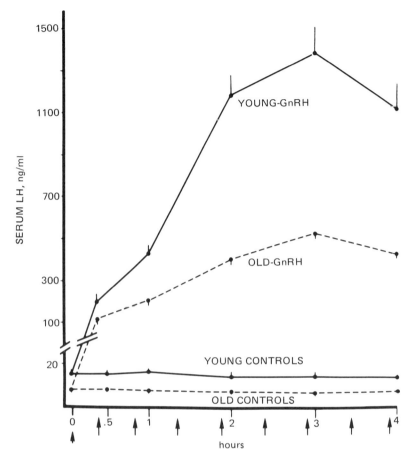

Fig. 5. Effects of multiple GnRH (50 ng/100 g body weight) injections on serum LH levels. See Fig. 4 for details. (From Bruni *et al.*, 1977.)

Basal and LHRH-induced LH release has also been shown to be reduced by the pituitary *in vitro* after removal from old rats (Riegle *et al.*, 1977). The data indicate that the old rat pituitary may not be able to sustain supraphysiologic LH output, but the problem of whether the old rat pituitary, when stimulated by physiological levels of LHRH, can continue to secrete sufficient LH and FSH to maintain normal testicular function, has not been addressed. It therefore, cannot be determined whether the hypothalamus, the pituitary, or both, are responsible for the age-related decline in gonadotropin secretion.

4. Aging of Male Sex Accessory Organs

Since the accessory sex organs in the male are dependent on androgenic stimulation for their development, growth, and functional integrity, a reduced release of androgens and an increased release of prolactin in aging rats may lead to functional deterioration in these organs. The most constant change in male sex accessory organs in the aging rat is deposition of pigment granules in the epithelial cells of the prostate, seminal vesicles, and epididymis (Brandes and Garcia-Bunuel, 1978). These pigment granules retain some morphological and histological properties of lysosomes, as well as lipofucsin and autophagic vascules. Deposition of lipofucsin in prostatic epithelial cells of young rats appears in the supranuclear region. In older rats, the deposition becomes more diffuse and extends to other regions of the cytoplasm, including the basal area. A similar phenomenon occurs in the epithelial cells of the seminal vesicle and epididymis during aging (Brandes, 1966). The cause and the functional significance of lipofucsin deposition in the general economy of the cell is not well understood.

The ventral prostatic epithelial cells in older rats vary in height in different parts of the same organ, and ultrastructurally they show the presence of a developed secretory apparatus such as well-developed Golgi body and abundant rough endoplastic reticulum. They also show signs of a depressed secretory activity, involving occasional emiocytosis of apical secretory vascules and a paucity of condensing vascules in the Golgi region. Further, they are characterized by the frequent occurrence of supra- and paranuclear pleomorphic lysosomes (Brandes and Groth, 1974; Ichihara and Kawamura, 1979).

The uptake of testosterone by the ventral prostate of old rats was much less than that of young rats. The ventral prostate of older male rats also showed a lower RNA and DNA content, but similar activity of acid or alkaline phosphate (Ghanadian and Fotherby, 1975). There was a marked decrease in the rise of phosphofructokinase activity in response to testosterone in the prostate and seminal vesicle of old rats (Singhal, 1967).

Shain and co-workers have published a series of papers on the function of the prostate and incidence of prostatic cancers in aging AXC rats. They found a decreased cytoplasmic and nuclear-androgen receptor content in the ventral prostate of aging rats, as well as a diminished capacity to synthesize 5α-dihydrotestosterone. In contrast, the capacity to produce Δ^4-androstenedione was increased. The changes in production of testosterone metabolites by the prostate of old AXC rats were partly due to a shift to increased oxidative and diminished reductive metabolism (Shain and Axelrod, 1973; Shain and Boesel, 1977; Shain and Nitchuk, 1979). A reduction of L-ornithine decarboxylase and S-adenosyl-L-methionine decarboxylase activities also was found in the prostate of AXC aging rats (Shain and Moss, 1981).

Specific prolactin binding sites in the prostate and seminal vesicle of rats were reduced with advancing age (Cesare and Friesen, 1975; Boesel and Shain, 1980). This decrease in prolactin receptors was un-related to blood prolactin level and was partially reversible by acute treatment with testosterone (Boesel and Shain, 1980). Specific glucocorticoid bindings also decrease in the ventral prostate of rats after 13 months of age (Roth, 1974). Since prolactin and possibly glucocorticoids may enhance testosterone action on the accessory sex organs, diminished receptors for these hormones could explain the diminished effect of testosterone (Bartke, 1980).

Shain and his co-workers have reported that the ventral prostate of old AXC rats (30–46 months) develops spontaneous adenocarcinomas with a frequency of 70%. In the tumor-affected prostate gland, proliferating epithelial cells are arranged in a cribriform pattern. The neoplastic epithelium is thickened and often obliterates much of the luminal space. Extensive neoplastic growth causes glandular enlargement and is associated with focal accumulations of necrotic debris and hemorrhage. The neoplastic cells have enlarged pleomorphic nuclei with prominent solitary or multiple nucleoli. Focal interglandular invasion is observed with larger neoplastic masses, but distinct metastases have not been demonstrated (Shain *et al.*, 1977). These spontaneous neoplasms are transplantable to isogenic hosts, yielding transplantable adenocarcinomas which demonstrate morphologic features very similar to the primary neoplasms. Testosterone metabolism by the spontaneous and transplantable ventral prostate adenocarcinoma demonstrates increased Δ^4-androstenedione synthetic capacity and diminished 5α-dihydrotestosterone synthetic capacity relative to lesion-free ventral prostate of old AXC rats. The senescent changes of ventral prostate cell function, indicated by diminished cytoplasmic androgen receptors and altered testosterone metabolism, may be pathogenetic of prostatic neoplasia (Shain *et al.*, 1977). Spontaneous prostatic tumors have also been found in aging-retired male Copenhagen breeder rats and old Wistar rats (Dunning, 1963; Pollard, 1973).

Very little attention has been paid to the aging of seminal vesicles and epididymides of rats. Kruszel (1967) investigated the fructose and citric acid concentrations in the seminal vesicles of rats from puberty to 80 weeks of age and found that fructose levels did not change. However, citric acid, which is believed to be a sensitive indicator of hormonal stimulation of the gland, reached a maximum level at 12–20 weeks and decreased gradually.

The mitotic activity in the epithelium of the epididymis of 2.5-, 4- and 12-month-old rats was observed by Clermont and Flannery (1970). They noted that the labeling indices of 2.5-month-old animals injected with [³H]thymidine was 2.2% in principal cells and 1.4% in basal cells. This dropped to 0.18% in principal cells and 0.42% in the basal cells of 12-month-old rats. These results suggest that the epidymis grows slowly during adult life, with little evidence of cell renewal.

5. Summary and Conclusions

The reproductive axis of the male rat shows only a slight decrement in function with age, in marked contrast to that of the female of the species. Changes in testicular gametogenic and steroidogenic function with age are well documented, but are not usually severe enough to induce infertility. Only when a pathological condition occurs, such as development of Leydig cell tumors frequently seen in the aging F344 rat, or prostatic carcinoma seen in the aging AXC rat, does reproductive function normally cease.

The small to moderate decrease in serum testosterone levels with age probably is due to decreased gonadotropin levels which, in turn, are most likely due to changes in hypothalamic neurotransmitter dynamics. The aging male rat pituitary probably functions normally, although this has not been conclusively proven.

ACKNOWLEDGMENT. We wish to thank Dr. A. I. Frankel for providing us with a preprint of the publication of which he is co-author (Frankel and Mock, 1982).

6. References

Bartke, A., 1980, Role of prolactin in reproduction in male mammals, *Fed. Proc.* **39**:2577–2581.

Boesel, R. W., and Shain, S. A., 1980, Aging in the AXC rat: Androgen regulation of prostate prolactin receptors, *J. Androl.* **1**:269–273.

Brandes, D., 1966, The fine structure and histochemistry of prostatic glands in relation to sex hormones, *Int. Rev. Cytol.* **20**:207–276.

Brandes, D., and Garcia-Bunuel, G., 1978, Aging of the male sex accessory organs, in: *The Aging Reproductive System* (E. L. Schneider, ed.), Raven Press, New York, pp. 127–157.

Brandes, D., and Groth, D. P., 1974, Hormonal regulation of fine structure of male accessory organs, in: *Male Accessory Sex Organs* (D. Brandes, ed.), Academic Press, New York, pp. 183–222.

Bruni, J. F., Huang, H. H., Marshall, S., and Meites, J., 1977, Effects of single and multiple injections of synthetic GnRH on serum LH, FSH and testosterone in young and old male rats, *Biol. Reprod.* **17**:309–312.

Cesare, A., and Friesen, H., 1975, Specific prolactin binding sites in the prostate and testis of rats, *Endocrinology* **97**:677–684.

Chen, G. C. C., Lin, T., Murono, E., Osterman, J., Cole, B. T., and Nankin, H., 1981, The aging Leydig cell: 2. Two distinct populations of Leydig cells and the possible site of defective steroidogenesis, *Steroids* **37**(1):63–72.

Clermont, Y., and Flannery, J., 1970, Mitotic activity in the epithelium of epididymis in young and old adult rats, *Biol. Reprod.* **3**:283–292.

Coleman, G. L., Barthold, S. W., and Osbaldiston, G. W., 1977, Pathological changes during aging in barrier-reared Fischer 344 male rats, *J. Gerontol.* **32**:258–278.

Conn, P. M., Cooper, R., McNamara, C., Rogers, D. C., and Shoenhardt, L., 1980, Qualitative change in gonadotropin during normal aging in the male rat, *Endocrinology* **106**(5):1549.

Dunning, W. F., 1963, Prostate cancer in the rat, *Natl. Cancer Inst. Monogr.* **12**:351–369.

Forman, L. J., Sonntag, W. E., Ramos, T., Miki, N., and Meites, J., 1981, Comparison of the effect of central acting drugs on prolactin release in young and old male rats, *Proc. Soc. Exp. Biol. Med.* **167**:354–358.

Frankel, A. I., and Mock, E. J., 1982, Testis vein testosterone falls in the aging rat: Refutation of the "dilution" hypothesis, *J. Androl.* **3**:113–116.

Ghanadian, R., and Fotherby, K., 1975, Testosterone uptake by prostatic tissue from young and old rats, *Gerontologia* **21**:211–215.

Ghanadian, R., Lewis, J. G., and Chisholm, G. D., 1975, Serum testosterone and dihydrotestosterone changes with age in rat, *Steroids* **25**:753–762.

Gray, G. D., 1978, Age-related changes in penile erections and circulating testosterone in middle-aged male rats. *Adv. Exp. Med. Biol.* **113**:149–158.

Gray, G. D., and Wexler, B. C., 1980, Estrogen and testosterone sensitivity of middle-aged female rats in the regulation of LH, *Exp. Gerontol.* **15**:201–207.

Gray, G. D., Smith, E. R., and Davidson, J. M., 1980, Gonadotropin regulation in middle-aged male rats, *Endocrinology* **107**:2021–2026.

Harman, S. M., Danner, R. L., and Roth, G. S., 1978, Testosterone secretion in the rat in response to chorionic gonadotropin: Alterations with age, *Endocrinology* **102**:540–544.

Huang, H. H., Steger, R. W., Campbell, G. A., and Meites, J., 1979, Reduced testosterone metabolic clearance rate in old male rats, *Conference on the Endocrine Aspects of Aging*, Bethesda, Maryland, October 18–20.

Humphreys, P. N., 1977, The histology of the testis in aging and senile rats, *Exp. Gerontol.* **12**:27–34.

Ichihara, I., and Kawamura, H., 1979, The fine structure of ventral prostatic secretory epithelial cells in older rats, *Cell Tissue Res.* **203**(2):181–188.

Kaler, L. W., and Neaves, W. B., 1981a, The androgen status of aging male rats, *Endocrinology* **108**(2):712–719.

Kaler, L. W., and Neaves, W. B., 1981b, The steroidogenic capacity of the aging rat testis, *J. Gerontol.* **36**:398–404.

Kruszel, T., 1967, Fructose and citric acid concentration in the seminal vesicles of rats in relationship to age, *Endokrynol. Polska* **18**:128–147.

Leathem, J. H., and Albrecht, E. D., 1974, Effect of age on testis Δ^5-3βhydroxysteroid dehydrogenase in the rat, *Proc. Soc. Exp. Biol. Med.* **145**:1212–1214.

Lin, T., Murono, E., Osterman, J., Allen, D. O., and Nankin, H. R., 1980, The aging Leydig cell, *Steroids* **35**(6):653–664.

Meites, J., Steger, R. W., and Huang, H. H., 1980, Relation of neuroendocrine system to the reproductive decline in aging rats and human subjects, *Fed. Proc.* **39**:3168–3171.

Peng, M. T., Pi, W. P., and Peng, Y. M., 1974, The hypothalamic-pituitary-testicular function of the old rat, *J. Formosan Med. Assoc.* **72**:495–502.

Pirke, K. M., Geiss, M., and Sintermann, R., 1978a, A quantitative study on feedback control of LH by testosterone in young adult and old male rats, *Acta Endocrinol.* **89**(4):789–795.

Pirke, K. M., Vogt, H. J., and Geiss, M., 1978b, *In vitro* and *in vivo* studies on Leydig cell function in old rats, *Acta Endocrinol.* **89**:393–398.

Pirke, K. M., Bolfilias, I., Sintermann, R., Langhammer, H., Wolf, I., and Pabst, H. W., 1979a, Relative capillary blood flow and Leydig cell function in old rats, *Endocrinology* **105**:842–845.

Pirke, K. M., Krings, B., and Foyt, H. G., 1979b, Further studies on hypothalamic-pituitary-testicular functions in old rats, *Acta Endocrinol.* **92**(2):358–369.

Pollard, M., 1973, Spontaneous prostate adenocarcinoma in aged germ free Wistar rats, *J. Natl. Cancer Inst.* **51**:1235–1241.

Prisco, C. L., and Dessi-Fulgheri, F., 1980, Endocrine and behavioral modifications in aging male rats, *Horm. Res.* **12**(3):149–160.

Riegle, G. D., and Meites, J., 1976, Effects of aging on LH and prolactin after LHRH, L-DOPA, methyl dopa and stress in male rats, *Proc. Soc. Exp. Biol. Med.* **151**:507–511.

Riegle, G. D., and Miller, A. E., 1978, Aging effects on the hypothalamic-hypophyseal-gonadal control system in the rat, in: *The Aging Reproductive System* (E. L. Schneider, ed.), Raven Press, New York, pp. 159–192.

Riegle, G. D., Meites, J., Miller, A. E., and Wood, S. M., 1977, Effect of aging on hypothalamic LH-releasing and prolactin inhibiting activities and pituitary responsiveness to LHRH in the male laboratory rat, *J. Gerontol.* **32**:13–18.

Roth, G. S., 1974, Age-related changes in specific glucocorticoid binding by steroid-responsive tissues of rats, *Endocrinology* **94**:82–90.

Saksena, S. K., and Lau, I. F., 1979, Variations in serum androgens, estrogens, progestins, gonadotropins and prolactin level in male rats from prepubertal to advanced age, *Exp. Aging Res.* **5**(3):179–194.

Saksena, S. K., Lau, I-F., and Chang, M-C., 1979, Age-dependent changes in the sperm population and fertility in the male rat, *Exp. Aging Res.* **5**:373–381.

Shaar, C. J., Fuker, J. S., Riegle, G. D., and Meites, J., 1975, Effects of castration and gonadal steroids on serum LH and prolactin in old and young rats, *J. Endocrinol.* **66**:45–51.

Shain, S. A., and Axelrod, L. R., 1973, Reduced high affinity 5α-hydrotestosterone receptor capacity in the ventral prostate of the aged rats, *Steroids* **21**(6):801–812.

Shain, S. A., and Boesel, R. W., 1977, Aging-associated diminished rat prostate androgen receptor content concurrent with decreased androgen dependence, *Mech. Ageing Dev.* **6**:219–232.

Shain, S. A., and Moss, A. L., 1981, Aging in the AXC rat: Differential effects of chronic testosterone treatment on restoration of diminished prostate L-ornithine decarboxylase and S-adenosyl-1-methionine decarboxylase activities, *Endocrinology* **109**: 1184–1191.

Shain, S. A., and Nitchuk, W. M., 1979, Testosterone metabolism by the prostate of the aging AXC rat, *Mech. Ageing Dev.* **11**:9–22.

Shain, S. A., McCullough, B., Mitchuk, M., and Boesel, R. W., 1977, Prostate carcinogenesis in the AXC rat, *Oncology* **34**:114–122.

Simpkins, J. W., Kalra, P. S., and Kalra, S. P., 1981, Alterations in daily rhythms of testosterone and progesterone in old male rats, *Exp. Aging Res.* **7**:25–32.

Singhal, R. L., 1967, Effects of age on phosphofructokinase induction in rat prostate and seminal vesicle, *J. Gerontol.* **22**(3):343–347.

Steger, R. W., 1981, Age-related changes in the control of prolactin secretion in the female rat, *Neurobiol. Aging* **2**:119–123.

Steger, R. W., 1982, Age-dependent changes in the responsiveness of the reproductive system to pharmacological agents, *Pharmacol. Ther.* **17**:1–64.

Steger, R. W., Peluso, J. J., Bruni, J. F., Hafez, E. S. E., and Meites, J., 1979, Gonadotropin binding and testicular function in old rats, *Endokrinologie* **73**:1–5.

Steger, R. W., Huang, H., and Meites, J., 1981, Reproduction, in: *CRC Handbook Series on Aging* (E. Masoro, ed.), CRC Press, Boca Raton, Florida, pp. 333–382.

Turek, F. W., and Desjardins, C., 1979, Development of Leydig cell tumors and onset of changes in the reproductive and endocrine systems of aging F344 rats, *J. Natl. Cancer Inst.* **63**:969–975.

CHAPTER 9

Hormonal Influences on Hypothalamic Sensitivity during Aging in Female Rodents

CALEB E. FINCH and CHARLES V. MOBBS

1. Introduction

The regulation of gonadotropins by ovarian steroids in laboratory rats and mice becomes progressively impaired during aging, as exemplified by the diminished LH surge observed by 8–14 months at proestrus, or in animals which were ovariectomized and treated with steroids to induce an LH surge. Apparently, similar impairments in the LH surge can be precociously induced in young adult female rodents by intensive exposure to estradiol. Since some impairments of gonadotropin regulation can be delayed by chronic ovariectomy, a major mechanism in reproductive aging may involve the long-term, possibly cumulative impact of estradiol or other hormones on the hypothalamus. We will discuss these phenomena with particular focus on the early stages of reproductive senescence. We do not discuss here the significant literature describing alterations of hypothalamic neurotransmitters with age in female rodents, e.g., Simpkins *et al.* (1977); Reymond and Porter (1981); Demarest *et al.* (1982).

Attempts to determine the etiology in processes of senescence are often complicated by interactions with other physiological changes with age. Moreover, some age changes may represent responses to the pathologic lesions common in aging mammals, in which individuals can vary greatly in the distribution of lesions (tumors, glomerulonephritis, lung

CALEB E. FINCH and CHARLES V. MOBBS ● Andrus Gerontology Center, Department of Biological Sciences, University of Southern California, Los Angeles, California 90007.

spots); such "pathogeric" changes (Finch, 1972) should, in principle, be distinguished from other non-disease-related "eugeric" changes. Very different conclusions about age changes may be drawn than if healthy subgroups are not defined, e.g., age changes in male mouse plasma testosterone are associated with a diseased subpopulation, whereas the healthy subgroup of old mice had normal values of testosterone (Nelson *et al.*, 1975). Similar effects are implied from recent studies on humans in which older men carefully selected for good health showed little or no change in plasma testosterone (Harman and Tsitouras, 1980), whereas other samplings showed major age-correlated decreases (Vermeulen *et al.*, 1972). The widespread changes and disease correlated with aging thus make it difficult to sort out "cause and effect" in older groups. Because reproductive functions completely cease in most female mammals by middle age (Talbert, 1977) when pathologic conditions are rare and when most other physiological functions remain robust, female reproductive senescence is attractive as a model for the aging of neuroendocrine systems. However, even at midlife, reproductive aging may be confounded by such age-correlated changes as increases in body weight and fat, which can influence steroid metabolism (Schindler *et al.*, 1972), steroid compartmentalization, and pituitary microadenomas (Schechter *et al.*, 1981) which are putative precursors of large pituitary tumors. Thus, experimental paradigms in young animals which produce select aspects of reproductive senescence may be valuable in analyzing age-correlated changes. Martin (1978) has aptly designated selectively accelerated aging phenomena as "segmental progerias."

2. Overview of Rodent Reproductive Senescence

2.1. Phenomenology

Some characteristics are generally observed during reproductive senescence in laboratory mice and rats. First is lengthening of estrous cycles, commonly determined from the patterns of vaginal smears (Nelson *et al.*, 1981; Talbert, 1977). Longitudinal studies of C57Bl./6J mice show that 4-day cycles become less frequent after 6–8 months, and are replaced by 5-day cycles and then by longer cycles (Nelson *et al.*, 1982). Then, there is a loss of cycling marked by various senescent acyclic anovulatory states, most commonly "persistent vaginal cornification" (PVC; Nelson *et al.*, 1981, 1982; Lu *et al.*, 1977). Other acyclic states which generally follow PVC include those with leukocytic vaginal smears, "persistent diestrus," sometimes associated with repetitive pseudopregnancy and the atrophic, thin "anestrus" smears often associated with atrophic ovaries, large pituitary tumors, and often elevated plasma prolactin (Lu *et al.*, 1979; Nelson *et al.*, 1980b). In 2-year-old C57BL/6J mice with persistent diestrus smears, plasma estradiol (E_2) is at castrate levels, whereas plasma luteinizing hormone (LH) is spontaneously elevated (Gee *et al.*, 1983); these changes are very similar to those which occur at menopause. The events in C57BL/6J mice are illustrated in Fig. 1. Variations in the distributions of different acyclic states are observed within and between various laboratory populations. Genotype, diet, season, and reproductive experience may be important variables in reproductive aging, reviewed in Nelson (1981). The use of inbred rodents may minimize some aspects of variation, but even C57BL/6J mice, inbred since 1936 (Staats, 1976), show striking variations within a cohort (Finch *et al.*, 1980) and between cohorts (Nelson *et al.*, 1982). Some sources of this variation are discussed below.

The cornified vaginal cells of anovulatory rodents in PVC indicate

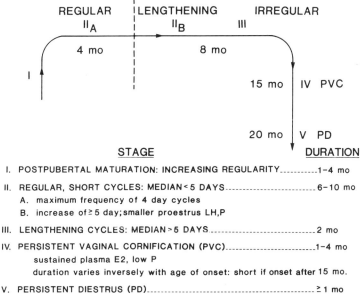

Fig. 1. A schematic representation of alterations in vaginal cytology typical during maturation and aging in C57BL/6J mice. Based on data in Nelson *et al.* (1981, 1982), Nelson (1981), and Flurkey *et al.* (1982). By 24 months, most mice have grossly visible pituitary tumors (Felicio *et al.*, 1980; Schechter *et al.*, 1981). Elevated plasma LH occurs in old mice with persistant diestrous(anestrus)-like smears, if pituitary tumors are absent (Gee *et al.*, 1983).

the continued secretion of estrogens, presumably by cohorts of growing ovarian follicles. In PVC, the plasma E_2:P (estradiol:progesterone) ratio is generally high, due to near-castrate levels of plasma P (Lu et al., 1979; Nelson et al., 1981). Plasma LH remains low during PVC in C57BL/6J mice (Flurkey et al., 1982). FSH levels in the related strain, C57BL/6, are also low during PVC (Parkening et al., 1980), as expected from the "inhibin" activities produced by the pool of growing but anovulatory follicles. Eventually, at later ages when mice leave PVC, plasma LH tends to rise towards castrate levels (Gee et al., 1983).

The follicular populations in PVC have potentially great bearing on the interpretations of reproductive senescence. The irreversible loss of ovarian oocytes and primary follicles after birth is an apparently universal feature of reproductive aging in mammals. By puberty, less than 50% of the original endowment of oocytes typically remain, and by the climacteric in rodents and humans only a small pool remains (Talbert, 1977). Most oocytes and primary follicles which enter the pool of growing follicles are lost through the still obscure process of atresia; ≤1% of the original neonatal store typically achieves maturity and ovulation. In C57BL/6J mice, aged 13–14 months, PVC is associated with a smaller average number of oocytes than mice of the same age that were still cycling (Fig. 1). Some mice are clearly approaching ovarian exhaustion with < 100 oocytes, whereas another subpopulation has entered PVC with more oocytes than mice of the same age that are still cycling and ovulating (Gosden et al., 1983). The subgroup of mice with imminent ovarian exhaustion may be a model for the transition to human menopause, in which a small pool of oocytes remains in the primary state, despite major elevations of gonadotropins. In human, there is also evidence for occasional ovulation and corpora lutea formation after menopause (Costoff and Mahesh, 1975; Novak, 1970).*

The functionality of the oocytes and follicles present at PVC are shown in many studies. The ovaries of aging mice which have recently entered in PVC continue to be responsive to injected gonadotropins which can induce ovulation (Mobbs et al., 1981). Ovulatory cycles can be transiently reactivated in PVC rodents by adrenergic drugs, tyrosine-rich diets, and other treatments (reviewed in Finch, 1978; Cooper and Linnoila, 1980). Moreover, ovaries from rodents shortly after the onset

* It may be possible to define a threshold number of ovarian oocytes, below which the production of steroids is insufficient to drive the cyclic release of gonadotropins. In mice, the threshold may be about 50 oocytes, in humans, about 1000. The numbers of oocytes found in young mice vary strikingly, over a five-fold range (Fig. 2). This variation could be the basis for later age differences in the numbers of oocytes. In any case, most mice in PVC retain a sizable resource of primary follicles.

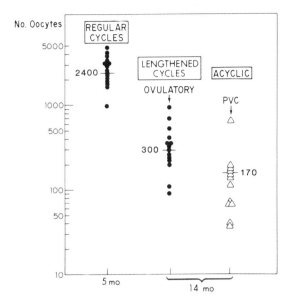

Fig. 2. The number of primary ovarian follicles and oocytes in 5-month-old regularly cycling C57BL/6J mice and in 14-month-old mice which were still cycling with verified ovulation or which were anovulatory and in persistent vaginal cornification (PVC; Gosden *et al.*, 1983).

of PVC will often support some estrous cycles when transplanted into young hosts (Peng and Huang, 1972; Aschheim, 1976; Felicio *et al.*, in preparation).* Lastly, transplantation of young, functional ovaries into older rodents which have already ceased to exhibit estrous cycles usually continues their anovulatory state (Aschheim, 1976; Peng and Huang, 1972; Nelson *et al.*, 1980a; Mobbs *et al.*, 1982a).

2.2. Effects of Altered E₂:P Ratios

The altered regulation of gonadotropins in rodents which have entered PVC is widely considered to indicate age-correlated changes in extra-ovarian reproductive loci (studies of altered positive and negative feedback of LH in aging rodents after ovariectomy are discussed below).

---

* The failure of some transplanted old ovaries to cycle in young hosts may be due to graft rejection in partially inbred rodents. Alternatively, loss of remaining oocytes can occur through transplantation trauma (Krohn, 1977). This possibility is shown for 13–14-month-old C57BL/6J mice, where some still cycling mice as well as those in PVC may be on the verge of ovarian exhaustion (Fig. 2).

In most studies, acyclic rodents in PVC or other acyclic states were compared to young cycling controls. However, the PVC state is associated with a two-fold elevated ratio of plasma E_2:P, without elevations of LH (Lu *et al.*, 1979; Nelson *et al.*, 1981; Fig. 3). The elevated E_2:P lead to impairments of neuroendocrine function *independently* of age. For example, in young ovariectomized rats given E_2 implants for 30 days, the ensuing persistently elevated E_2 with low P reduces the size of a subsequent E_2-P induced LH surge (Lu *et al.*, 1981). Conversely, prolonged ovariectomy of PVC rodents before surge induction leads to considerable recovery of the steroid-induced LH surge, e.g., in rats ovariectomized for 30 days (Lu *et al.*, 1981) or in mice ovariectomized for 30–60 days (Mobbs *et al.*, 1982b). These variations in hypothalamic-pituitary response as a function of steroid history resemble the "desensitization" by chronic treatment with drugs which are neurotransmitter agonists, and the recovery from desensitization after removal of the agonist. These are familiar phenomena in the regulation of receptors for neurotransmitters (Gnegy and Costa, 1980; Randall *et al.*, 1981). An altered plasma E_2:P ratio in still-cycling aging rodents could also be important. The plasma E_2:P ratio tends to increase with age on proestrus in C57BL/6J

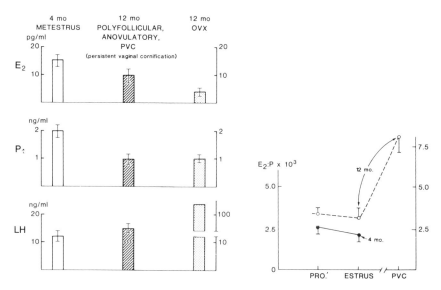

Fig. 3. The hormonal status of 12–16-month-old C57BL/6J mice in persistent vaginal cornification PVC as compared with young mice in metestrus and ovariectomized older mice. (From data in Nelson *et al.*, 1981, and Flurkey *et al.*, 1982). The PVC hormonal state is clearly distinct from that following ovariectomy (Gee *et al.*, 1983).

mice largely as a consequence of the normal E_2 levels at proestrus, but with smaller elevations of P during the surge (Nelson *et al.*, 1981; Flurkey *et al.*, 1982; Fig. 4). Thus, a major problem in the etiology of cycle lengthening and cessation in aging rodents is how to resolve if the disturbances in gonadotropin regulation are secondary to disturbances of steroids in still-cycling animals.

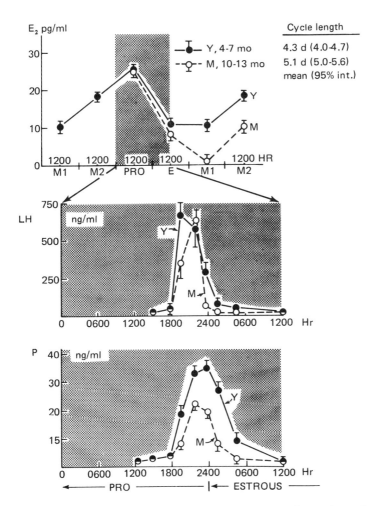

Fig. 4. The hormonal status of regularly cycling young (Y, 4–7 months) and middle-aged (M, 10–13 months) C57BL/6J at various days of the estrous cycle. Plasma estradiol (E_2) was measured in a different sample of mice (Nelson *et al.*, 1981) than plasma LH and progesterone (P; Flurkey *et al.*, 1982).

2.3. Negative Feedback

In young controls, ovariectomy leads to dramatic increases in LH due to the removal of the inhibitory effect of E_2 (Fig. 4). The elevations of LH after ovariectomy generally become smaller with age: in middle-aged (8- to 14-month-old) rats which were previously cycling regularly (Gray et al., 1980; Gray and Wexler, 1980), cycling irregularly (Steger et al., 1980) or in the PVC state (Steger et al., 1980; Howland and Preiss, 1975; Peluso et al., 1977; Shaar et al., 1975; Gee et al., 1983). However, not all studies detected impairments, e.g., in rats aged 14 months vs. 3 months 5 days after ovariectomy (McPherson et al., 1977). Firm conclusions about the set points or the gain of E_3-LH feedback controls cannot be drawn, because plasma steroid levels are not known in most studies of feedback. Even in ovariectomized rodents, the adrenal cortex can produce some aromatizable steroids. Hypothetically, an extragonadal production of estrogens by adipose tissue (Schindler et al., 1972) might be greater in older rodents which often have more body fat. A direct functional assay for extragonadal estrogens would be the number of nuclear bound E_2 receptors in the pituitary and hypothalamus. Similarly, the response of the depressed postovariectomy LH controls needs investigation under conditions of defined plasma E_2 in conjunction with measurements of nuclear bound E_2 receptors. A series of E_2 implants followed with their time course could lead to valuable information on whether reproductive aging influences the sensitivity of LH regulation to E_2 as a function of plasma E_2 ($\delta LH/\delta E_2$).

2.4. Positive Feedback

A 30–50% smaller preovulatory proestrous surge of LH is widely observed in aging rodents, and occurs in rats with 4-day estrous cycles (Cooper et al., 1980) as well as in aging rodents with 5-day or longer cycles: C57BJ/6J mice (Fig. 4; Flurkey et al., 1982) and rats (Miller and Riegle, 1980; Gray et al., 1980). Since plasma E_2 at proestrus midday was normal in 12-month-old mice (Nelson et al., 1981) which also showed in a separate study impaired LH surges (Fig. 4), we provisionally conclude that the responsiveness of hypothalamic-pituitary functions related to LH is reduced with age. This view is supported by numerous studies showing impaired LH surges in aging rodents after ovariectomy and steroid injections to induce LH surges which were vigorous in young rodents (Lu et al., 1979, 1981; Steger et al., 1980; Finch et al., 1980; Gosden and Bancroft, 1976; Howland, 1976; Peluso et al., 1977). Studies of a series of ages suggest that the LH surge becomes progressively impaired in still-cycling mice (Mobbs *et al.*, 1982b). The maintenance of a normal sized LH surge in some samples of "regularly cycling" 11-month-old mice (Lu and Kledzik, 1981) suggest that impairments of LH regulation are gradual and are not tightly linked to chronologic age.

The effects of aging on the gain of negative feedback could be related to the alterations in the E_2-induced LH surge. Two studies of young mice showed an "upper limit" of effective priming E_2 doses, above which a subsequent surge inducing implant or injection then failed to induce a surge (Flurkey *et al.*, 1980; Bronson, 1981). Thus, the possibility arises that the inhibitory phase of negative feedback from E_2 on LH might have a higher gain in older rodents. For example, two-year-old male rats appear to be *more* sensitive than the young testosterone implants, as deduced by a lower plasma testosterone threshold for the triggering of "compensatory" postcastration elevations of LH (Pirke *et al.*, 1978). If the gain of negative feedback increased with age in females, then the same levels of plasma E_2 might cause them to exceed the "upper limit" for effective priming. Age changes are documented in the gain of another hypothalamic system; the output of vasopressin as a function of increased plasma osmolality which increases about two-fold during aging in humans (Robertson and Rowe, 1980).

Because the proestrous LH surge can be smaller and delayed in 10.5-month-old rats with 4-day cycles (Cooper *et al.*, 1980), it seems possible that the lengthening of the estrous cycle is a subsequent and *separate* event from the reduced LH surge. More detailed studies are needed to resolve if impaired regulation of gonadotropins [prolactin (PRL) and follicle-stimulating hormone (FSH) as well as luteinizing hormone (LH)] precedes the lengthening of cycles. This issue is critical because a lengthening of cycles in the presence of normal gonadotropin regulation could implicate ovarian aging, e.g., reduced numbers of growing follicles, as an early cause, perhaps the first event, in a cascade of hypothalamic-pituitary dysfunctions. The slower rise of plasma E_2 in aging mice to the same proestrous levels as in the young suggested the hypothesis that the cycle was lengthened because of the slower E_2 rise (Nelson *et al.*, 1981).

Although the steroid-induced LH and FSH surges are critical for ovulation and maintenance of estrous cycles, it is generally agreed that only a small fraction ($< 25\%$) of the proestrous LH surge is required for ovulation (see Turgeon, 1979). Nonetheless, the deficits of LH and FSH at proestrus may influence follicular development, e.g., LH is required for the induction of LH receptors on ovarian granulosa cells (Ireland and Richards, 1978). Since the secretion of midcycle E_2 from developing follicles is dependent on the presence of LH (Ely and Schwartz,

1971), the slower rise of plasma E_2 in older mice with extended cycles (Fig. 4) could be a consequence of fewer ovarian LH receptors, and in turn, consequent to the smaller LH surge at proestrus. Analysis of the populations of growing follicles in aging rodents with lengthening cycles and their responses to gonadotropins *in vitro* or after transplantation to young hosts may resolve whether the lengthening of cycles is due to impaired hypothalamic-pituitary regulation or whether it results from impending ovarian depletion with a reduced pool of growing follicles.

2.5. Prolactin and Pituitary Responsiveness

The elevations of plasma prolactin which are a characteristic of acyclic rodents (Shaar *et al.*, 1975; Reymond and Porter, 1981; Demarest *et al.*, 1982) raise a theoretically important issue: since hyperprolactinemia is well-known to impair LH secretion and some of its gonadal actions (Hodson *et al.*, 1980; reviewed in Clemens *et al.*, 1978; Evans *et al.*, 1982), could the onset of cycle irregularities be associated with elevated prolactin? A further rationale for investigating this issue comes from the reactivation of estrous cycles in aging rats by dopaminergic agonists which also suppress elevated prolactin (Clemens *et al.*, 1978). However, in 12-month-old C57BL/6J mice with 4- or $\geqslant$ 5-day cycles, the proesterous prolactin surge was about 50% smaller than in the young (Fig. 5). Only in a subpopulation of mice with sizable pituitary tumors

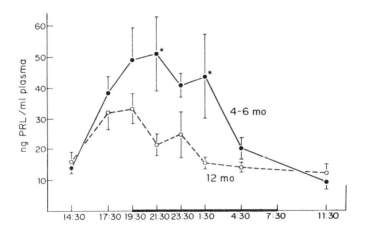

Fig. 5.   The prolactin surge at proestrus in C57BL/6J mice aged 4–6 and 12 months.

was prolactin elevated (Nelson *et al.*, 1980b). Pituitary tumors are rare until after cycles cease in C57BL/6J mice (Felicio *et al.*, 1980). These data appear to minimize the possibility that elevated prolactin is an early cause of reduced hypothalamic sensitivity during cycle lengthening. Furthermore, in older rats whose prolactin was reduced by treatment with lergotrile (dopaminergic agonist) the steroid-induced LH surge remained impaired (Clemens *et al.*, 1978). However, subtle age changes in prolactin regulation still could have important influences on hypothalamic-pituitary functions.

The responsiveness of the female rodent's pituitary to LHRH has not given clear cut effects of age. Some studies find no effects during the reproductive transitions before tumor incidence increases greatly (Wise and Ratner, 1980). The responsiveness of LHRH can show all effects as a function of cycle stage (Smith *et al.*, 1982). However, rats 2 years or older often show greatly reduced response (Watkins *et al.*, 1975). Contrarily, *in vitro* responses of pituitary monolayer cultures (9 vs. 31 months) did not have major age effects in LH output at different LHRH concentrations; the enhanced release from dibutyryl cyclic AMP or by E_2 decreased markedly in the old cells (Tang and Tang, 1981), suggesting important cell alterations at advanced ages which can persist during 4 days of culture. More *in vitro* studies of responses to LHRH over a wider dynamic range to including exposure to pulsatile LHRH are needed.

2.6. Progesterone-LH Interactions at Proestrus

The analysis of plasma P and LH during the proestrous surge suggests two causes of their smaller elevations. First, plasma P and LH were positively correlated during the ascending phase of the surge in the age group (Fig. 6). This correlation extends previous findings that LH is a direct and immediate stimulus for ovarian P secretion at proestrus in the rat (Ichikawa *et al.*, 1972). Although older mice had lower P and LH values during the ascending phase, the regressions of P on LH were identical. Moreover, by analysis of covariance, age does not have a significant effect on P, independently of LH (Flurkey *et al.*, 1982).

The smaller elevations of P in aging mice could contribute to their truncated LH surge. Effects are known on two levels: (1) there is a short term (3 hr) facilitation by P on the pituitary response to LHRH *in vitro* (Turgeon and Waring, 1981), and (2) as an acceleration of norepinephrine turnover in the arcuate nucleus within several hours after implantation of P in E_2-primed ovariectomized rats (Wise *et al.*, 1981).

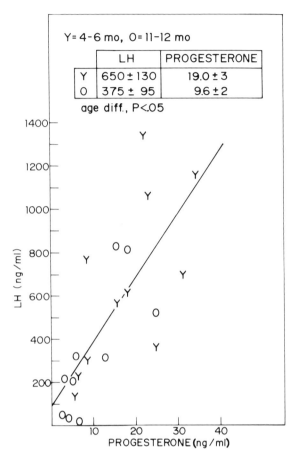

Fig. 6. Correlations between plasma progesterone (P) and LH measured in the same plasma sample during the ascending phase of the proestrus LH surge. The regressions of P and LH were indistinguishable in both age groups (Flurkey *et al.*, 1981, 1982).

3. Effects of Ovariectomy on Manifestations of Neuroendocrine Aging

3.1. Long-Term Ovariectomy and Ovarian Transplants

Almost 20 years ago Pierre Aschheim discovered that 2-year-old rats, ovariectomized when 6–12 months of age, could support regular reproductive cycles with bilateral grafts of young ovaries beneath their kidney capsules (Aschheim, 1965). This finding suggests that some aspects of neuroendocrine aging might be dependent on continued ovarian functions and, in turn, might be slowed by ovariectomy. Subsequent evidence continues to support this view.

First, we have repeated Aschheim's basic finding with young ovarian grafts given to long-term ovariectomized C57BL/6J mice, aged 18 and 26 months. Inbred mice have important advantages for transgenerational grafting studies because risk of graft rejection is minimal as the result of inbreeding for histocompatability loci. In our laboratory, $\geq$ 90% of grafts in young mice cycle for 4 months or more; moreover histologic examination shows that normal numbers of Graafian follicles are produced and apparently normal ova are shed into the space between the ovary and the kidney capsule (Gosden, unpublished). Mice ovariectomized at 6 months and given young ovarian grafts at 18 months then support regular cycles during the same 4- to 6-month-long post-transplantation period as in the "young to young" control transplants (Felicio *et al.*, in preparation.)

Secondly, the experimentally-induced LH surge is maintained at close to young levels by long-term ovariectomy (Elias *et al.*, 1978; Mobbs *et al.*, 1982c). This result is consistent with the ovarian transplant experiments. Nonetheless, since a relatively small fraction of the proestrus LH surge ($< 30\%$) suffices to cause ovulation (Turgeon, 1979), the induction of regular cycles with young ovarian grafts in long-term ovariectomized hosts does not eliminate the possibility of concurrent, but subcritical neuroendocrine impairments.

Finally, morphologic changes in the arcuate nucleus of the hypothalamus are found in the aging female rodent which can be in large part retarded by long-term ovariectomy. Similar hypothalamic damage was first described in young rats by James Brawer and colleagues. Experimental treatments which induced a prolonged polyfollicular ovarian status (E_2 valerate injections, see Section 4.4; constant light, see Section 4.5) lead after 3–6 months to a hyperactivity of astroglia and microglia in the dorsolateral zones of the arcuate nucleus (Brawer *et al.*, 1978, 1980a). Subsequently, similar glial changes were found in 14-month-old female Wistar rats and in 13-month-old female C57BL/6J mice obtained from this laboratory (Schipper *et al.*, 1981). In striking parallel with the effects of long-term ovariectomy on ovarian-graft functioning, mice and rats ovariectomized by 3 months and examined at 13–14 months showed much less glial hyperactivity. Since the old control (intact) rodents had probably experienced extensive cycle irregularity by the age of examination, we cannot distinguish the contribution of irregular cycles with their expected alterations in E_2:P ratio vs. a possible contribution from the cumulative effects of E_2 or other steroids during regular cycling.

The meaning of glial hyperactivity also remains to be clarified in these studies. Although glial activity is often associated with neuronal degeneration as in Parkinsonism and Huntingtonism (Bernheimer *et al.*, 1973), no altered neuronal cell bodies have yet been identified. The reported decrease of neurons in the arcuate and other hypothalamic regions in aging female rats (Hsu and Peng, 1978) is of major interest in this regard.

3.2. Long-Term Ovariectomy and Pituitary Tumors

Grossly visible pituitary tumors are rare in C57BL/6J mice before 12–14 months, but increase rapidly in most mice by 24 months (Felicio *et al.*, 1980; Nelson *et al.*, 1980b). These tumors contain hyperplastic but not invasive nests of lactotrophes (Schechter *et al.*, 1981; Clayton *et al.*, in preparation), and are sometimes associated with elevated plasma prolactin, particularly in mice with the largest tumors (Nelson *et al.*, 1980a). We have hypothesized that the increase of tumors is secondary to elevated plasma E_2:P associated with the lengthening of cessation of cycles since long-term ovariectomy greatly reduced tumor incidence (Nelson *et al.*, 1980b, 1981) and since pituitary tumors are very rare in male C57BL/6J mice at all ages (Finch, 1973).

3.3. Ovarietomy of Noncycling Rodents

John Lu and colleagues observed that the steroid-induced LH surge was greater in old rats that were in the low E_2 state of persistent diestrus vs. those in PVC before ovariectomy for surge induction (Lu *et al.*, 1980). A subsequent study showed that a single steroid-induced LH surge could be induced in old PVC rats if 30 days lapsed between ovariectomy and surge induction (Lu *et al.*, 1981). We have confirmed and extended these findings with 16-month-old C57BL/6J mice. First, the increased size of the E_2-induced LH surge 30 days after ovariectomy of PVC mice can increase at least twofold more in amplitude by 60 days after ovariectomy (Mobbs *et al.*, 1982c) (although the increased LH surge at 16 months is significantly increased.) Other studies also show that complete "rejuvenation" has not occurred. If mice in PVC, aged 16 months, are ovariectomized for 2 months and then given ovarian transplants, most mice will transitorily begin to cycle (Mobbs *et al.*, 1982a). However, cycles are less frequent and cease earlier than the young-to-young controls (Mobbs *et al.*, in preparation). This study emphasizes that the size of the steroid-induced LH peak does not indicate the extent of potential for cyclic neuroendocrine functions in aging rodents.

Thus, the effects of long-term ovariectomy on delaying some manifestations of neuroendocrine aging and on partially reversing changes
indicate considerable experimental opportunities for manipulating a major aging process. Such studies may eventually permit quantitative statements on the steroid dose and time requirements to produce specific
degrees of neuroendocrine aging. For further discussion of the hypothesis relating cumulative effects of estradiol on the hypothalamus to reproductive aging, see Finch *et al.* (1980).

4. Postnatal Steroidal Influences

Some anovulatory syndromes in young rodents have been proposed
as experimental models for reproductive senescence. The criteria for
such models include that the anovulatory state be due at least partially
to extra-ovarian loci, and that the anovulatory state be stable, that is, not
sporadic. The five experimental paradigms considered below will be
useful in evaluating the steroid requirements for reproductive aging in
the female rodent.

4.1. The Neonatal Anovulatory Syndrome

Long-lasting consequences of postnatal steroids on reproduction in
female rodents were first shown for the early postnatal period. Large
doses of testosterone or other "aromatizable" steroids, if injected during
the first 2–10 postnatal days, e.g., > 30 μg testosterone on postnatal day
2 in rats, subsequently cause permanent infertility, i.e., the "full anovulatory" syndrome in adult females, which is characterized by loss of
ovulatory cycles and steroid-induced LH surges, and by polyfollicular,
anovulatory ovaries. With sufficiently large injections, gonadotropins can
induce ovulation (Uilenbrock and van der Werff ten Bosch, 1972).
Transplantation of these ovaries into young controls also yields many
regular cycles (Mobbs *et al.,* 1981). In most cases, those early postnatal
steroid treatments "masculinize" the female brain, resulting in a refrac-
toriness to the induction of female-type sex behavior with E_2 and P, and
its replacement by male-type responsiveness to testosterone. For example, the synaptic populations in the preoptic region (Raisman and
Field, 1973) of females given neonatal steroid treatments resemble those
of males. However, the adult male characteristic of several-fold larger
preoptic region than in females (Gorski *et al.,* 1980) is not completely
acquired by postnatal steroid treatment of females, but can be achieved

if testosterone is injected in the late prenatal period (Coquelin *et al.*, 1981).

4.2. The Delayed-Anovulatory Syndrome

If smaller doses of aromatizable steroids are given in the first 10 days, e.g., 10 μg testosterone on day 5 in rats, then animals will initiate a series of normal ovulatory cycles after puberty, but will subsequently become anovulatory, e.g., by day 10 at this dose (Harlan and Gorski, 1977). Gorski (1968) introduced the widely used term "delayed-anovulatory syndrome" (DAS) to describe these phenomena. Unlike the neonatal-anovulatory syndrome resulting from complete neonatal androgenization, rats in the DAS retain lordosis responses when ovariectomized and injected with E_2 and P (Harlan and Gorski, 1978). Early observations of DAS lead to the intriguing question of its similarity to normal reproductive aging. For example, Swanson and van der Werff ten Bosch (1964) raised the possibility " . . . that the influence of aging on the ovaries is partially due to aging of the central nervous system, and that the presence of androgen shortly after birth promotes the later process." Alternatively, Gorski (1968) suggested that " . . . the [delayed]-anovulation syndrome develops . . . because of a subsequent and independent modification of a neonatally partially differentiated system. This modification presumably is produced by postpubertal ovarian steroid feedback. . . ." At present, no choice between the two possibilities for mechanisms of the DAS is strongly indicated with respect to the control of the gonadotropin surge. Aging, anovulatory rodents (Peng *et al.*, 1977) as well as those in DAS (Hendricks *et al.*, 1977) retain lordosis responses and ovulation can be induced in aging (Mobbs *et al.*, 1981) and in DAS rats (see above) by exogenous gonadotropins. Thus, there does not appear to be a "delayed-anestrous syndrome" (Hendricks *et al.*, 1977). Although aging, as well as the DAS could be considered as a "sectorial masculinization," it cannot yet be concluded that the failure of the steroid-induced gonadotropin surge results from long-lasting steroid effects at the *same* anatomic locus in both conditions. For example, experimental lesions at different loci in the preoptic or anterior hypothalamus can impair steroid-induced LH surges; moreover, lesions in distinct hypothalamic regions can differentially affect LH regulation as induced by injections of E_2 or of P (Kawakami *et al.*, 1978; Wiegand *et al.*, 1980).

An important similarity of the DAS to reproductive aging is the required presence of the ovaries for subsequent impairments of the LH surge. In most studies, ovariectomy at various times after weaning postponed the impairments of the gonadotropin surge (Arsi, 1971; Harlan and Gorski, 1978). However, Hendricks *et al.* (1977) failed to observe this effect of ovariectomy; moreover, the long-term ovariectomized, lightly androgenized rats in that study seemingly were even more impaired than the intact controls. This anomaly could result from uncontrolled prenatal factors or genotypic differences. For example, the DAS developed somewhat more rapidly when mice were injected with T on day 3 than on day 5 (Hendricks *et al.*, 1977). This finding raises two issues in such studies of neonates: (1) that postnatal age may not accurately characterize developmental age, since successful parturition can occur within a 2-day range depending on litter size and maternal age (Holinka *et al.*, 1978), and (2) that the steroid levels in plasma and brain are unknown and body weights of injected pups are not usually given. Since increased adrenal production of estrogens occurs in some mouse strains after ovariectomy (Frantz and Kirschbaum, 1949), studies on the effect of ovariectomy can not be critically evaluated without data on plasma-steroid levels. These difficulties may limit the precision and reproducibility of studies in neonates.

4.3. Long-Lasting Steroid Effects in the Postweaning Period

In some studies of DAS, sham-injected neonates were given steroids, but with sometimes heterogeneous outcomes. It might be expected that injection of adolescent or young adult rodents could accelerate some aging changes in gonadotropin regulation. For example, if rats (not given any neonatal treatment) are ovariectomized at 75 days (young adults) and then injected with testosterone, 1 mg/day for 30 days followed by 30 days without hormones, the subsequent E_2, P-induced LH surge was greatly impaired (Harlan *et al.*, 1977). The 30-day-period between the last testosterone injection and the LH-surge test should have sufficed to clear the injected steroids from circulation, but carry-over effects remain to be investigated in such studies. In contrast, these same investigators obtained different results with a generally similar procedure (Harlan and Gorski, 1978). Rats were ovariectomized at 30 days (just before puberty) and were injected with E_2 (5 μg/day) or testosterone (0.1 mg/day) from 35-days to 95 days. After 30 days without steroids, LH surges were induced by two procedures; in the E_2-induced LH surge on day 125, the E_2 and testosterone injected rats were markedly *more* responsive than in controls (not injected during days 30–95), whereas on day 128 the E_2, P-induced LH surge was similar in all groups. The lightly androgenized rats showed the expected DAS-like response, with smaller LH surges (Harlan and Gorski, 1978). In their discussion, Harlan and Gorski comment, "It remains to be seen, however, if this effect is really permanent, although it is reproducible [based on unpublished results]. The relationship between the masculinizing effect of steroids given post-pubertally in lightly androgenized rats and the feminizing effect in normal rats is unknown at this time." These divergent effects of steroids in rats of generally similar age groups suggest that age, steroid dose, and duration of treatment are critical variables in the outcome of steroid manipulations. For example, the first study (Harlan *et al.*, 1977) involved E_2 treatment from 75–105 days, whereas in the second study (Harlan and Gorski, 1978) rats were treated for 35 to 95 days. Moreover, treatment of neonates with exogenous steroids could conceivably "androgenize" *different* loci than do endogenous steroids during normal development.

Clarification of these issues may await a better understanding of neural responses to steroids. The absence of a steroid-induced LH surge could result from single or multiple changes in a complex series of neuronal events, which cannot be presumed identical throughout diverse treatments, even though the endpoint of these various histories may yield a polyfollicular, anovulatory condition with impaired LH surges. For example, compare rodents neonatally androgenized with the various doses used (30 μg to 12,500 μg testosterone), or lightly androgenized with various steroids and examined as adults, or given various steroid manipulations as adults. Also prenatal exposure to sex steroids can vary with the sex of the neighboring fetus (Meisel and Ward, 1981; vom Saal and Bronson, 1978). There is a need for tests of alterations on the various, presently obscure control points in the LH-surge mechanism. Elucidation of the details of the surge mechanism will probably emerge from future studies of the interrelations between the various neurotransmitters which directly or indirectly influence LHRH release and pituitary responses, e.g., dopamine, norepinephrine, serotonin, acetylcholine, GABA, opioids, etc.

4.4. Estradiol-Induced Adult Anovulatory Syndrome

Long-lasting effects of exogenous E_2 in young postpubertal rodents are now well established and clearly extend the age for differentiation-like effects of steroids on the CNS into the adult phase of rodents. An early study showing long term effects of a single E_2 injection was that of Brown-Grant (1974) who found that 2–5 mg E_2-benzoate injected into 50- to 70-day-old rats induced "a prolonged period of persistent vaginal cornification" with anovulatory ovaries lasting beyond 110 days. Eventually, most rats became ovulatory, by 160–220 days of age. Testosterone proprionate (25 mg) produced transient diestrous smears with subsequent return to "regular 4-day cycles. . . . maintained until. . . . 220 days of age." In another protocol, a single large injection of E_2-valerate, e.g., 2–8 mg/kg body weight, rapidly causes the loss of regular ovulatory cycles and the onset of PVC in young adult mice and rats (Brawer et al., 1978; Mobbs et al., 1981). In C57BL/6J mice, plasma E_2 levels are extremely high on the day after injection (2000 pg/ml, about 50-fold above the normal range), but subside to a physiologic range of 15–30 pg/ml during the next 6 weeks (Mobbs and Finch, unpublished). The noncycling PVC state continues indefinitely, and is so far hormonally indistinguishable from the polyfollicular anovulatory state of the neonatally androgenized rodent or rodents with age-correlated PVC. We even find that after 4 months, the ovary retains some potential for normal function, as assayed by its ability to produce normal numbers of ova in response to an injection of gonadotropins (hCG) or by the regular cycles the ovary supports after transplantation to young controls (Mobbs et al., 1981). Hypothalamic functions, however, become impaired at some time after the initial injection of E_2-valerate, as assayed by the E_2-induced LH surge, the smaller postcastration elevations of LH, or by the failure of young ovarian transplants to cycle in the treated mice (Mobbs and Finch, unpublished). In these studies mice were compared at least 30 days after ovariectomy to "wash out" short-term effects of the injected or endogenous steroids. Hypothalamic impairments are also implied by smaller LH surges induced by electrochemical stimulation of the preoptic region in E_2-valerate treated rats as compared to controls in proestrus (Brawer et al., 1980b). There is no evidence for major impairments at the pituitary level as assayed by responses to injected luteinizing hormone-releasing hormone (LHRH) (Brawer et al., 1980a; Mobbs et al., 1981), although the single injections of LHRH do not generate as large an LH output as during the E_2-P induced LH surge. Thus, a fuller dynamic range of LHRH levels and time course need study before it can be concluded that the pituitary is unimpaired.

Brawer and colleagues described a glial hyperactivity in the arcuate nucleus several months after the initial estrogen injection, which resembles that found in normal aging rodents (Brawer et al., 1978). Such glial hyperactivity is usually associated with neuronal degeneration, which in this case seems to involve the neuronal processes rather than cell death (Brawer et al., 1980b). The effects of these steroid treatments on neuronal synapses and their regional localization are not yet known.

It is intriguing that these effects of E_2-valerate depend on the presence of the ovary, if ovariectomy precedes the single injection of E_2-valerate then long-term effects are decreased, as evaluated by the normal cycling obtained with ovarian transplants into these mice (unpublished) and by the absence of glial hyperactivity (Schipper *et al.,* 1981). The hypothalamic damage from E_2-valerate thus appears to require a prolonged exposure to the polyfollicular state, which involves modest but sustained levels of plasma E_2 and low levels of plasma P.

We hypothesize that the initial high levels of E_2 "desensitize" subsequent hypothalamic positive feedback responses to E_2 and that the desensitization is maintained by the polyfollicular (PVC) state once the injected E_2 has cleared, after about 1 month. As an example of desensitization, young rats given E_2 implants for 30 days, had reduced E_2-P induced LH surges (Lu *et al.,* 1981). Eventually, the continued PVC with elevated plasma E_2:P might cause hypothalamic changes which could not be readily reversed.

Consistent with the view that prolonged exposure to moderate levels of E_2 is the major cause of hypothalamic damage after E_2-valerate injections is the pioneering study of Kawashima (1960). Daily injections of E_2 in the minute amount of .02 μg/day caused the loss of regular cycles with intermittent PVC after about 100 days, even though the E_2 injections did not initially alter cycles, nor cornify vaginal smears in ovariectomized controls. Taken together these studies clearly demonstrate that low sustained levels of E_2 can exert long-term, possible cumulative and irreversible effects on neuroendocrine functions in adult female rodents.

The specificity for effects of chronic steroids on the adult brain is partly known. P does not have these long-term effects when given at 500 μg/day (Kawashima, 1960). Moreover, the injection of P (25 mg/wk) after the single injection of 2 mg E_2-valerate will suppress the glial activity which results from the E_2-valerate alone (Brawer and Finch, 1982). Testosterone given in daily injections (Kawashima, 1960) or in one large injection each month for 4 months (Brawer and Finch, 1982) did not interrupt cycles. If estrogens are the active agents, the absence of effects of injected testosterone is puzzling because of the well-known conversion of testosterone to estrogens by hypothalamic aromatases (Naftolin *et al.,* 1976). Direct information of tissue steroid levels might resolve this issue.

Such effects of estrogens on the adult brain also appear in sheep which graze on types of clover which contain estrogenic isoflavones, "phytoestrogens." Several years of exposure to phytoestrogens can lead to a permanent infertility syndrome, clover disease, which is associated with mild glial hyperactivity and shrinkage of hypothalamic neurons (Adams, 1976, 1977). These hypothalamic correlates of clover disease closely resemble some effects of exogenous estrogens in rodents and raise the possibility that adult brains of a variety of mammals may be subject to long-term effects of E_2 and possibly other hormones. There is as yet no evidence for such effects in primates.

Finally, another example of E_2-related desensitization is found in the daily, late afternoon LH surges which are induced in young adult rats by large E_2 implants leading to supraphysiologic plasma E_2. The surges gradually grow smaller and usually cease by 2 weeks (Legan *et al.*, 1975).

4.5. Light-Induced Anovulatory Syndrome

Exposure of female rodents to constant light interrupts estrous cycles and leads to vaginal smear patterns similar to those seen in the above anovulatory syndromes (e.g., Damassa and Davidson, 1973), the light-induced anovulatory syndrome. Although the stability of the light-induced anovulatory syndrome after resumption of normal light is not well studied, this paradigm has some physiological correlates similar to those seen in the senescent anovulatory syndrome, and which are clearly neurally mediated.

5. Mechanisms

We can merely speculate on the molecular mechanisms by which ovarian secretions or exogenous E_2 cause long-lasting, possibly cumulative hypothalamic changes in adult rodents. First, the possibility must be considered that the effects of endogenous or exogenous E_2 on the hypothalamus are mediated indirectly through other molecules. For example, E_2 acts on the rodent brain and other organs to induce heat-labile non-dialyzable factors which enhance growth of tumor cells *in vitro* (Sirbasku, 1978). Such steroid-induced growth factors could influence neural or glial functions independently of the classic "steroid-receptor" mechanism. Moreover, E_2 has well-known influences on prolactin, among other hormones which act on the hypothalamus. In many situations glial hyperactivity, particularly for microglia, is strongly correlated with neuronal degeneration (Matthews and Kruger, 1973; Bernheimer *et al.*, 1973). Nonetheless, some steroids can act directly on glia, e.g., glucocorticoids, which induce glucose-6-phosphate dehydrogenase (de Vellis *et al.*, 1974) or E_2 which induces nerve growth factor (Perez-Polo *et al.*, 1977).

An appealing mechanism for the effects of ovarian steroids is through an effect on neuronal synapses. Many studies show influences of E_2 on synapses and neuritic growth, e.g., of neonatal hypothalamic explants (Toran-Allerand, 1980) or in the response of the arcuate nucleus to differentiation in adult rats (Matsumoto and Arai, 1981). The elevated

E_2-P ratios during the PVC state or at proestrus in the aging rodent can be considered in terms of the long known antagonism of E_2 and P (discussed in Section 2.2). There is now strong evidence in uterine cells that the translocation of the P-receptor to the nucleus results in an early exit of the E_2-receptor from the nucleus of that same cell (Okulicz et al., 1981); injection of P at proestrus reduced the amount of E_2-R in uterine nuclei. Conversely, these results would suggest that the reduced P levels at proestrus in aging rodents (see Section 2.6) could result in prolonged retention of the E_2-receptor in the nucleus. P ratios of the PVC state might also perpetuate a continuous supranormal nuclear retention of the E_2-receptor. Effects of P on E_2 receptors in the hypothalamus have not been investigated at a molecular level, but could also account for the antagonism of neonatal androgenization by P (Kincl and Maqueo, 1965). In the uterus, the duration of nuclear residency by the E_2-receptor is strongly correlated with uterine growth (Anderson et al., 1975). Two major classes of uterine nuclear E_2-receptors can be distinguished by differential extraction with 0.3–0.4 M KCl (Ruh and Baudendistel, 1977; Clark et al., 1980). The salt-resistant nuclear receptors are strongly correlated with the extent of uterine growth. The fraction of receptors translocated merits separate consideration, since there is some proportionality between the numbers of translocated receptors and the extent of response as shown by the transcription of conalbumin messenger RNA in the chick oviduct (Mulvihill and Palmiter, 1977). Another issue concerns the "spare receptors" of some steroid target cells. Even at proestrus when the maximum physiological translocation of E_2-receptors occurs in the hypothalamus and pituitary, a considerable fraction (circa 50%) of the total E_2-receptors remain in the cytoplasm and a large injection of E_2 can then double the numbers of translocated receptors above that at proestrus (McGinnis et al., 1981). The effects of this supranormal translocation are unknown, as are the distribution of these receptors in different nuclear binding classes. Unfortunately, few molecular markers for the immediate effects of sex steroid receptor translocation are known in the brain, e.g., hypothalamic tyrosine hydroxylase and choline acetyltransferase increase modestly a day or so after treatment with E_2 (Luine et al., 1975, 1977), in contrast to the uterus or oviduct where effects of E_2 on RNA and on the synthesis of specific proteins can be demonstrated in 30–60 min. The availability of more molecular markers for effects of E_2 and other steroids on the genome of hypothalamic neurons would be valuable for analysis of aging phenomena and for study of reproductive neuroendocrinology.

In the uterus, sustained modest elevators of estrogens through estrogen replacement therapy for menopause are associated with increased risk of endometrial cancer (Shapiro, 1980). A common speculation is that "unopposed" estrogens are the underlying disturbance, i.e., the absence of the normal cyclic variations of E_2 and P. We have raised a similar issue in relation to E_2-induced and spontaneous age-related pituitary tumors (Felicio et al., 1980; Nelson et al., 1981). The possibility then arises that disturbances of cyclic hormonal stimulae may have adverse consequences on a variety of target cells. The "aging" or finite proliferative capacity of human diploid fibroblasts in vitro may also be considered in this context, since cultured cells are obviously not exposed to circadian and ultradien variations of growth hormone, insulin, glucocorticoids, and many other endogenous hormones. Could the absence of cyclically varying hormones in cell cultures be a factor in the finite proliferation of diploid fibroblasts and some other diploid cells in vitro? Some evidence supports this view: supplement of media with hormones can increase the proliferate potential, e.g., hydrocortisone in WI-38 lung fibroblasts (Rosner and Cristofalo, 1981) and fibroblast growth factor in bovine aortic endothelial cells (Johnson and Longenecker, 1982). It would be of interest to consider studies of diploid cell proliferative capacities with diffusion chambers which implanted in a large mammal to permit some normal cyclic variations of hormones.

6. References

Adams, N. R., 1976, Pathological changes in the tissue of infertile ewes with clover disease, *J. Comp. Pathol.* **86:**29–35.

Adams, N. R., 1977, Morphological changes in the organs of ewes grazing on oestrogenic subterranean clover, *Res. Vet. Sci.* **22:**216–221.

Anderson, J. N., Peck, E. J., and Clark, J. H., 1975, Estrogen-induced uterine responses and growth: Relationship to receptor binding by uterine nuclei, *Endocrinology* **96:**160–167.

Arai, Y., 1971, Possible process of the secondary sterilization: Delayed anovulation syndrome, *Experientia* **27:**463–464.

Aschheim, P., 1965, Resultats fournis par la greffe hétérochrone des ovaries dans l'étude de la régulation hypothalamus-hypophyso-ovarienne de la ratte sénile, *Gerontologia* **10:**65–75.

Aschheim, P., 1976, Aging in the hypthalamic-hypophyseal-ovarian axis in the rat, in: *Hypothalamus, Pituitary and Aging,* Chap. 19 (A. V. Everitt and J. A. Burgess, eds.), C. C. Thomas, Springfield, Illinois, pp. 376–418.

Bernheimer, H., Birkmayer, W., Hornykiewicz, O., Jellinger, K., and Seitelberger, F., 1973, Brain dopamine and the syndrome of Parkinson and Huntington. Clinical, morphological and neurochemical correlations, *J. Neurol. Sci.* **20:**415–455.

Brawer, J. R., and Finch, C. E., 1982, Normal and experimentally altered aging processes in the rodent hypothalamus and pituitary, in: *Experimental and Clinical Interventions in Aging* (R. F. Walker and R. L. Cooper, eds.), Dekker, New York (in press).

Brawer, J. R., Naftolin, F., Martin, J., and Sonnenschein, C., 1978, Effects of a single injection of estradiol valerate on the hypothalamic arcuate nucleus, and on reproductive function in the female rat, *Endocrinology* 103:501–512.

Brawer, J. R., Ruf, K. B., and Naftolin, F., 1980a, The effects of estradiol-induced lesions of the arcuate nucleus on gonadotropin release in response to preoptic stimulation in the rat, *Neuroendocrinology* 30:144–149.

Brawer, J. R., Schipper, H., and Naftolin, F., 1980b, Ovary-dependent degeneration in the hypothalamic arcuate nucleus, *Endocrinology* 107:274–279.

Bronson, F. H., 1981, The regulation of luteinizing hormone secretion by estrogen: Relationships among negative feedback, surge potential, and male stimulation in juvenile, peripubertal, and adult female mice, *Endocrinology* 108:506–516.

Brown-Grant, K., 1974, On "critical periods" during the postnatal development of the rat, Int. Symp. on Sexual Endocrinology of the Perinatal Period, *INSERM* 32:357–376.

Clark, J. H., Markaverich, B., Upchurch, S., Eriksson, H., Hardin, J. W., and Peck, E. J., Jr., 1980, Heterogeneity of estrogen binding sites: Relationship to estrogen receptors and estrogen responses, *Rec. Prog. Horm. Res.* 36:89–134.

Clemens, J. A., Fuller, R. W., and Owen, N. V., 1978, Some neuroendocrine aspects of aging, in: *Parkinson's Disease-II. Aging and Neuroendocrine Relationships* (C. E. Finch, D. E. Potter, and A. D. Kenny, eds.), Plenum, New York.

Cooper, R. L., and Linnoila, M., 1980, Effects of centrally and systemically administered L-tyrosine and L-leucine on ovarian function in the old rat, *Gerontology* 26:270–275.

Cooper, R. L., Conn, P. M., and Walker, R. F., 1980, Characterization of the LH surge in middle-aged female rats, *Biol. Reprod.* 23:611–615.

Coquelin, A., Döhler, K. D., Gorski, R. A., and Shryne, J. E., 1981, Experimental sex reversal of the sexually dimorphic nucleus in the preoptic area of the female rat, *Soc. Neurosci. Abstr.* 7:286.

Costoff, A., and Mahesh, V. B., 1975, Primordial follicles with normal oocytes in the ovaries of postmenopausal women, *J. Am. Geriatr. Soc.* 23:193–196.

Damassa, D., and Davidson, J. M., 1973, Effects of ovariectomy and constant light on responsiveness of estrogen in the rat, *Horm. Behav.* 4:269–279.

Demarest, K. T., Moore, K. E., and Riegle, G. D., 1982, Dopaminergic neuronal function, anterior pituitary dopamine content and serum concentrations of prolactin, luteinizing hormone, and progesterone in the aged female rat, *Brain Res.* 247:347–354.

de Vellis, J., McEwen, B. S., Cole, R., and Inglish, D., 1974, Relations between glucocorticoid nuclear binding, cytosol receptor activity and enzyme induction in a rat glial cell line, *J. Steroid Biochem.* 5:392–393.

Elias, K. A., Huffman, L. J., Blake, C., 1979, Age of ovariectomy affects subsequent plasma LH responses in old age rats, *61st Annual Meeting of the Endocrine Society*, p. 106 (abstr.).

Ely, C. A., and Schwartz, N. B., 1971, Elucidation of the role of luteinizing hormone in estrogen secretion and ovulation by use of antigonadotropic sera, *Endocrinology* 89:1103–1108.

Evans, W. F., Cronin, M. J., and Thorner, M. O., 1982, Hypogonadism in hyperprolactinemia: proposed mechanisms. in: *Frontiers in Neuroendocrinology*, (W. F. Ganong, and L. Martini, eds.), pp. 77–114, Raven Press, New York.

Felicio, L. S., Nelson, J. F., and Finch, C. E., 1980, Spontaneous pituitary tumorigenesis in aging female C57BL/6J mice, *Exp. Gerontol.* 15:139–142.

Finch, C. E., 1972, Enzyme activities, gene function, and aging in mammals (review), *Exp. Gerontol.* 7:53–67.

Finch, C. E., 1973, Catecholamine metabolism in the brains of aging male mice, *Brain Res.* 52:261–276.

Finch, C. E., 1978, Reproductive senescence in rodents: Factors in the decline of fertility and loss of regular estrous cycles, in: *The Aging Reproductive System, Aging*, Vol. 4 (E. L. Schneider ed.), Raven Press, New York, pp. 193–212.

Finch, C. E., Felicio, L. S., Flurkey, K., Gee, D. M., Mobbs, C., Nelson, J. F., and Osterburg, H. H., 1980, Studies in ovarian-hypothalamic-pituitary interactions during reproductive aging in C57BL/6J mice, *Peptides* (Suppl. 1) **1:**163–176.

Flurkey, K., Gee, D., and Finch, C. E., 1980, Estradiol regulation of LH in aging mice. *The Geronotologist* **20:**104 (abstr.).

Flurkey, K., Gee, D. M., and Finch, C. E., 1981, Age changes in progesterone and its relationship to LH during proesterus in C57BL/6J mice, in: *Dynamics of Ovarian Function* (N. B. Schwartz, and M. Hunzicker-Dunn, eds.), Raven Press, New York, pp. 297–301.

Flurkey, K., Gee, D. M., Sinha, Y. N., and Finch, C. E., 1982, Age effects on luteinizing hormone, progesterone, and prolactin in proestrous and acyclic C57BL/6J mice, *Biol. Reprod.* **26:**835–846.

Frantz, M. J., and Kirschbaum, A., 1949, Sex hormone secretion by tumors of the adrenal cortex of mice, *Cancer Res.* **9:**257–266.

Gee, D. M., Flurkey, K., and Finch, C. E., 1983, Aging and the regulation of leuteinizing hormone in C57BL/6J mice: impaired elevations after ovariectomy and spontaneous elevations at advanced ages. *Biol. Reprod.* **28:**598–607.

Gnegy, M. E., and Costa, E., 1980, Catecholamine receptor supersensitivity and subsensitivity in the central nervous system, in: *Essays in Neurochemistry and Neuropharmacology.* (M. B. H. Youdim, W. Lovenberg, D. F. Sharman, and F. R. Lagnado, eds.), Wiley and Sons, New York, pp. 249–282.

Gorski, R. A., 1968, Influence of age on the response to paranatal administration of a low dose of androgen, *Endocrinology* **82:**1001–1104.

Gorski, R. A., Gordon, J. H., Shryne, J. E., and Southam, A. M., 1980, Evidence for the existence of a sexually dimorphic nucleus in the preoptic area of the rat, *J. Comp. Neurol.* **193:**529–539.

Gosden, R. G., Bancroft, L., 1976, Pituitary function in reproductively senescent female rats, *Exp. Gerontol.* **11:**157–160.

Gosden, R. C., Liang, S. C., Felicio, L. S., Nelson, J. F., and Finch, C. E., 1983, Imminent oocyte exhaustion and reduced follicular recruitment mark the climacteric in aging mice, *Biol. Reprod.* **28:**255–260.

Gray, G. D., and Wexler, B. C., 1980, Estrogen and testosterone sensitivity of middle-aged female rats in the regulation of LH, *Exp. Gerontol.* **15:**201–207.

Gray, G. D., Tennent, B., Smith, E. R., and Davidson, J. M., 1980, Luteinizing hormone regulation and sexual behavior in middle-aged female rats, *Endocrinology* **107:** 187–194.

Harlan, R. E., and Gorski, R. A., 1977, Steroid regulation of luteinizing hormone secretion in normal and androgenized rats at different ages, *Endocrinology* **101:**741–749.

Harlan, R. E., and Gorski, R. A., 1978, Effects of postpubertal ovarian steroids on reproductive function and sexual differentiation of lightly androgenized rats, *Endocrinology* **102:**1716–1724.

Harlan, R. E., Nance, D. M., Shryne, J. E., and Gorski, R. A., 1977, Effects of septal lesions and testosterone on lordosis behavior and luteinizing hormone release in female rats, *Brain Res. Bull.* **2:**389–392.

Harman, S. M., and Tsitouras, P. D., 1980, Reproductive hormones in aging men. Measurement of sex steroids, basal luteinizing hormone, and Leidig cell response to human chorionic gonadotropin, *J. Clin. Endocrinol. Metabol.* **51:**35.

Hendricks, S. E., McArthur, D. A., and Pickett, S., 1977, The delayed anovulation syndrome: influence of hormones and correlation with behaviour, *J. Endocrinol.* **75:** 15–22.

Hodson, C. A., Simpkins, J. W., Pas, K. A., Aylsworth, C. F., Steger, R. W., and Meites, J., 1980, Effects of a prolactin-secreting pituitary tumor on hypothalamic, gonadotropic, and testicular function in male rats, *Neuroendocrinology* **30:**7–10.

Holinka, C. F., Tseng, Y-C., and Finch, C. E., 1978, Prolonged gestation, elevated preparturitional plasma progesterone, and reproductive aging in C57BL/6J mice, *Biol. Reprod.* **19:**807–816.

Howland, B. E., 1976, Reduced gonadotropin release in response to progesterone or gonadotropin releasing hormone (GnRH) in old female rats, *Life Sci.* **19:**219–224.

Howland, B. E., and Preiss, C., 1975, Effects of aging on basal levels of serum gonadotropins, ovarian compensatory hypertrophy, and hypersecretion of gonadotropins after ovariectomy in female rats, *Fertil. Steril.* **26:**271–276.

Hsu, H. K., and Peng, M. T., 1978, Hypothalamic neurone number of old female rats, *Gerontology* **24:**434–440.

Ichikawa, S., Morioka, H., and Sawada, T., 1972, Acute effects of gonadotropins on the secretion of progestins by the rat ovary, *Endocrinology* **90:**1356–1362.

Ireland, J. J., and Richards, J. S., 1978, A previously undescribed role for luteinizing hormone (LH:hCG) on follicular cell differentiation; *Endocrinology* **102:**1458–1465.

Johnson, L. K., and Longenecker, J. P., 1982, Senescence of aortic endothelia cells *in vitro:* Influence of culture conditions and preliminary characterization of the senescent phenotype, *Mech. Ageing Dev.* **18:**1–18.

Kawakami, M., Yoshioka, E., Konda, N., Arita, J., and Visessuvan, S., 1978, Data on the sites of stimulatory feedback action of gonadal steroids indispensible for luteinizing hormone release in the rat, *Endocrinology* **102:**791–798.

Kawashima, S., 1960, Influence of continued injections of sex steroids on the estrous cycle in the adult rat, *Annot. Zool. Japon.* **33:**226–232.

Kincl, F. A., and Maqueo, M., 1965, Prevention by progesterone of steroid-induced sterility in neonatal male and female rats, *Endocrinology* **77:**859–862.

Krohn, P. L., 1977, Transplantation of the ovary, in: *The Ovary,* Vol. 2 (S. Zuckerman and B. J. Weir, eds.), Academic Press, New York, pp. 101–128.

Legan, S., Coon, G., and Karsch, F., 1975, Role of estrogen and initiator of daily LH surges in the ovariectomized rat, *Endocrinology* **96:**50–56.

Lu, J. H. K., and Kledzik, G. S., 1981, Chronological changes in ovarian function and morphology in aging rats and their relation to neuroendocrine responses, in: *Dynamics of Ovarian Function* (N. B. Schwartz and M. Hunzicker-Dunn, eds.), Raven Press, New York, pp. 291–296.

Lu, K. H., Huang, H. H., Chen, II. T., Kurcz, M., Mioduszewski, R., and Meites J., 1977, Positive feedback by estrogen and progesterone on LH release in old and young rats, *Proc. Soc. Exp. Biol. Med.* **154:**82–85.

Lu, K. H., Hopper, B. R., Vargo, T. M., and Yen, S. S. C., 1979, Chronologic changes in sex steroid, gonadotropin, and prolactin secretion in aging female rats displaying different reproductive states, *Biol. Reprod.* **21:**193–203.

Lu, J. H. K., Damassa, D. A., Gilman, D. P., Judd, H. L., and Sawyer, C. H., 1980, Differential patterns of gonadotropin responses to ovarian steroids and the LH releasing hormone between constant estrous and pseudopregnant states in aging rats, *Biol. Reprod.* **23:**345–351.

Lu, J. K. H., Gilman, D. P., Meldrum, D. R., Judd, H. L., and Sawyer, C. H., 1981, Relationship between circulating estrogens and the central mechanisms by which ovarian steroids stimulate luteinizing hormone secretion in aged and young female rats, *Endocrinology* **108:**836–841.

Luine, V. N., Khylchevskaya, R. I., and McEwen, B. S., 1975, Effect of gonadal steroids on activities of monoamine oxidase and choline acetylase in rat brain, *Brain Res.* **86:**293–306.

Luine, V. N., McEwen, B. S., and Black, I. B., 1977, Effect of 17B-estradiol on hypothalamic tyrosine hydroxylase activity, *Brain Res.* **120:**188–192.

Martin, G. M., 1978, Genetic syndromes in man with potential relevance to the pathobiology of aging. *Birth Def.* (Original Article Series) **14**(1)**:**5–39.

Matsumoto, A., and Arai, Y., 1981, Neuronal plasticity in the deafferented hypothalamic arcuate nucleus of adult female rats and its enhancement by treatment with estrogen, *J. Comp. Neurol.* **197:**197–205.

Matthews, M. R., and Kruger, L., 1973, Electron microscopy of nonneuronal cellular changes accompanying neuronal degeneration in thalamic nuclei of the rabbit. II. Reactive elements within the neurophil, *J. Comp. Neurol.* **148:**313–346.

McGinnis, M. Y., Krey, L. C., MacLusky, N. J., and McEwen, B. S., 1981, Steroid receptor levels in intact and ovariectomized estrogen-treated rats: An examination of quantitative, temporal and endocrine factors influencing the efficacy of an estradiol stimulus, *Neuroendocrinology* **33:**158–165.

McPherson, J. C., III, Costoff, A., Mahesh, V. B., 1977, Effects of aging on the hypothalamic-hypophyseal-gonadal axis in female rats, *Fertil. Steril.* **28:**1365–1370.

Miesel R. L., and Ward, I. L., 1981, Fetal female rats are masculinized by male littermates located caudally in the uterus, *Science* **213:**239–242.

Miller, A. E., and Riegle, G. D., 1980, Temporal changes in serum progesterone in aging female rats, *Endocrinology* **106:**1579–1583.

Mobbs, C., Flurkey, K., Gee, D. M., and Finch, C. E., 1981, Estradiol-induced acyclicity in mice: A model of reproductive aging? *63rd Annual Meeting of the Endocrine Society,* p. 159 (abstr.).

Mobbs, C., Gee, D. M., and Finch, C. E., 1982a, Ovariectomy partially restores neuroendocrine reproductive functions in aging female mice as assayed by ovarian grafts, *64th Annual Meeting of the Endocrine Society,* p. 114 (abstr.).

Mobbs, C., Gee, D. M., and Finch, C. E., 1982b, Partial restoration of LH regulation in aging C57BL/6J female mice, *Programs and Abstracts, 35th Annual Scientific Meeting, The Gerontological Society of America* (abstr.).

Mobbs, C., Gee, D., and Finch, C. E., 1982c, Delay and partial reversal of age-correlated neuroendocrine reproductive impairments in C57BL/6J female mice. *Programs and Abstracts, 12th Annual Meeting, Society for Neuroscience* (abstr.).

Mulvihill, E. K., and Palmiter, R. D., 1977, Relationships of nuclear estrogen receptor levels to the induction of ovalbumin and conalbumin in RNA in chick oviduct, *J. Biol. Chem.* **252:**2060–2068.

Naftolin, F., Ryan, K. J., and Davies, I. J., 1976, Androgen aromatization by neuroendocrine tissues, in: *Subcellular Mechanisms in Reproductive Neuroendocrinology* (F. Naftolin, K. J. Ryan, and I. J. Davies, eds.), Elsevier, Amsterdam, pp. 347–355.

Nelson, J. F., 1981, Patterns of reproductive aging in C57BL/6J mice: Estrous cycles, gonadal steroids, and uterine estradiol receptors, Ph.D. Thesis, The University of Southern California, Los Angeles.

Nelson, J. F., Latham, K. R., and Finch, C. E., 1975, Plasma testosterone levels in C57BL/6J male mice: Effects of age and disease, *Acta Endocrinol.* **80:**744-752.

Nelson, J. F., Felicio, L. S., and Finch, C. E., 1980a, Ovarian hormones and the etiology of reproductive aging in mice, in: *Aging—Its Chemistry* (A. A. Dietz, ed.), Am. Assoc. Clin. Chemists, Washington, D.C., pp. 64–81.

Nelson, J. F., Felicio, L. S., Sinha, Y. N., and Finch, C. E., 1980b, An ovarian role in the spontaneous pituitary tumorigenesis, *Gerontologist* (abstr.) **20**(5):171.

Nelson, J. F., Felico, L. S., Osterburg, H. H., and Finch, C. E., 1981, Altered profiles of estradiol and progesterone associated with prolonged estrous cycles and persistent vaginal cornification in aging C57BL/6J mice. *Biol. Reprod.* **24**:784–794.

Nelson, J. F., Felicio, L. S., Randall, P. K., Simms, C., and Finch, C. E., 1982, A longitudinal study of estrous cyclicity in aging C57BL/6J mice: I, cycle frequency, length, and vaginal cytology, *Biol. Reprod.* **27**:327–339.

Novak, E. R., 1970, Ovulation after 50, *Obstet. Gynecol.* **36**:903–910.

Okulicz, W. C., Evans, R. W., and Leavitt, W. W., 1981, Progesterone regulation of the occupied form of the nuclear estrogen receptor, *Science* **213**:1503–1505.

Parkening, T. A., Collins, T. J., and Smith, E. R., 1980, A comparative study of prolactin levels in five species of aged female laboratory rodents, *Biol. Reprod.* **22**:513–518.

Peluso, J. J., Steger, R. W., and Hafez, E. S. E., 1977, Regulation of LH secretion in aged female rats, *Biol. Reprod.* **16**:212–215.

Peng, M. T., and Huang, H. O., 1972, Aging of hypothalamic-pituitary-ovarian function in the rat, *Fertil. Steril.* **23**:535–542.

Peng, M. T., Choung, C. F., and Peng, Y. M., 1977, Lordosis response of senile female rats, *Neuroendocrinology* **24**:317–324.

Perez-Polo, J. R., Hall, K., Livingston, K., and Westlund, K., 1977, Steroid induction of nerve growth factor synthesis in cell culture, *Life Sci.* **21**:1535–1544.

Pirke, K. M., Geiss, M., and Sintermann, R., 1978, A quantitative study on feedback control of LH by testosterone in young adult and old female rats, *Acta Endocrinol.* **89**:789–795.

Raisman, G., and Field, P., 1973, Sexual dimorphism in the neurophil of the preoptic area of the rat and its dependence on neonatal androgen, *Brain Res.* **54**:1–29.

Randall, P. K., Severson, J. A., and Finch, C. E., 1981, Aging and the regulation of striatal dopaminergic mechanisms in mice, *J. Pharmacol. Exp. Ther.* **219**:696–700.

Reymond, M. J., and Porter, J. C., 1981, Secretion of hypothalamic dopamine into pituitary stalk blood of aged female rats, *Brain Res. Bull.* **7**:69–73.

Robertson, G. L., and Rowe, J., 1980, The effect of aging on neurohypophyseal function, *Peptides* **1**(1):159–162.

Rosner, B. A., and Cristofalo, V. J., 1981, Changes in specific dexamethasone binding during aging in WI-38 cells, *Endocrinology* **108**:1965–1971.

Ruh, T. S., and Baudendistel, L. J., 1977, Different nuclear binding sites for antiestrogen and estrogen receptor complexes, *Endocrinology* **100**:420–426.

Schechter, J., Felicio, L. S., Nelson, J. F., and Finch, C. E., 1981, Pituitary tumorigenesis in aging female C57BL/6J mice: Electron microscopy, *Am. J. Anat.* **199**:423–432.

Schindler, A. E., Ebert, A., Friederich, E., 1972, Conversion of androstenedione to estrone by human fat tissue, *J. Clin. Endocrinol. Metabol.* **35**:627.

Schipper, H., Brawer, J. R., Nelson, J. F., Felicio, L. S., and Finch, C. E., 1981, The role of gonads in the histologic aging of the hypothalamic arcuate nucleus, *Biol. Reprod.* **25**:413–419.

Shaar, C. J., Euker, J. S., Riegle, G. D., and Meites, J., 1975, Effects of castration and gonadal steroids on serum luteinizing hormone and prolactin in old and young rats, *J. Endocrinol.* **66**:45–51.

Shapiro, S., 1980, Recent and past use of conjugated estrogens in relation to adeno-carcinoma of the endometrium, *N. Engl. J. Med.* **303**:485–489.

Simpkins, J. W., Mueller, G. P., Huang, H. H., and Meites, J., 1977, Evidence for depressed catecholamine and enhanced serotonin metabolism in aging male rats: Possible relation to gonadotropin secretion, *Endocrinology* **100**:1672–1678.

Sirbasku, D. A., 1978, Estrogen induction of growth factors specific for hormone-responsive mammary, pituitary, and kidney tumor cells, *Proc. Natl. Acad. Sci. USA* **75**:3786–3790.

Smith, W. A., Cooper, R. L., and Conn, M. P., 1982, Altered pituitary responsiveness to gonadotropin-releasing hormone in middle-aged rats with 4-day estrous cycles. *Endocrinology* **111**:1843–1848.

Staats, J., 1976, Standardized nomenclature for inbred strains of mice: Sixth listing, *Cancer Res.* **36**:4333–4377.

Steger, R. W., Huang, H. H., Chamberlain, D. S., and Meites, J., 1980, Changes in control of gonadotropin secretion in the transition period between regular cycles and constant estrous in aging female rats, *Biol. Reprod.* **22**:595–603.

Swanson, H. E., and van der Werff ten Bosch, J. J., 1964, The early-androgen syndrome: Its development and the response to hemi-spaying, *Acta Endocrinol.* **45**:1–12.

Talbert, G. B., 1977, Aging of the reproductive system, in: *Handbook of the Biology of Aging* (C. E. Finch and L. Hayflick, eds.), pp. 318–350.

Tang, L. K., and Tang, F. Y., 1981, LH responses to LHRH, DBcAMP, and 17β-estradiol in cultures derived from aged rats, *Am. J. Physiol.* **240** (*Endocrinol. Metabol.* 3):E510–E518.

Toran-Allerand, C. D., 1980, Sex steroids and the development of the newborn mouse hypothalamus and preoptic area *in vitro.* II. Morphological correlates and hormonal specificity, *Brain Res.* **189**:413–427.

Turgeon, J. L., 1979, Estradiol-luteinizing hormone relationship during the proestrous gonadotropin surge, *Endocrinology* **105**:731–736.

Turgeon, J., and Waring, D. W., 1981, Acute progesterone and 17β-estradiol modulation of luteinizing hormone secretion by pituitaries of cycling rats superfused in vitro, *Endocrinology* **108**:413–419.

Uilenbrock, I. T. J., and van der Werff ten Bosch, J. J., 1972, Ovulation induced by pregnant mare serum gonadotropin in the immature rat treated with a low or a high dose of androgen, *J. Endocrinol.* **55**:533–538.

Vermeulen, A., Reubens, R., and Verdonck, L, 1972, Testosterone secretion and metabolism in male senescence, *J. Clin. Endocrinol. Metabol.* **34**:730.

vom Saal, F. S., and Bronson, F. H., 1978, *In utero* proximity of female mouse fetuses to males: effect of reproductive performance during later life, *Biol. Reprod.* **19**:842.

Watkins, B. E., Meites, J., and Riegle, G. D., 1975, Age-related changes in pituitary responsiveness to LHRH in the female rat, *Endocrinology* **97**:543–548.

Wiegand, S. J., Terasawa, E., Bridson, W. E., and Goy, R. W., 1980, Effects of discrete lesions of preoptic and suprachiasmatic structures in the female rat, *Neuroendocrinology* **31**:147–157.

Wise, P. M., and Ratner, A., 1980, LHRH-induced LH and FSH responses in the aged female rat, *J. Gerontol.* **35**:506–511.

Wise, P. M., Rance, N., and Barraclough, C. A., 1981, Effects of estradiol and progesterone on catecholamine turnover rates in discrete hypothalamic regions in ovariectomized rats, *Endocrinology* **108**:2186–2193.

CHAPTER 10

Pathophysiology of Menopausal Hot Flushes

HOWARD L. JUDD

1. Introduction

In women, the most common and characteristic symptom of the climacteric is an episodic disturbance consisting of sudden flushing and perspiration, referred to as a "hot flush or flash." It has been observed in 65–76% of women who go through the physiological menopause or have a bilateral ovariectomy (Hannan, 1927; Neugarten and Kraines, 1965; Jaszmann *et al.*, 1969; Thompson *et al.*, 1973; McKinlay and Jeffreys, 1974). Of those having flushes, 82% will experience the disturbance for more than 1 year (Jaszmann *et al.*, 1969) and 25–50% will complain of the symptom for more than 5 years (Neugarten and Kraines, 1965; Thompson *et al.*, 1973). Although hot flushes occur in millions of women, there have been few attempts to understand the pathophysiology of this symptom until recently.

In 1927, Hannan (1927) provided an excellent description of the subjective symptoms associated with hot flushes. This description was based on personal interviews with 131 of his patients at the time of their menopause. A majority of these women complained that the episodes began with a sensation of pressure in the head, much like a headache. This increased in intensity until the actual flush occurred. Sometimes heart palpitations were also experienced. Hannan termed this a "premonitory phase." The actual flush usually commenced in the region of the head and neck, then passed to other parts of the body, often in waves

HOWARD L. JUDD ● Department of Obstetrics and Gynecology, University of California at Los Angeles School of Medicine, Los Angeles, California 90024.

over the entire body. Only a few subjects indicated the disturbance was limited to the head, neck, and breasts. The flush was characterized by a feeling of heat or burning in the affected areas. This was followed immediately by an outbreak of perspiration which affected the entire body, but was particularly prominent over the head, neck, upper chest, and back. Other symptoms were also experienced including weakness, fatigue, faintness, and vertigo, but these were noted less frequently.

Since this description, other observers have reported the duration of the subjective discomfort to range from 30 sec to 5 min (mean 4 min; Fig. 1), while the frequency varies from as often as 24 min to as seldom as 1–2 per week. In subjects with severe flushes the mean frequency is 54 min (Meldrum *et al.*, 1979).

Associated with the flush are alterations in behavior. Patients will attempt to dissipate body heat, by fanning themselves, standing by a window, in a draft, or in front of an air conditioner. They will loosen or take off articles of clothing and throw off blankets if the flush occurs while they are in bed.

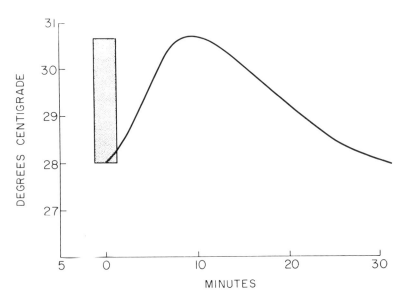

Fig. 1. Mean characteristics and typical configuration of finger temperature fluctuations associated with hot flushes. The shaded area delineates the period from the mean beginning to completion of subjective flushing. (From Meldrum *et al.*, 1979, with permission.)

2. Physiological Studies

Because of the subjective nature of the complaint, the actual existence of hot flushes has been questioned, and papers have been published suggesting the basis of the condition is psychosomatic. Recently, several investigators have begun to characterize the physiological changes associated with hot flushes. These researchers have found that profound changes do occur, indicating that some major disturbance in basic function is responsible for these events.

Initially, limited attempts were made to define changes in physiological function. Albeaux-Fernet and Deribreux (1946) observed perspiration and alterations of central temperature in a single, symptomatic patient. Collett (1949) found increases of oxygen consumption and cheek temperature in several women with the disturbance. Reynolds (1941) reported increases in finger volume (vasodilation) and face temperature during flushes in one woman, and King (1926) showed no change in basal metabolic rate after removal of the ovaries.

The first in depth study was reported by Molnar (1975). He measured skin temperature of the fingers, toes, and forehead, and central temperature at the tympanic membrane and within the rectum, in a woman with frequent hot flushes. Since then, several other investigators have conducted similar studies in groups of patients (Sturdee et al., 1978; Meldrum et al., 1979; Molnar, 1979; Sturdee and Reece, 1979; Tataryn et al., 1980, 1981).

At first, these reports described a prodromal period between the onset of the subjective feeling and the first recordable change in physiological function. With development of better methods to assess changes of physiological function, it was reported that the physiological changes actually precede the onset of the subjective feeling. The first measurable sign of the attack is an increase in cutaneous vasodilation (Mashchak et al., 1982). This has been measured using either a digital plethysmograph or a skin thermosensor to record increases in skin temperature. The vasodilation, as measured by the plethysmograph, begins approximately 1 min before the onset of the subjective flush and continues for approximately 8 min. The skin temperature rise, which reflects cutaneous vasodilation, begins on the average 90 sec after the initiation of the subjective flush (Molnar, 1975; Sturdee et al., 1978; Meldrum et al., 1979; Tataryn et al., 1980, 1981), reaches its maximum by 9 min and returns to baseline after 40 min (Fig. 2). The magnitude of the skin temperature rise is variable, depending on which area of the body is tested, with the fingers and toes showing the greatest increases (Molnar, 1975). This

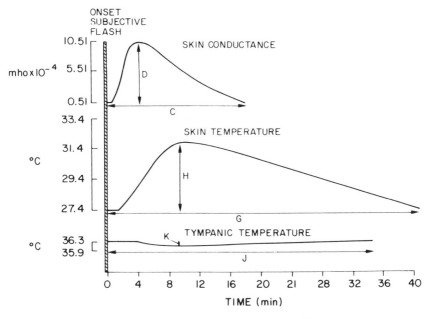

Fig. 2. Characteristics of the changes in skin conductance, skin temperature, and tympanic membrane temperature based on observations of 25 hot flushes. All measurements are referenced to the signal by the patient at the onset of the subjective flush. (From Tataryn *et al.*, 1980, with permission.)

observation indicates the cutaneous vasodilation is generalized and not limited to the upper trunk and head. Temperature changes on the forehead, where the symptomatic flush is experienced, are of lesser magnitude probably because of the perspiration and evaporation that occur in this area (Molnar, 1975). For the finger, the average change in temperature is about 4°C with the maximum being 9°C (Tataryn *et al.*, 1980). The magnitude of the rise shows an indirect correlation with the resting skin temperature (temperature prior to the flush; Fig. 3). In other words, the lower the resting skin temperature the greater the rise will be. During the increase, the skin temperature does not exceed core temperature, but because of cutaneous vasodilation, it reflects the central temperature.

The next measurable sign is a decrease in skin resistance, a measurement of perspiration (Fig. 2). This begins on the average 45 sec after the onset of the subjective flush, reaches its maximum within 4 min and returns to baseline in 18 min.

As heat is lost from the body, by cutaneous vasodilation and perspiration, a decline in core temperature occurs (Fig. 2). This commences about 4 min after the onset of the subjective symptoms, and returns to baseline in about 30 min (Meldrum *et al.*, 1979, Tataryn *et al.*, 1980). The average decrease in core temperature, as measured at the tympanic membrane, is 0.2°C. Alterations of pulse rate also occur during flushing with increases of 13–20% being reported (Sturdee *et al.*, 1978; Fig. 4). Fluctuations of the baseline recording of the electrocardiogram are seen, probably reflecting changes in skin resistance (Molnar, 1975; Sturdee *et al.*, 1978). Alterations of either heart rhythm or blood pressure have not been observed with flushes (Molnar, 1975; Sturdee *et al.*, 1978).

These changes in physiological function do not correspond identically to the subjective symptoms. As mentioned previously, the subjective symptoms begin approximately 1 min after the onset of the first recordable change in cutaneous vasodilation and only last for an average of 4 min (Meldrum *et al.*, 1979; Mashchak *et al.*, 1982; Fig. 1). Thus, the physiological signs continue many minutes after the subjective symptoms have ceased.

The exact mechanism responsible for hot flushes is not known. Early

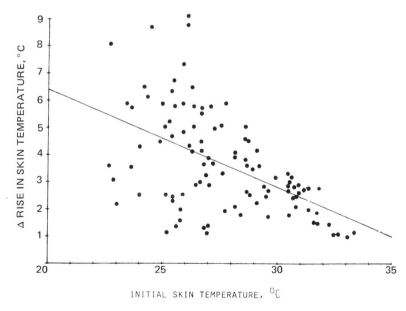

Fig. 3. Relationship of the rise in skin temperature to the initial skin temperature in 275 flushing episodes.

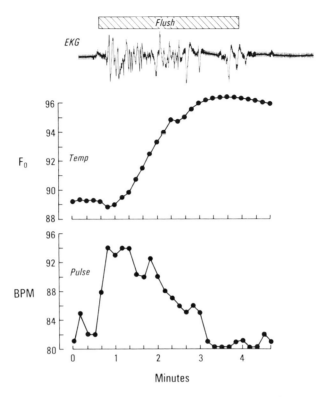

Fig. 4. Increases of fluctuations of baseline recording of EKG, skin temperature, and pulse rate during hot flush. (From S. S. C. Yen, by permission.)

investigators believed that an imbalance of the autonomic nervous system was somehow responsible, and this could occur because of central or peripheral instability of this system. Based on the physiological data presented above, it would appear that the menopausal hot flush is the result of a defect in central thermoregulatory function. There are three indications to support this conclusion.

First, the two major physiological changes associated with hot flushes are the result of different peripheral sympathetic functions. Excitation of sweat glands is by sympathetic cholinergic fibres (Venables, 1967), while cutaneous vasoconstriction is under the exclusive control of tonic α-adrenergic fibres (Greenfield, 1963). It is difficult to envision some peripheral event, resulting in cholinergic effects on sweat glands and α-adrenergic blockade of cutaneous vessels. However, these are the two basic mechanisms triggered by central thermoregulatory centers to lower core temperature. Thus, a hot flush appears to be a normal thermo-regulatory event, occurring at an inappropriate time.

Second, during a hot flush, central temperature decreases following cutaneous vasodilation and perspiration. If hot flushes were the result of some peripheral mechanism, then one would expect the body's regulatory mechanisms to prevent a decrease in core temperature.

The third indication is the change in behavior associated with the symptom. Women have a conscious desire to try and cool their bodies. They will remove clothing, throw off bedcovers, stand by open windows and doors, etc. All these feelings occur in the face of a normal central temperature. An analogous dissociation between perception and central temperature is found at the onset of a fever, when the individual feels cold or a "chill" prior to any change of central temperature. Because of this "chill" subjects will modify behavior to conserve heat. This assists in elevating the central temperature, thus the fever.

Most investigators working in the field of temperature regulation consider a fever to be the result of an elevation of the set point of central thermoregulatory centers, particularly those in the rostral hypothalamus (Snell and Atkins, 1968; Bligh, 1973; Kluger, 1978). Pyrogen elevates the central set point and the febrile organism, whether it be shellfish or human, actively raises the central body temperature, using both physiological (cutaneous vasoconstriction and shivering) and behavioral mechanisms (curling in a ball, putting on more clothes, drinking hot liquids, etc. (Cooper *et al.*, 1964; Reynolds *et al.*, 1974). This continues until the core temperature reaches the new set point.

Employing all these observations it is suggested that the menopausal hot flush is triggered by a sudden downward setting of the central, hypothalamic thermostats (Fig. 5). Subsequently, heat loss mechanisms are activated to bring the core temperature in line with the new set point resulting in the fall of core temperature.

3. Hormonal Studies

Since hot flushes occur after the spontaneous cessation of ovarian function or following ovariectomy, it has been presumed that the underlying mechanism responsible is endocrinological, and has something to do with enhancement of pituitary gonadotropin secretion or reduction of ovarian estrogen secretion. Based on this, attempts have been made to correlate hot flushes with urinary or circulating hormones, particularly gonadotropins and estrogens.

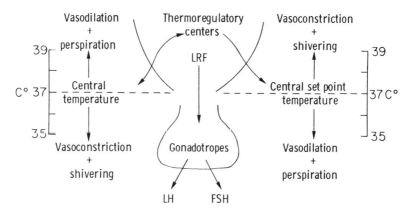

Fig. 5. Proposed mechanism of hot flushes is a sudden downward setting of central set point temperature in hypothalamic thermoregulatory centers. Since central temperature would be higher, this would trigger vasodilation and perspiration (hot flush) to dissipate heat.

3.1. Gonadotropin Studies

Several types of studies have been performed to determine if a relationship exists between gonadotropins and hot flushes. Aitken *et al.* (1974) found a negative correlation between the frequency and severity of hot flushes and urinary LH levels, while Abe *et al.* (1977) observed a positive correlation between the occurrence of the symptom and LH levels in premenopausal women between 35–39 years of age. Aksel *et al.* (1976) found no difference in LH and FSH levels in women with or without flushes studied 10 days following ovariectomy, while Hunter *et al.* (1977) observed parallel increases in the incidence of hot flushes and LH and FSH levels following ovariectomy with the maximal increases of the three occurring approximately 6 weeks after surgery.

Of particular interest are the studies correlating the occurrence of hot flushes with pulsatile LH release. Tataryn *et al.* (1979) measured hot flushes in six women using continuous finger temperature recordings (Figs. 6 and 7). Blood samples were drawn at 15-min intervals before and at 5-min intervals following the commencement of each flush. During 48 hr of study, 34 flushes were recorded. Fluctuations of LH levels were also observed. Pulses of LH were defined as increases of hormone concentration of at least 20% over a nadir. Based on this definition, 31 pulses of LH secretion were seen and 26 (84%) had a close temporal

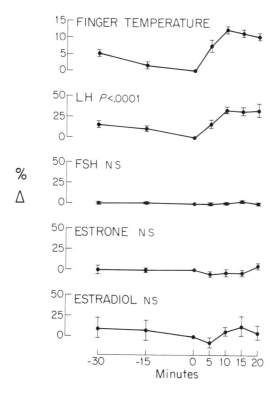

Fig. 6. The mean (± SE) percent change of finger temperature and serum LH, FSH, estrone, and estradiol levels before and after objectively measured hot flushes. Temperature and hormone levels are related to the measurements immediately preceding the onset of the temperature rises (time 0) and are plotted with these as the reference point. (From Meldrum *et al.*, 1980, with permission.)

relationship to the occurrence of hot flushes. There was a strong correlation between LH levels and finger skin temperature in five of the six subjects. Independently, Casper *et al.* (1979) made similar observations at the same time (Fig. 8). Since these reports, several groups of investigators have confirmed this association (Mashchak *et al.*, 1982). These results strongly suggest there is a close temporal relationship between the pulsatile release of LH and the occurrence of hot flushes. Tataryn *et al.* (1979) and Casper and co-workers (1979) also assessed the relationship of pulsatile FSH release with hot flushes with one finding and the other not observing an association.

    The close temporal relationship between pulsatile LH release and

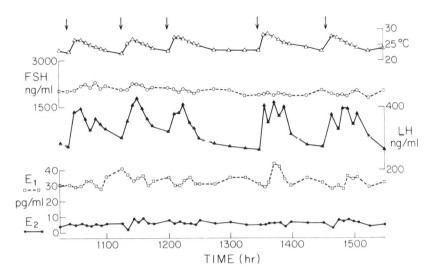

Fig. 7. Serial measurements of finger temperature and serum FSH, LH, estrone, and estradiol in an individual subject. Arrows mark the onset of the temperature rises. (From Meldrum *et al.*, 1980, with permission.)

hot flushes suggests LH or the factors that initiate pulsatile LH release is/are involved with triggering these thermoregulatory events. It is doubtful that LH itself, or increased pituitary activity is responsible, since subjectively measured hot flushes have been described in patients following a surgical hypophysectomy (Mulley and Mitchell, 1976; Mulley *et al.*, 1977; Larsen, 1977). The observations of Meldrum *et al.* (1981) also support this conclusion. These investigators objectively measured

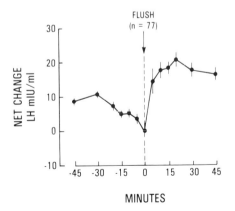

Fig. 8. Mean ne + change of serum LH with onset of flushes.(From S. S. C. Yen, by permission.)

hot flushes in two patients with hypoestrogenism secondary to surgically induced pituitary insufficiency (Fig. 9). In each patient, gonadotropins were low with no pulsatile release. However, hot flushes were observed in both women. The episodes were similar to those experienced by normal postmenopausal subjects in regard to mean interval between flushes, magnitudes of the skin temperature and resistance changes, and relationships of these changes to the onset of subjective flushes.

Further support that the relationship between these two events is not related to pulsatile LH release itself, is the finding of Casper and Yen (1982) that administration of a potent agonist of gonadotropin hormone-releasing hormone (GnRH-a) to postmenopausal women obliterates the pulsatile release of LH, but not the occurrence of hot flushes (Fig. 10). A similar observation also has been made in premenopausal subjects given the same analog (DeFazio *et al.*, 1982). In subjects with normal menstrual cycles, the daily administration of analog for 1 month blocked the pulsatile release of LH from the pituitary presumably through pituitary desensitization. Ovarian function was also obliterated with estrone and estradiol levels falling to concentrations seen in postmenopausal women. Within 3 weeks of initiation of analog administration hot

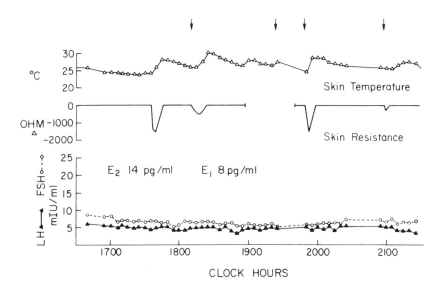

Fig. 9. Serial measurements of skin temperature, skin resistance, and serum LH and FSH levels in a woman following partial resection, cryotherapy, and irradiation of a chromophobe adenoma of the pituitary. Arrows mark the onsets of subjective flushes. (From Meldrum *et al.*, 1981, with permission.)

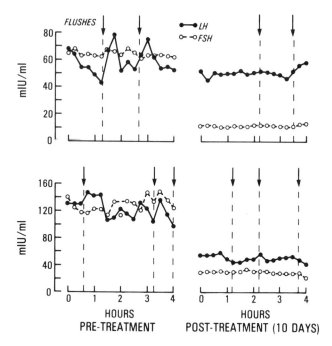

Fig. 10. Serum LH and FSH levels in two postmenopausal women before and after administration of a potent GnRh-agonist. Arrow marks occurrence of a hot flush (Caspar *et al.,* 1981, with permission).

flushes were induced in three of five subjects (60%). This incidence of occurrence was similar to the 76% incidence observed in 25 premenopausal women who underwent surgical castration. The characteristics of the flushes induced with GnRH-a were also similar to the events observed in the women following surgical oophorectomies.

Based on these findings, it seems likely that a suprapituitary mechanism must initiate hot flushes and is somehow influenced by the hypothalamic factors responsible for pulsatile LH release. In rats and monkeys the hypothalamic hormone, GnRH, fluctuates in the hypophysial portal vein blood, and these fluctuations are thought to be responsible at least partially for pulsatile LH release from the pituitary (Carmel *et al.,* 1976; Eskay *et al.,* 1977). The observation by Elkind-Hirsch *et al.* (1981) that serum GnRH levels rise prior to the onset of hot flushes, suggests GnRH or the factors which influence its secretion from the hypothalamus may trigger these abnormal thermoregulatory events.

In monkeys, the site governing the pulsatile release of GnRH is within the arcuate nucleus of the hypothalamus (Krey *et al.,* 1975; Plant *et al.,* 1978). The secretion of GnRH is governed by neurotransmitter input to GnRH-secreting neurons. Factors such as norepinephrine, dopamine, endogenous opioids, and prostaglandins have been shown to influence gonadotropin release from the pituitary, presumably through effects on GnRH release from the hypothalamus (Bhattacharya *et al.*, 1972; LeBlanc *et al.*, 1976; Pang *et al.*, 1977; Linton *et al.*, 1979). Thus, GnRH or the factors that influence its release may somehow alter the set point of the thermoregulatory centers to trigger hot flushes. Since an animal model of hot flushes has not been identified, classical lesioning experiments of hypothalamic function cannot be performed to define which of the above factors trigger flushes. Thus, experiments must be confined to the study of women with spontaneously occurring defects in hypothalamic function.

To address this issue Gambone *et al.* (1982a) studied five subjects with isolated gonadotropin deficiency, who had received exogenous estrogens for hormone replacement for at least one year. These subjects were used as a model of a spontaneously occurring defect of GnRH synthesis and/or release. This assumption was based on the findings of pathological changes in the hypothalamus in patients with this defect (DeMorsier and Gauthier, 1963) and the stimulation of gonadotropin release from the pituitary of patients with repetitive injections of GnRH (Crowley and McArthur, 1980). In four of the five subjects studied, Gambone *et al.* (1982a) observed objectively recorded hot flashes after one month of discontinuation of exogenous estrogen administration. Since these subjects with defects in GnRH synthesis and/or release had flushes, it was presumed that GnRH, itself, is probably not involved in triggering these thermoregulatory episodes.

These investigators also studied five patients with hypothalamic amenorrhea. These women were considered to be models of a defect of neurotransmitter input to GnRH neurons. This assumption was based on the observations that patients with this syndrome have limited or no pulsatile release of gonadotropins (Yen *et al.*, 1973), and have evidence of increased dopaminergic and opioid activity in the hypothalamus (Quigley *et al.*, 1980). This abnormal, neurotransmitter activity is thought to contribute to the reduced release of GnRH from the hypothalamus resulting in amenorrhea and hypogonadism.

The studies of the patients with hypothalamic amenorrhea were conducted within 1 year of disease onset and were limited to patients with hypoestrogenism equivalent to that seen following surgical castration. In these subjects no objectively measured hot flushes were recorded. This finding in these hypoestrogenic women suggests that the mechanism responsible for hypothalamic amenorrhea inhibits the occurrence of hot flushes. Since abnormal neurotransmitter input to GnRH neurons has been reported in this disease, this finding suggests that the hypothalamic factors responsible for GnRH release and not GnRH itself, may somehow alter the set point of thermoregulatory centers of the hypothalamus resulting in the initiation of hot flushes. The close proximity of some of the GnRH neurons with the thermoregulatory centers in the preoptic anterior hypothalamus is consistent with this concept (Lomax and Knox, 1973; Krey *et al.*, 1975; Kobayashi *et al.*, 1978; Plant *et al.*, 1978; Reaves and Hayward, 1979). However, experimental evidence has shown that thermoregulatory responses to neurotransmitters are not precisely localized to the anterior hypothalamus. Destruction of the preoptic anterior hypothalamic nuclei in rats enhances the hypothermic response to norepinephrine injected into the third ventricle, indicating that the site of action of this catecholamine in regard to thermoregulation may be in other areas of the hypothalamus (Satinoff and Cantor, 1975).

The observations that catecholamines play roles in both central thermoregulatory function and GnRH release is also consistent with the hypothesis that neurotransmitter metabolism in the hypothalamus is responsible for the simultaneous occurrence of pulsatile LH release and hot flushes (Cox and Lomax, 1977; Crowley *et al.*, 1978; Simpkins and Kalra, 1979). The finding that clonidine partially blocks the occurrence of objectively measured flushes also supports this possibility (Laufer *et al.*, 1982). The effect of clonidine on flushes could be exerted through peripheral or central mechanisms. Clonidine is an α-adrenergic receptor agonist that stimulates postsynaptic α-adrenergic receptors in the depression site of the vasomotor center of the medulla oblongata (Houston, 1981). In addition, it may also influence supra bulbar structures such as α-adrenergic receptors in the hypothalamus.

3.2. Estrogen Studies

For estrogens, three types of studies have been performed. First, investigators have compared circulating estrogen levels in perimenopausal women with and without the symptom. Aksel *et al.* (1976) found no difference of total estrogen concentrations, while Chakravarti *et al.* (1976) observed lower estradiol levels in patients with the symptom. This latter observation suggests perimenopausal women begin to experience hot flushes when endogenous estrogen levels start to fall. Second, estrogen levels have been measured before, during, and after the occurrence of objectively measured flushes. Meldrum *et al.* (1980) quantitated circulating estrone and estradiol levels at 5–15 min intervals before and after flushes, and found no association (Figs. 6 and 7). Third, comparisons of circulating estrogen levels in postmenopausal women with or without hot flushes have been conducted. Again, Aksel *et al.* (1976) found no difference of total estrogen levels and Stone *et al.* (1975) observed no differences of estrone or estradiol levels in ovariectomized patients with and without the symptom. However, this latter study must be questioned because the estrogen levels reported, particularly estrone, were notably higher than most other investigators have found in ovariectomized subjects (Judd, 1976).

The most extensive study of this type was published by Erlik and co-workers (1982). These investigators compared the physical characteristics and serum estrogen levels of 24 women complaining of frequent, severe hot flushes with those observed in an equal number of postmenopausal women who had never experienced the symptom (Figs. 11 and 12). The women with severe hot flushes were found to have significantly

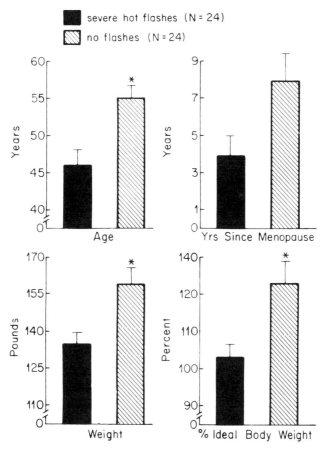

Fig. 11. Mean ± SE age, years since menopause, weight, and percent ideal weight in 24 women with severe hot flushes compared with an equal number of postmenopausal subjects who had never experienced the symptom. * = significantly different from asymptomatic subjects. (From Erlik *et al.*, 1982, with permission.)

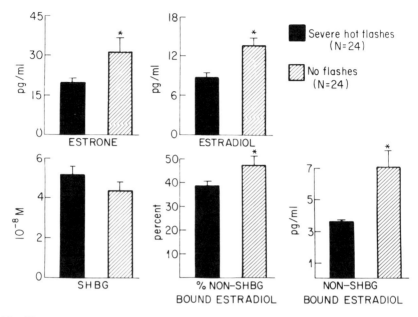

Fig. 12. Mean ± SE levels of estrone, estradiol, sex hormone-binding globulin (SHBG) percent non-SHBG bound estradiol, and non-SHBG-bound estradiol in 24 with severe flushes and an equal number of asymptomatic subjects. * = significantly different from asymptomatic subjects. (From Erlik *et al.*, 1982, with permission.)

lower mean body weight, percent ideal weight, and levels of total estrone and estradiol than the asymptomatic women. The occurrence of hot flushes in the symptomatic women was confirmed objectively. Subsets of the two groups of women matched for age, years since menopause, and ovarian status showed similar differences, excluding possible effects of these variables on the experimental findings. These data support the concept that body size and its effect on endogenous estrogen metabolism may be a factor responsible for the occurrence of hot flushes in some postmenopausal women and not others.

As previously mentioned, hypothalamic dysfunction plays a key role in the genesis of hot flushes. With minor exceptions, the hypothalamus is behind the blood brain barrier, which can exclude circulating substances which freely diffuse across other capillary beds. Thus, the fraction of circulating estrogens that could influence hypothalamic function should be that portion that is transported across the blood brain barrier.

Using an *in vivo* model to determine the fraction of circulating steroids which crosses the blood brain barrier of the rat, Pardridge and

Mietus (1979) have observed that the portion of estradiol not bound to the plasma protein, sex hormone-binding globulin (SHBG), is the fraction which is transported into the brain. These investigators have termed this measurement the Brain Uptake Index. This fraction of circulating estradiol, which includes the portion bound to albumin and not bound to plasma proteins, can also be assessed using an *in vitro* technique that measures the percent non-SHBG bound estradiol (Gambone *et al.*, 1982b). Using sera from 50 postmenopausal women, these investigators observed a significant linear correlation between the values obtained by the *in vitro* (percent non-SHBG bound estradiol) and the *in vivo* (Brain Uptake Index of Estradiol) assays with an *r* value of 0.895 (Fig. 13).

Based on this correlation, Erlik *et al.* (1982) measured the concentration of non-SHBG bound estradiol, and found the mean level in women who had never experienced a hot flush to be twice the mean concentration observed in women complaining of frequent, severe symptoms. This suggested this fraction of circulating estradiol may be a major factor influencing the occurrence of this disturbance.

Androstenedione is the major, if not exclusive, precursor of circulating estrogens in postmenopausal women (Siiteri and MacDonald, 1973; Judd *et al.*, 1982). Differences in the production rate of androstenedione could account for the differences of circulating estrogens present in these two groups of subjects. Studies have shown that the ovary after menopause continues to secrete a small amount of androstenedione and a substantial amount of testosterone (Judd, 1976). Erlik *et al.* (1982) matched

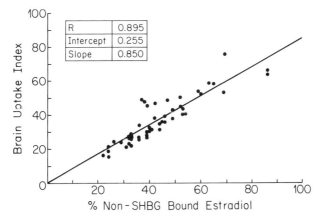

Fig. 13. Correlation of *in vitro* assay (% non-SHBG bound estradiol) with *in vivo* assay (Brain Uptake Index) of fraction of circulating estradiol available for transport across blood brain barrier. Samples tested were drawn from 50 postmenopausal women.

18 pairs of subjects for the presence of ovaries, and no significant differences were noted between the mean androstenedione levels in the women with or without hot flushes. Since the circulating level of androstenedione reflects its production rate (Bardin and Lipsett, 1967), these data do not support the concept that differences in the production rate of this androgen account for the differences in circulating estrogens observed in the two groups.

3.3. Adrenal Studies

The relationship of adrenal medullary function to hot flushes has been studied. Casper *et al.* (1979) found no change in the levels of dopamine, norepinephrine, or epinephrine before, during, or after flushes (Fig. 14). These findings were confirmed by Mashchak *et al.* (1982). These observations provide further support that hot flushes are triggered by central and not peripheral mechanisms. The relationship of adrenal

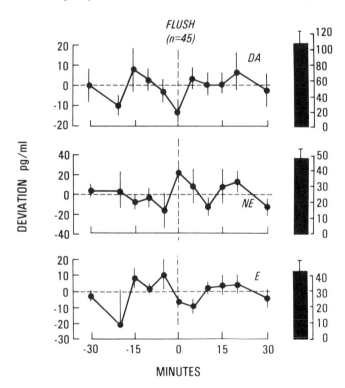

Fig. 14.   Correlation of onset of flushes with mean levels of dopamine (DA), norepinephrine (NE) and epinephrine. (From S. S. C. Yen, with permission.)

cortical function to hot flushes has also been examined. Meldrum *et al.* (1980) found significant increases of cortisol, dehydroepiandrosterone, and androstenedione occurring at the time of flushes (Fig. 15). A borderline significant rise ($P = 0.051$) of progesterone was also noted. The maximal increases of these hormones occurred 20, 15, 20, and 20 min after the onset of the subjective flushes for cortisol, dehydroepiandrosterone, androstenedione, and progesterone, respectively. Since these hormones are principally adrenal in origin, it was felt their pulsatile release represented enhanced adrenal secretion.

This apparent increase in adrenal cortical activity at the time of a flush could be explained by several possible mechanisms. First, perception of the discomfort of the flush could stimulate the hypothalamic-pituitary-adrenal axis as a manifestation of stress. Second, alterations of hypothalamic neurotransmitters could directly stimulate release of corticotropin-releasing hormone from the hypothalamus. Third, sudden ruminal cooling of the hypothalamus of the goat (Illner *et al.*, 1977) has

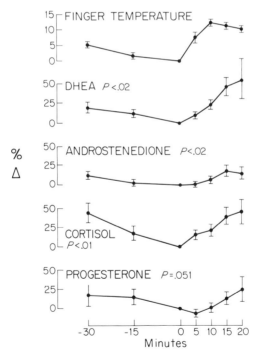

Fig. 15. Mean percentage changes of finger temperature and serum dihydroepiandrosterone, androstenedione, cortisol, and progesterone levels before and after objective flushes. (From Meldrum *et al.*, 1980, with permission.)

been shown to stimulate ACTH release. A similar mechanism may occur with a hot flush. Finally, changes in blood flow within the adrenal during a hot flush could affect steroidogenesis at a local level. Enhanced blood flow through the adrenal gland increases steroid secretion (Eik-Nes 1964; Porter and Klaiber, 1965). Further studies are needed to define this mechanism.

4. Sleep Studies

Hot flushes are a greater disturbance than most physicians have recognized. Patients experiencing the symptom frequently complain of "night sweats" and insomnia. To examine the relationship between hot flushes and sleep, Erlik *et al.* (1981b) recorded sleep stages using polygraphic techniques and the occurrence of hot flushes using objective methods. Patients with frequent, severe flushes were studied in a sleep laboratory after 2 nights of conditioning to the laboratory. In nine post-

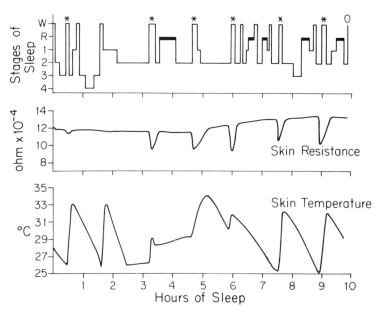

Fig. 16. Sleepgram and recordings of skin resistance and temperature in postmenopausal subject with severe flushes. Each * marks occurrence of objectively measured hot flush. Open circle indicates arousal of patient by investigator at end of study. (From Erlik *et al.*, 1981b, with permission.)

menopausal women, 45 of 47 objectively measured hot flushes which occurred during sleep and were associated with a waking episode within 5 min before or after the onset of the flush (Fig. 16). Although most hot flushes were associated with waking episodes, 40% of waking episodes were not associated with flushes. The onset of the waking episodes usually preceded any measurable change in perspiration or cutaneous vasodilation (Fig. 17). These findings suggest that hot flushes can lead to a chronic sleep disturbance in symptomatic women and that the onset of waking is due to a central disturbance rather than to the discomfort associated with cutaneous perspiration or vasodilation.

In five premenopausal controls, two simultaneous changes of skin temperature and resistance (objective criteria for a hot flush) were recorded and neither was associated with a waking episode (Fig. 18). This finding provided further support of the association between flushes and waking episodes in the symptomatic women.

Administration of estrogen to four of the patients significantly reduced the number of flushes and waking episodes (Fig. 19). With the use of randomized, prospective, double-blind studies, investigators have shown estrogen administered to postmenopausal women reduces the occurrence of hot flushes (Coope, 1976; Campbell and Whitehead, 1977), and improves certain aspects of sleep in comparison to placebo (Thomp-

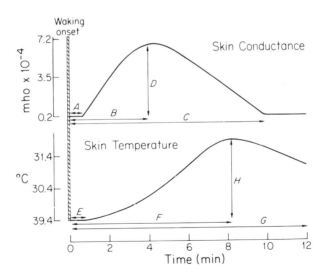

Fig. 17.   Mean interval and changes of skin conductance and temperature during 25 hot flushes that were associated with waking episodes. Data are plotted in reference to onset of awakening (hatched bar). (From Erlik *et al.*, 1981b, with permission.)

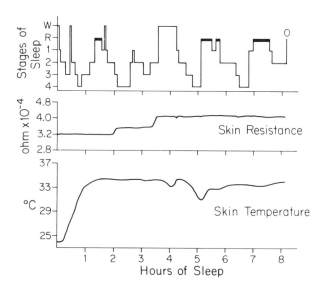

Fig. 18.   Sleepgram and skin resistance and temperature recordings of premenopausal subject. (From Erlik *et al.*, 1981b, with permission.)

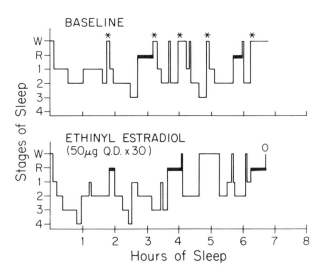

Fig. 19.   Sleepgram measured in symptomatic patient before and after 30 days administration of ethinyl estradiol, 50 µg/daily. (From Erlik *et al.*, 1981b, with permission.)

son and Oswald, 1977; Schiff *et al.*, 1979). Beneficial effects include decreases in insomnia, sleep latency and the number and duration of episodes of wakefulness, and increases in the length of sleep and the amount of rapid eye movement sleep. These actions are different from those observed with most sleeping pills. Hypnotic agents reduce both sleep latency and the time of rapid eye movement sleep (Kales *et al.*, 1975). Since a chronic sleep disturbance, as seen with hot flushes, can lead to disturbances of psychological function, the above findings provide a plausible explanation for the improvement of affective and cognitive functions that have been observed with estrogen administration in post-menopausal women experiencing severe flushes (Campbell and White-head, 1977).

5. Treatment

Because of the number of women experiencing the symptom, and the subjective nature of the complaint, it is not surprising that numerous agents have been used in an attempt to relieve hot flushes and many have been reported to be effective. Adding to the confusion are the observations of several investigative teams that marked placebo effects occur when double-blind studies are employed to evaluate various medications (Coope, 1976; Campbell and Whitehead, 1977). This latter problem has been alleviated with the use of objective measurement of flushes. When these techniques have been employed, no placebo effects have been noted in studies using single or double-blind study designs (DeFazio *et al.*, 1982; Laufer *et al.*, 1982).

Estrogen has been the principal medication utilized to relieve hot flushes. Although its efficacy has been questioned recently (Mulley and Mitchell, 1976), there are good randomized, prospective, double-blind, cross-over studies showing beneficial effects. Utian (1972) reported a reduction in symptomatic flushes with short-term estrogen replacement, using a single-blind, cross-over study design. Other investigators (Coope, 1976; Coope *et al.*, 1975; Campbell and Whitehead, 1977) also showed significant reductions of subjective flushing with estrogen with the investigative teams testing the daily administration of 1.25 mg of conjugated equine estrogens.

Estrogen not only blocks the subjective sensation but also the physiological changes. Meldrum *et al.* (1979) showed a significant reduction in the number and amplitude of finger temperature elevations in postmenopausal women given 50 μg of ethinyl estradiol for 30 days (Fig. 20).

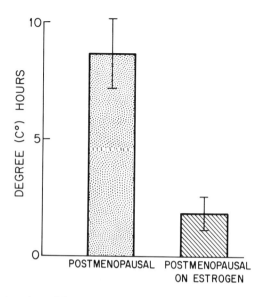

Fig. 20. Total elevation of finger temperature per 8-hr recording in postmenopausal women before and after estrogen treatment. (From Meldrum *et al.*, 1979, with permission.)

Although estrogen appears to be effective in preventing this symptom, there has been concern about the use of the medication because of possible side effects. These include endometrial cancer (Antunes *et al.*, 1979), hypertension (Pfeffer and Van den Noort, 1976; Stern *et al.*, 1976), and gallbladder disease (Boston Collaborative Drug Surveillance Program, 1974). Consequently, other medications have been tested with varying success.

Monthly, intramuscular injections of 150 mg of medroxyprogesterone acetate have been associated with a 90% reduction of flushes, which was significantly more than placebo (Bullock *et al.*, 1975). Daily, oral administration of 250 μg of *d*-norgestrel also has been shown to be more effective than placebo, but less efficacious than estrogen (Dennerstein *et al.*, 1978).

Progestational agents have also been shown to block objectively measured flushes. Erlik *et al.* (1981a) observed significant reductions of hot flushes with the daily administration of 20, 40, and 80 mg of megestrol acetate (Fig. 21), and Albrecht *et al.* (1981) reported significant decreases of objectively recorded flushes with 10 mg of medroxyprogesterone acetate.

Nonsteroidal medications also have been tried. Dithiocarbamoyl-hydrazine, a mild tranquillizer, was shown to effectively reduce subjec-

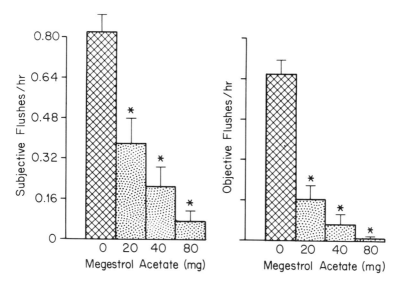

Fig. 21.   The mean ($\pm$ SE) subjective and objective flushes per hour before and following the oral administration of various doses of megestrol acetate. * = significantly different ($P < 0.01$) from baseline. (From Erlik *et al.*, 1981a, with permission.)

tively measured flushes with a double-blind study design (Ferriman and Purdie, 1965). As mentioned previously, clonidine, an α-adrenergic agonist, has been found to be partially effective in some but not all studies, (Clayden *et al.*, 1974; Barr, 1975; Bolli and Simpson, 1975; Lindsay and Hart, 1978; Laufer *et al.*, 1982); while propranolol, an α-adrenergic antagonist, does not appear to be more effective than placebo (Coope and Patterson, 1978). Numerous other compounds, including Vitamins E and K, mineral supplements, belladonna alkaloids in combination with mild sedatives, tranquillizers, sedatives, and antidepressants have all been used for the relief of the symptom, but their actual effectiveness have not been critically evaluated.

6.   References

Abe, T., Fuguhashi, N., Yamaya, Y., Wada, Y., Hoshiai, A., and Suzuki, M., 1977, Correlation between climacteric symptoms and serum levels of estradiol, progesterone, follicle-stimulating hormone, and luteinizing hormone, *Am. J. Obstet. Gynecol.* **123**:65–67.

Aitken, J. M., Davidson, A., England, P., Govan, A. D. T., Hart, D. M., Kelly, A., Lindsay, R., and Moffatt, A., 1974, The relationship between menopausal vasomotor symptoms and gonadotropin excretion in urine after oophorectomy, *J. Ob/Gyn. Brit. Commun.* **81**:150–154.

Aksel, S., Schomberg, D. W., Tyrey, L., and Hammond, C. B., 1976, Vasomotor symptoms, serum estrogens, and gonadotropin levels in surgical menopause, *Am. J. Obstet. Gynecol.* **126:**165–169.

Albeaux-Fernet, M., and Deribreux, J., 1946, La bouffee de chaleur symptome majeur de la menopause, *Semaine Hop. (Paris)* **22:**1500–1502.

Albrecht, B. H., Schiff, I., Tulchinsky, D., and Ryan, K. J., 1981, Objective evidence that placebo and oral medroxyprogesterone acetate therapy diminish menopausal vasomotor flushes, *Am. J. Obstet. Gynecol.* **139:**631–635.

Antunes, C. M., Stolley, P. D., Rosenshein, N. B., Davies, J. L., Tonascia, J. A., Brown, C., Burnett, L., Rutledge, A., Pokempner, M., and Garcia, R., 1979, Endometrial cancer and estrogen use, *N. Engl. J. Med.* **300:**9–13.

Bardin, C. W., and Lipsett, M. B., 1967, Testosterone and androstenedione blood production rates in normal women and women with idiopathic hirsutism or polycystic ovaries, *J. Clin. Invest.* **46:**891–902.

Barr, W., 1975, Problems related to postmenopausal women, *S. Afr. Med. J.* **49:**437–439.

Bhattacharya, A. N., Dierschke, D. J., Yamaji, T., and Knobil, E., 1972, The pharmacologic blockade of the circhoral mode of LH secretion in the ovariectomized rhesus monkey, *Endocrinology* **90:**778–786.

Bligh, J., 1973, *Temperature Regulation in Mammals and Other Vertebrates*, North-Holland Publishing, Amsterdam.

Bolli, P., and Simpson, F. O., 1975, Clonidine in menopausal flushing: A double blind trial, *New Zealand Med. J.* **82:**196–197.

Boston Collaborative Drug Surveillance Program, Boston University Medical Center, 1974, Surgically confirmed gallbladder disease, venous thromboembolism, and breast tumors in relation to postmenopausal estrogen therapy, *N. Engl. J. Med.* **290:**15–19.

Bullock, J. L., Massey, F. M., and Gambrell, R. D., Jr., 1975, Use of medroxyprogesterone acetate to prevent menopausal symptoms, *Obstet. Gynecol.* **46:**165–168.

Campbell, S., and Whitehead, M., 1977, Estrogen therapy and the postmenopausal syndrome, *Clin. Obstet. Gynecol.* **4:**31–47.

Carmel, P. W., Araki, S., and Ferin, M., 1976, Pituitary stalk portal blood collection in rhesus monkeys: Evidence for pulsatile release of gonadotropin-releasing hormone (GnRH), *Endocrinology* **99:**243–248.

Casper, R. F., and Yen, S. S. C., 1981, Menopausal flushes: Effect of pituitary gonadotropin desensitization by a potent luteinizing hormone-releasing factor agonist, *J. Clin. Endocrinol. Metabol.* **53:**1056–1058.

Casper, R. F., Yen, S. S. C., and Wilkes, M. M., 1979, Menopausal flushes: A neuroendocrine link with pulsatile luteinizing hormone secretion, *Science* **205:**823–825.

Chakravarti, S., Collins, W. P., Forecast, J. D., Newton, J. R., Oram, D. H., and Studd, J. W. W., 1976, Hormonal profiles after the menopause, *Brit. Med. J.* **2:**784–787.

Clayden, J. R., Bell, J. W., and Pollard, P., 1974, Menopausal flushing: Double-blind trial of a non-hormonal medication, *Brit. Med. J.* **1:**409–412.

Collett, M. E., 1949, Basal metabolism at the menopause, *J. Appl. Physiol.* **1:**629–639.

Coope, J., 1976, Double-blind cross-over study of estrogen replacement therapy, in: *The Management of the Menopausal and Postmenopausal Years* (S. Campbell, ed.), Baltimore University Park Press, Baltimore, pp. 159–168.

Coope, J., and Patterson, J. S., 1978, A study of the effectiveness of propanolol in menopausal hot flushes, *Brit. J. Obstet. Gynecol.* **85:**472–475.

Coope, J., Thomson, J. M., and Poller, L., 1975, Effects of "natural oestrogen" replacement therapy on menopausal symptoms and blood clotting, *Brit. Med. J.* **4:**139–143.

Cooper, K. E., Cranston, W. I., and Snell, E. S., 1964, Temperature regulation during fever in man, *Clin. Sci.* **27:**345–356.

Cox, B., and Lomax, P., 1977, Pharmacologic control of temperature regulation, *Annu. Rev. Pharmacol. Toxicol.* **17:**341–353.

Crowley, W. F., Jr., and McArthur, J. W., 1980, Simulation of the normal menstrual cycle in Kallman's Syndrome by pulsatile administration of luteinizing hormone-releasing hormone (LHRH), *J. Clin. Endocrinol. Metabol.* **51:**173–175.

Crowley, W. R., O'Donohue, T. L., Wachslicht, H., and Jacobowitz, D. M., 1978, Effects of estrogen and progesterone on plasma gonadotropins and on catecholamine levels and turnover in discrete brain regions of ovariectomized rats, *Brain Res.* **154:**345–357.

DeFazio, J., Meldrum, D., Laufer, L., Vale, W., Rivier, J., Lu, J., and Judd, H., 1982, Induction of hot flashes in premenopausal women treated with a long acting GnRH agonist, *Proc. 29th Annual Meeting Soc. Gynecol. Invest.* (Abst. 142), Dallas, Texas, March 24–27.

DeMorsier, G., and Gauthier, G., 1963, La dysplasie olfacto-genitale, *Pathol. Biol. (Paris)* **11:**1267–1272.

Dennerstein, L., Burrows, G. D., Hyman, G., and Wood, C., 1978, Menopausal hot flushes: A double-blind comparison of placebo, ethinyl oestradiol and norgestrel, *Brit. J. Obstet. Gynecol.* **85:**852–856.

Eik-Nes, K. B., 1964, On the relationship between testicular blood flow and secretion of testosterone in anesthetized dogs stimulated with human chorionic gonadotropins, *Can. J. Physiol. Pharmacol.* **42:**671–677.

Elkind-Hirsch, K. E., Ravnikar, V., Schiff, I., Tulchinsky, D., and Ryan, K. J., 1981, Determinations of endogenous immunoreactive LHRH levels in the plasma of postmenopausal women, *Proc. 28th Annual Meeting Soc. Gynecol. Invest.* (Abst. 20), St. Louis, Missouri, March 18–21.

Erlik, Y., Meldrum, D. R., Lagasse, L. D., and Judd, H. L., 1981a, Effect of megestrol acetate on flushing and bone metabolism in postmenopausal women, *Maturitas* **3:**167–172.

Erlik, Y., Tataryn, I. V., Meldrum, D. R., Lomax, P., Bajorek, J. G., and Judd, H. L., 1981b, Association of waking episodes with menopausal hot flushes, *J. Am. Med. Assoc.* **245:**1741–1744.

Erlik, Y., Meldrum, D. R., and Judd, H. L., 1982, Estrogen levels in postmenopausal women with hot flashes, *Obstet. Gynecol.* **59:**403–407.

Eskay, R. L., Mical, R. S., and Porter, J. C., 1977, Relationship between luteinizing hormone releasing hormone concentration in hypophysial blood and luteinizing hormone release in intact, castrated and electrochemically-stimulated rats, *Endocrinology* **100:**263–270.

Ferriman, D., and Purdie, A. W., 1965, Mechanism of menopausal hot flushes indicated by the effect of a dithiocarbamoylhydrazine, *J. Endocrinology* **31:**173–174.

Gambone, J., Meldrum, D., Laufer, L., Chang, J., Lu, J., and Judd, H., 1982a, Further delineation of hypothalamic dysfunction responsible for menopausal hot flashes, *Proc. 29th Annual Meeting Soc. Gynecol. Invest.* (Abst. 60), Dallas, Texas, March 24–27.

Gambone, J. C., Pardridge, W. A., Lagasse, L. D., and Judd, H. L., 1982b, *In vivo* availability of circulating estradiol in postmenopausal women with and without endometrial cancer, *Obstet. Gynecol.* **59:**416–421.

Greenfield, A. D., 1963, The circulation through the skin, *Handbook Physiol. Sect.* **2:**1325–1351.

Hannan, J. H., 1927, *The Flushings of the Menopause*, Bailliere, Tindall and Cox, London, pp. 1–22.

Houston, M., 1981, Clonidine hydrochloride: Review of pharmacologic and clinical aspects, *Prog. Cardiovasc. Dis.* **23**(5):337–350.

Hunter, D. J. S., Julier, D., Franklin, M., and Green, E., 1977, Plasma levels of estrogen, luteinizing hormone, and follicle stimulating hormone following castration and estradiol implant, *Obstet. Gynecol.* **49:**180–185.

Illner, P., Marques, P., Williams, D. D., Steiner, R. A., Green, W. L., Davis, S. L., Kendall, J. W., Johnson, D. G., and Gale, C. C., 1977, Endocrine responses to ruminal cooling in goats, in: *Proceedings of the Third Symposium on the Pharmacology of Thermoregulation* (K. E. Cooper and P. Lomax, eds.), Karger, Basel, pp. 58–61.

Jaszmann, L., Van Lith, N. D., and Zaat, J. C. A., 1969, The perimenopausal symptoms, *Med. Gynecol. Soc.* **4:**268–276.

Judd, H. L., 1976, Hormonal dynamics associated with the menopause, *Clin. Obstet. Gynecol.* **19:**775–788.

Judd, H. L., Shamonki, I. M., Frumar, A. M., and Lagasse, L. D., 1982, Origin of serum estradiol in postmenopausal women, *Obstet. Gynecol.* **59:**680–686.

Kales, A., Kales, J. D., Bixler, E. O., and Scharf, M. B., 1975, Effectiveness of hypnotic drugs with prolonged use: Flurozepan and pentobarbital, *Clin. Pharmacol. Ther.* **18:**356–363.

King, J. R., Jr., 1926, Observations on the menopause I. The basal metabolism after the artifical menopause, *Bull. Johns Hopkins Hosp.* **39:**281–303.

Kluger, M. J., 1978, The evolution and adaptive value of fever, *Ann. Sci.* **66:**38–43.

Kobayashi, R. M., Lu, K. H., Moore, R. Y., and Yen, S. S. C., 1978, Regional distribution of hypothalamic luteinizing hormone-releasing hormone in proestrous rats: Effects of ovariectomy and estrogen replacement, *Endocrinology* **102:**98–105.

Krey, L. C., Butler, W. R., and Knobil, E., 1975, Surgical disconnection of the medial basal hypothalamus and pituitary function in the rhesus monkey. I. Gonadotropin secretion, *Endocrinology* **96:**1073–1087.

Larsen, I. F., 1977, Hot flashes after hypophysectomy, *Brit. Med. J.* **2:**1356.

Laufer, L. R., Erlik, Y., Meldrum, D. R., and Judd, H. L., 1982, Effect of clonidine on hot flashes in postmenopausal women, *Obstet. Gynecol.,* (in press).

Leblanc, H., Lachelin, G. C. L., Abu-Fadil, S., and Yen, S. S. C., 1976, Effects of dopamine agonists on LH release in women, *J. Clin. Endocrinol. Metabol.* **44:**728–732.

Lindsay, R., and Hart, D. M., 1978, Failure of responses of menopausal vasomotor symptoms to clonidine, *Maturitas* **1:**21–25.

Linton, E. A., Bennet, G. W., and Whitehead, S. A., 1979, Prostaglandins and the release of LHRH from hypothalamic synaptosomes, *Neuroendocrinology* **28:**394–401.

Lomax, P., and Knox, G. V., 1973, The sites and mechanisms of action of drugs affecting thermoregulation, in: *The Pharmacology of Thermoregulation,* Karger, Basel, pp. 146–154.

Mashchak, C. A., Kletzky, O. A., Artel, R., and Mishell, D. R., Jr., 1982, Postmenopausal vasomotor perfusion changes investigated by digital plethysmography and plasma catecholamine levels, *Proc. 29th Annual Meeting Soc. Gynecol. Invest.* (Abst. 277), Dallas, Texas, March 24–27.

McKinlay, S., and Jeffreys, M., 1974, The menopausal syndrome, *Brit. J. Prev. Soc. Med.* **28:**108–115.

Meldrum, D. R., Shamonki, I. M., Frumar, A. M., Tataryn, I. V., Chang, R. J., and Judd, H. L., 1979, Elevations in skin temperature of the finger as an objective index of postmenopausal hot flashes: Standardization of the techniques, *Am. J. Obstet. Gynecol.* **135:**713–717.

Meldrum, D. R., Tataryn, I. V., Frumar, A. M., Erlik, Y., Lu, K. H., and Judd, H. L., 1980, Gonadotropins, estrogens, and adrenal steroids during the menopausal hot flash, *J. Clin. Endocrinol. Metabol.* **50:**685–689.

Meldrum, D. R., Erlik, Y., Lu, J. H. K., and Judd, H. L., 1981, Objectively recorded hot flashes in patients with pituitary insufficiency, *J. Clin. Endocrinol. Metabol.* **52:**684–687.

Molnar, G. W., 1975, Body temperatures during menopausal hot flashes, *J. Appl. Physiol.* **38:**499–503.

Molnar, G. W., 1979, Investigation of hot flashes by ambulatory monitoring, *Am. J. Physiol.* **237:**R306–310.

Mulley, G., and Mitchell, J. R. A., 1976, Menopausal flushing: Does oestrogen therapy make sense, *Lancet* **1:**1397–1399.

Mulley, G., Mitchell, J. R. A., and Tattersall, R. B., 1977, Hot flushes after hypophysectomy, *Brit. Med. J.* **2:**1062.

Neugarten, B. L., and Kraines, R. J., 1965, Menopausal symptoms in women of various ages, *Psychosom. Med.* **27:**266–273.

Pang, C. N., Zimmermann, E., and Sawyer, C. H., 1977, Morphine inhibition of the preovulatory surges of plasma luteinizing hormone and follicle stimulating hormone in the rat, *Endocrinology* **101:**1726–1732.

Pardridge, W. M., and Mietus, L. J., 1979, Transport of steroid hormones through the rat blood-brain barrier: Primary role of albumin-bound hormone, *J. Clin. Invest.* **64:**145–154.

Pfeffer, R. I., and Van den Noort, S., 1976, Estrogen use and stroke risk in postmenopausal women, *Am. J. Epidemiol.* **103:**445–456.

Plant, T. M., Krey, L. C., Moossy, J., McCormack, J. T., Hess, D. L., and Knobil, E., 1978, The arcuate nucleus and the control of gonadotropin and prolactin secretion in the female rhesus monkey, *Endocrinology* **102:**52–62.

Porter, J. C., and Klaiber, M. S., 1965, Corticosterone secretion in rats as a function of ACTH input and adrenal blood flow, *Am. J. Physiol.* **209:**811–814.

Quigley, M. E., Sheehan, K. L., Casper, R. F., and Yen, S. S. C., 1980, Evidence for increased dopaminergic and opioid activity in patients with hypothalamic hypogonadotropic amenorrhea, *J. Clin. Endocrinol. Metabol.* **50:**949–954.

Reaves, T. A., and Hayward, J. M., 1979, Hypothalamic and extrahypothalamic thermoregulatory centers, in: *Body Temperature: Regulation, Drug Effects and Therapeutic Implications* (P. Lomax and E. Schonbaum, eds.), Dekker, New York, pp. 39–70.

Reynolds, S. R. M., 1941, Dermovascular action of estrogen, the ovarian follicular hormone, *J. Invest. Dermatol.* **4:**7–22.

Reynolds, W. W., Casterlin, M. E., and Covert, J. B., 1974, Behavioral fever in teleost fishes, *Nature* **259:**41–42.

Satinoff, E., and Cantor, A., 1975, Intraventricular norepinephrine and thermoregulation in rats, in: *Temperature Regulation and Drug Action* (P. Lomax, E. Schonbaum, and J. Jacob, eds.), Karger, Basel, pp. 103–110.

Schiff, I., Regestein, Q., Tulchinsky, D., and Ryan, K. J., 1979, Effects of estrogens on sleep and psychological state of hypogonadal women, *J. Am. Med. Assoc.* **242:**2405–2407.

Siiteri, P. K., and MacDonald, P. C., 1973, Role of extraglandular estrogen in human endocrinology, in: *Handbook of Physiology: Endocrinology,* Vol. 2(1), (R. O. Greep and E. Astwood, eds.), American Physiological Society, Washington, D.C., pp. 615–629.

Simpkins, J. W., and Kalra, S. P., 1979, Central site(s) of norepinephrine and LHRH interaction, *Fed. Proc.* **38:**1107.

Snell, E. S., and Atkins, E., 1968, *The Mechanisms of Fever, the Biological Basis of Medicine* (E. E. Bittar and N. Bittar, eds.), Academic Press, New York, pp. 397–419.

Stern, M. P., Brown, B. W., Haskell, W. L., Farquhar, J. W., Wehrle, C. L., and Wood, P. D. S., 1976, Cardiovascular risk and use of estrogens or estrogen-progestagen combinations, *J. Am. Med. Assoc.* **235:**811–815.

Stone, S. C., Mickal, A., and Rye, P. H., 1975, Postmenopausal symptomatology, maturation index, and plasma estrogen levels, *Obstet. Gynecol.* **45:**625–627.

Sturdee, D. W., and Reece, B. L., 1979, Thermography of menopausal hot flushes, *Maturitas* **1:**201–205.

Sturdee, D. W., Wilson, K. A., Pipili, E., and Crocker, A. D., 1978, Physiological aspects of menopausal hot flush, *Brit. Med. J.* **2:**79–80.

Tataryn, I. V., Meldrum, D. R., Lu, K. H., Frumar, A. M., and Judd, H. L., 1979, LH, FSH, and skin temperature during the menopausal hot flash, *J. Clin. Endocrinol. Metabol.* **49:**152–154.

Tataryn, I. V., Lomax, P., Bajorek, J. G., Chesarek, W., Meldrum, D. R., and Judd, II. L., 1980, Postmenopausal hot flushes: A disorder of thermoregulation, *Maturitas* **2:**101–107.

Tataryn, I. V., Lomax, P., Meldrum, D. R., Bajorek, J. G., Chesarek, W., and Judd, H. L., 1981, Objective techniques for the assessment of postmenopausal hot flashes, *Obstet. Gynecol.* **57:**340–344.

Thompson, J., and Oswald, I., 1977, Effect of estrogen on the sleep, mood and anxiety of menopausal women, *Brit. Med. J.* **2:**1317–1319.

Thompson, B., Hart, S. A., and Durno, D., 1973, Menopausal age and symptomatology in general practice, *J. Biol. Sci.* **5:**71–82.

Utian, W. H., 1972, The mental tonic effect of oestrogens administered to oophorectomized females, *S. Afr. Med. J.* **46:**1079–1082.

Venables, R., 1967, Methods in psychophysiology (C. C. Brown, ed.), Williams Wilkins, Baltimore, pp. 1–26.

Yen, S. S. C., Rebar, R., Vandenberg, G., and Judd, H., 1973, Hypothalamic amenorrhea and hypogonadotropinism: Responses to synthetic LRF, *J. Clin. Endocrinol. Metabol.* **36:**811–816.

CHAPTER 11

Relation of the Neuroendocrine System to Reproductive Decline in Men

S. MITCHELL HARMAN

1. Introduction

In contrast to the sharp landmark provided by the menopause in aging women, reproductive senescence in men appears to be a gradual process. In fact, there is still some question as to whether a true male climacteric occurs at all in normal men. Certainly, some human males retain full reproductive function into extreme old age. For example, Seymour, *et al.* (1935) documented successful paternity in a 94-year-old man. Nonetheless, considerable published data support the concept that men do show reduced reproductive capacity with age. This phenomenon may seem of little interest in the human male, since only rarely are new offspring desired by men past the age of 50. The subject of sexual function in older men, however, arouses lively interest because, in humans, sexual activity is not necessarily associated with procreation, but rather serves deeply felt personal needs, reinforces the permanence of pair-bonding, and hence is at the root of the stability of human families and, thus, societies. It is important to remember that the same hormones which regulate reproductive function also support and modulate sexual capacity and drive. Alterations in the secretion of these hormones, whether produced by aging or disease, can produce deleterious effects on sex drive and capacity which will be of concern to men of any age. Such

S. MITCHELL HARMAN • Endocrinology Section, Clinical Physiology Branch, Gerontology Research Center, National Institute on Aging, NIH, Baltimore City Hospital, Baltimore, Maryland 21224.

alterations could occur as a result of aging changes in the function of the testes themselves. They might result from alterations in the pituitary gland, which secretes the gonadotropic hormones LH and FSH. Finally, aging changes might occur primarily in the hypothalamus, which regulates pituitary gonadotropic function both by secretion of the stimulatory polypeptide, luteinizing hormone-releasing hormone (LHRH), and by release of the neurotransmitter, dopamine, which inhibits pituitary secretion of prolactin. Both LHRH and Dopamine are released by hypothalamic neurosecretory cells into capillaries of the ventral hypothalamus and hence into the pituitary portal circulation.

2. Testis

Besides germ cells, the testes produce the sex steroid hormones, the major one being the androgen, testosterone. Pedersen-Bjergaard and Jonnesen (1948) were the first investigators to demonstrate a decrease in androgens in aging men. They found that bioassayable androgen excreted in urine decreased after age 40, reaching very low levels by the eighth decade. Hollander and Hollander (1958) found similar aging changes in testosterone concentration in testicular vein blood obtained during surgery. Investigators using chromatographic, isotope dilution, and spectrophotometric methods (Coppage and Cooner, 1965; Kent and Acone, 1966; Gandy and Peterson, 1968) all failed to confirm a decrease in peripheral serum-testosterone level with age in men. Kirschner and Coffman (1968) did find a decrease in serum testosterone and Kent and Acone (1966) reported decreases in both testosterone production and metabolism rates in older men.

More recently, a large number of investigations using radioimmunoassay to quantify testosterone, have shown a decrease in plasma testosterone concentrations in men with age (Baker *et al.*, 1976; Frick, 1969; Mazzi *et al.*, 1974; Nieschlag *et al.*, 1973; Rubens *et al.*, 1974; Horton *et al.*, 1975; Stearns *et al.*, 1974; Pirke and Doerr, 1973; Vermeulen *et al.*, 1972; Lewis *et al.*, 1976; Forti *et al.*, 1974; Nankin *et al.*, 1981). In general, a decline in mean serum testosterone seemed to begin at about age 50 and to progress into the eighth or ninth decades. Although Vermeulen *et al.* (1972) reported a decrease with age in mean serum testosterone after age 50, they found a wide scatter of individual values, with many elderly men having normal testosterone levels, but also an increase with age in the number of men with testosterone levels in the frankly hypogonadal, i.e., pathologic, range (Fig. 1).

Since testosterone availability to target tissues is modulated by its

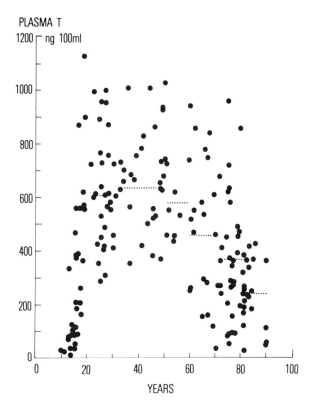

Fig. 1. Effect of aging on total serum testosterone concentrations in men. (From Vermeulen *et al.*, 1972.)

binding to a plasma globulin (SHBG), a number of investigators have inquired whether age-related alterations in binding might occur which would affect the free (bioavailable) testosterone fraction. These studies have generally resulted in the conclusion that SHBG capacity increases with age (Fig. 2) producing a decrease in the free testosterone fraction and hence in the plasma-free testosterone (Fig. 3). This decrease in indices of free testosterone appears more prominent than the decrease in total plasma testosterone in some studies (Baker *et al.*, 1976; Horst *et al.*, 1974; Kley *et al.*, 1974; Pirke and Doerr, 1973, 1975b; Vermeulen and Verdonck, 1972; Vermeulen *et al.*, 1972; Rubens *et al.*, 1974; Stearns *et al.*, 1974). A number of these workers have hypothesized that the increase in SHBG might be secondary to an increase in plasma estrogenic steroids, since it is known that estrogens promote synthesis of SHBG by the liver. Increased plasma concentrations of unconjugated estradiol and

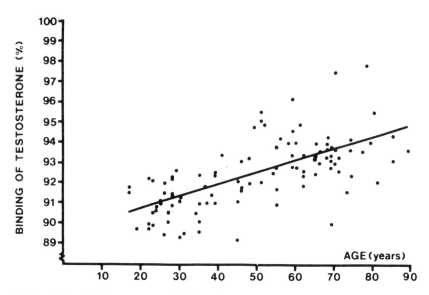

Fig. 2. Effect of aging on percent binding of testosterone to sex hormone binding globulin in sera of men. (From Kley *et al.*, 1974.)

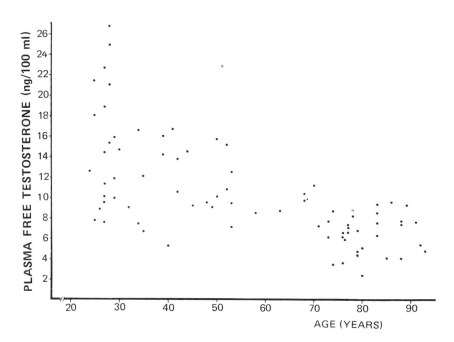

Fig. 3. Effect of aging on free testosterone index in sera of men. (From Pirke and Doerr, 1975b.)

estrone have indeed been demonstrated in older men in many of these same studies (Kley *et al.*, 1974; Pirke and Doerr, 1975b; Rubens *et al.*, 1974). This increase in estrogens did not appear to be simply a result of increased binding protein (SHBG also binds estrogens), since the free estrogen concentrations were also increased (Pirke and Doerr, 1975b; Rubens *et al.*, 1974). Other workers have not found altered plasma estrogen concentrations in older men (Stearns *et al.*, 1974; Zumoff *et al.*, 1982; Sparrow *et al.*, 1980; Nankin *et al.*, 1981; Lammers *et al.*, 1982).

Harman and Tsitouras (1980) have studied these issues in men in the Baltimore Longitudinal Study (BLS). These men are a group of healthy, well-educated, and prosperous volunteers, who report to the Gerontology Research Center of the NIA every 1–2 years for 2 days of extensive study by various investigative groups. Because they are ambulatory and in good health, they are less likely to show effects of variables other than aging *per se* on their endocrine function. As can be seen in Fig. 4A, in 69 men aged 25–90 there was no decrease in serum

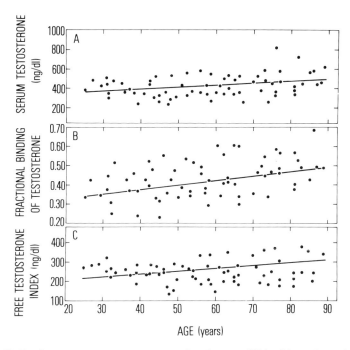

Fig. 4. (A) Total serum testosterone concentrations in sera of 69 healthy male participants in the BLS, aged 25–80; (B) fractional binding of testosterone to sex hormone-binding globulin in these same men; (C) free testosterone indices of the same men (percent binding × total testosterone concentration). (From Harman and Tsitouras, 1980.)

testosterone with age. Each point is the mean of duplicate determinations on four sera taken over a period of 1 hr. In Fig. 4B the fractional binding of serum testosterone to SHBG is shown to increase slightly but statistically significantly with age ($p < 0.05$). The free testosterone index, which is presumably correlated with the bioavailable serum T, shows no significant change with age (Fig. 4C). They also found no increase in the serum estrogens with age. Both estrone and estradiol remained stable, as can be seen in Fig. 5.

Most androgen target tissues reduce testosterone to 5α-dihydrotestosterone (DHT), which then binds to cytoplasmic androgen receptors. DHT is the intracellular active androgen, and can therefore be thought of as more potent than testosterone, while plasma testosterone may be considered a circulating reservoir of precursor androgen. DHT is also found in serum, coming about 20% from direct testicular secretion and 80% from peripheral reduction of testosterone in cells containing 5α-reductase followed by release from these (presumably target) cells into the circulation. Circulating DHT may thus be an indirect indicator of target tissue androgenic exposure. Giusti *et al.* (1975) reported reduced DHT as well as testosterone in testicular vein blood. Pirke and Doerr

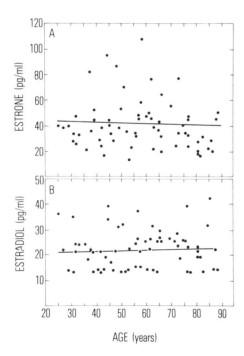

Fig. 5. (A) Serum estrone concentrations in BLS men aged 25–80; (B) serum estradiol concentrations in the same men. (From Harman and Tsitouras, 1980.)

(1975a), Pazzagli *et al.* (1975), and Lewis *et al.* (1976) all found somewhat decreased DHT in peripheral vein blood of aging men. Pirke and Doerr (1975b) reported no significant change in total serum DHT, but decreased free DHT and an increase in DHT/testosterone ratio, suggesting more efficient reduction of testosterone to DHT with advancing age. Harman and Tsitouras (1980), Zumoff *et al.* (1982), and Lammers *et al.* (1982) did not see any change in DHT concentrations with age, while Horton *et al.* (1975) reported a significant increase in plasma DHT in a group of older men with a high incidence of benign prostatic hyperplasia, despite a decrease in the precursor, testosterone.

The reasons for the wide variety of results obtained for plasma sex steroids of aging men in various studies is far from clear. It is possible that in some studies, altered sex steroid levels may represent effects of non-comparability of old and young study subjects for such variables as chronic illness, medications, obesity, alcohol intake, or environmental stress (all of which can affect plasma testosterone), rather than age *per se.*

In general, when special care is taken to exclude ill or debilitated subjects, as by Harman and Tsitouras (1980), Sparrow *et al.* (1980), and Lammers *et al.* (1982), little or no change in sex steroids has been observed. Exceptions to this generalization may be the studies of Nankin *et al.* (1981), in which a modest, but significant decrease in total serum testosterone was observed (474 vs. 651 ng/dl, $p < 0.05$) in six elderly men, and Purifoy *et al.* (1981), in which a decrease in total testosterone of only borderline significance ($0.1 < p < 0.05$) occurred with age, but a highly significant decline in free testosterone index occurred.

When only single blood samples are examined, variance is increased due to the considerable minute to minute variation of plasma testosterone, reflecting episodic secretion. In addition, there is a pattern of diurnal variation with a morning peak and lower afternoon plateau in plasma testosterone. A loss of the morning peak in older men could result in the appearance of reduced plasma testosterone with age when morning samples are examined and no reduction when afternoon samples are compared (as by Harman and Tsitouras, 1980). Bremner and Prinz (1981) did, in fact, find a loss of diurnal testosterone peak in elderly men, so that morning but not afternoon values appeared to decrease with age. In contrast, Murono *et al.* (1982) have found intact diurnal rhythm of testosterone in their older men, and the diurnal effect did not account for the observation of unchanged plasma testosterone in morning samples by Sparrow *et al.* (1980), Tsitouras *et al.* (1982), and Lammers *et al.* (1982). On the other hand, Zumoff *et al.* (1982) found significantly reduced 24-hr mean integrated plasma testosterone in older men, whom they describe as healthy and ambulatory. The issue is not yet settled.

A number of investigators have used human chorionic gonadotropin (hCG) stimulation to compare Leydig cell reserve capacity in men of various ages. Frick (1969), Longcope (1973), and Mazzi et al. (1974) all found that, although both baseline and peak testosterone levels were lower in older men, the percent response appeared unchanged with age. This finding is consistent with a reduced complement of normally responsive Leydig cells in older men. Rubens et al. (1974), Nieschlag et al. (1973), Nankin et al. (1981), and Lammers et al. (1982) all found reduced percent responses as well as absolute peak levels of testosterone after hCG stimulation. Nankin et al. (1981) state that both early and late testosterone response components were reduced in aging men and that younger men showed greater rises in 17-hydroxy-progesterone and estradiol as well as in testosterone.

Table 1 shows that when Harman and Tsitouras (1980) stimulated the testes of BLS men with hCG, 2000 IU/day for 2 days, there was a decrease in the responses of the older and to a lesser extent of the middle-aged men at 15 hr. By 39 hr the difference between young and middle-aged men was no longer significant, but the older men still remained about 50% less responsive. The results of hCG stimulation data favor the hypothesis that Leydig cell number and/or reserve secretory capacity is diminished with age in men.

Another consideration with regard to androgens and their effects is the question of whether target tissue sensitivity to these hormones may be altered with age. Although this question is difficult to answer in humans, the findings by Muta et al. (1981) that more testosterone is required to inhibit gonadotropin secretion in aged men and that by

Table 1. Serum Testosterone after Injection of hCG: Effect of Age on Response/Basal Ratio[a]

Group	Age	15-hr post hCG	39-hr post hCG
		Mean ± SEM	
A	25–49	1.98 ± 0.13	2.20 ± 0.13
B	50–69	1.53 ± 0.09[b]	1.86 ± 0.11
C	70–89	1.55 ± 0.11[c]	1.76 ± 0.13[d]

[a] Different from group A, $p < 0.01$.
[b] Different from group A, $p < 0.02$.
[c] Different from group A, $p < 0.05$.
[d] From Harman and Tsitouras, 1980.

Desleypere and Vermeulen (1981) that binding of DHT to sex hormone responsive skin is reduced in older men, suggest that androgen responsiveness may be decreased with age, perhaps as a result of diminished hormone receptor capacity.

3. Pituitary

A modest but significant increase in excretion of urinary gonadotropins in aging men was first recorded by Pedersen-Bjergaard and Jonnesen (1948) using bioassay methods. This was confirmed by Albert (1956) and by Christiansen (1972), who reported that although both LH and FSH were elevated, the increase in FSH was more prominent. More recent studies, using radioimmunoassay methods have nearly all demonstrated increased circulating gonadotropin concentrations in men after about age 50 (Haug *et al.*, 1974; Mazzi *et al.*, 1974; Rubens *et al.*, 1974; Snyder *et al.*, 1975; Baker *et al.*, 1976; Stearns *et al.*, 1974). Some subjects in their 80s and 90s had LH and FSH concentrations similar to those seen in postmenopausal women or castrate men. The elevations of plasma gonadotropin concentration appear to be due to increased secretion rather than diminished elimination of hormone, since the rate of clearance of LH from plasma appears to be age invariant (Kohler *et al.*, 1968; Pepperell *et al.*, 1975). This increase in gonadotropin secretion has been interpreted to be a secondary phenomenon due to a primary reduction in Leydig cell function with resulting decrease in sex steroid feedback inhibition of the hypothalamic-pituitary axis. It has been suggested that the greater increase in FSH than LH may represent the independent regulation of FSH secretion by a seminiferous tubular factor (inhibin) which becomes deficient as tubular function decreases with age (Baker *et al.*, 1976). This hypothesis is consistent with experiments showing significantly increased FSH but no increase in LH in healthy elderly men with unaltered (Sparrow *et al.*, 1980) or even moderately decreased (Zumoff *et al.*, 1982) plasma testosterone concentrations. In contrast, in similar subjects, Harman *et al.* (1982) measured increases in both serum FSH and LH levels, despite unchanged plasma sex steroid concentrations. The LH increase, they concluded, might represent compensation for a mild degree of Leydig cell failure (as demonstrated by decreased testosterone response to hCG), reduction in feedback sensitivity of the hypothalamic-pituitary axis (as suggested by Dilman and Anasimov, 1979), or a combination of both these factors. Direct evidence for an age-related alteration in the feedback control of gonadotropin secretion comes from work by Muta *et al.* (1981) showing greater steroid dose requirements for inhibition of gonadotropin secretion in young vs. old men.

On the other hand, the finding by Rubens *et al.* (1974) and others that plasma testosterone levels were decreased in their men despite demonstrated residual Leydig cell secretory capacity (in response to hCG injection), raises the question whether some limitation of gonadotropin responsiveness may develop in older men, since they failed to secrete enough LH to return plasma testosterone concentrations to normal. Ryan (1962) reported increased LH content of male human pituitaries with age, eliminating exhaustion of pituitary hormone stores as an explanation for submaximal gonadotropic response. Use of LHRH (lutropin) to test pituitary secretory reserve for LH and FSH has given various results. Rubens *et al.* (1974) and Hashimoto *et al.* (1973) found percent, but not absolute incremental LH and FSH responses, to be diminished in older men. This was due to elevated basal levels, i.e., an increased denominator with no increase in the numerator. Since in young men, LHRH responses increase roughly in proportion to basal gonadotropin levels, they interpreted their results to mean that some diminution of pituitary LHRH responsiveness did occur with age. Haug *et al.* (1974) and Snyder *et al.* (1975) both reported decreases in absolute as well as relative LHRH responses.

To evaluate the responsiveness of the pituitary gland of aged men, Harman *et al.* (1982) measured gonadotropins, both basal levels and responses to a 100-μg intravenous bolus of LHRH. They found that basal levels of LH were significantly higher in older men, but response peaks were not significantly different (Fig. 6, upper). On the other hand, percent responses were significantly reduced with age. They reported similar results for FSH basal levels and responses (Fig. 6, lower). Since it is known that as basal gonadotropin level increases, the magnitude of the response to LHRH also increases, but the percent response decreases, it was at first unclear to what extent the responses were altered as an effect of age, and to what extent they merely reflected the increase in basal gonadotropin levels. To get at this question, it was necessary to use repeated measures analysis of variance to correct response criteria for the effect of basal level. The finding of a highly significant interaction term in this analysis is consistent with the conclusion that these men had smaller LH and FSH responses to LHRH than would be expected for their (elevated) basal gonadotropin levels. Although providing evidence of some impairment of pituitary gonadotropin secretory response, all the above studies document the existence of some pituitary gonadotropic reserve capacity. Therefore, the question why, in those studies where

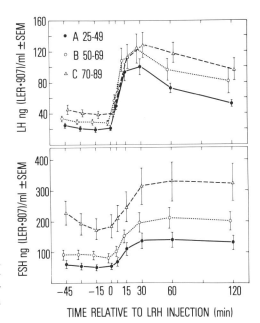

Fig. 6. Mean serum gonadotropin concentrations before and up to 120 min after intravenous injection of a 200-μg bolus of LHRH into 69 male BLS subjects of various ages (upper panel, LH; lower panel, FSH). (From Harman *et al.*, 1982.)

plasma testosterone was diminished, the LH production did not increase enough to return testosterone concentrations to "normal" is still moot. That such compensation may sometimes occur is suggested by the study of Harman and Tsitouras (1980), who found normal serum testosterone with elevated basal LH levels. Its failure to occur in other studies may represent suppression of LH secretion by other plasma steroids, e.g., estrogens or DHT), a resetting of the hypothalamic "steroidostat" to accept somewhat lower levels of testosterone as normal, or disturbance of the hypothalamic-hypophyseal response to diminished steroids due to concomitant illness, general debilitation, or aging itself.

4. Hypothalamus

Use of clomiphene citrate (an estrogen antagonist) to block hypothalamic-estrogen receptors and hence release gonadotropin secretion from steroid feedback inhibition is another way to test LH and FSH secretory reserve. Unlike LHRH infusion, clomiphene tests the hypothalamic as well as the pituitary secretory responses. When such tests have been done in elderly men (Mazzi *et al.*, 1974; Natoli *et al.*, 1972; Rubens *et al.*, 1974) a reduction in LH response has been consistently found. However, since only LH and FSH (not LHRH) were measured, the tests did not distinguish between alterations at the hypothalamic vs. the pituitary level (in the latter of which hyporesponsiveness is already documented).

The role of altered prolactin secretion as a cause and/or effect of age-related changes in reproductive hormone regulation is unclear. In men, Vekemans and Robyn (1975) have reported a modest rise in basal serum prolactin levels with age. Hossdorf and Wagner (1980) found no such change in basal levels, but demonstrated a significantly higher and later prolactin peak response to thyrotropin-releasing hormone (TRH) stimulation in older men. Murri *et al.* (1980) have found that the diurnal rhythm for prolactin, studied in 12 subjects aged 62–78, was similar to that in young men. Although clinical hyperprolactinemia is associated with hypogonadism and impotence (Carter *et al.*, 1978), the degree of change observed in the above studies of aging men is not sufficient to produce a decrease in reproductive capacity.

5. Sex Hormones and Sexual Function

At the time we began our studies, there was data from Kinsey *et al.* (1948) showing steady decrease in the frequency of intercourse in American men from age 30 on. The same study showed a rise in the overall incidence of impotence with age. Other investigators (Newman and Nichols, 1960; Pfeiffer and Davis, 1972) have reached similar conclusions. In more recent studies (Martin, 1977, 1981), Baltimore Longitudinal Study of Aging (BLS) men showed a similar decrease in level of sexual activity (defined as all events leading to orgasm) with age. These men reported that as they became older, the time span over which they were comfortable without sex increased and their awareness of erotic sensation from visual stimuli diminished. There was a clear tendency for men with higher levels of sexual activity in their youth to sustain higher levels into their sixties and seventies. Harman *et al.* (1979) have reported on their subjects' sexual activity levels, defined as the total number of events leading to orgasm in the year prior to interview. It was apparent that, despite their unaltered sex steroid concentrations, the number of sexual events per year fell precipitously from approximately 140 in the late 20's, to less than 20 events per year by age 70. When they tested the correlation of sexual activity with serum free testosterone index within each age group, a significant correlation ($p < 0.05$) was found only in the oldest men. It seemed, therefore, that in their elderly men, even though mean testosterone levels had not decreased, those who maintained the highest levels of sexual activity tended to have higher testosterone concentrations.

There are data to support the concept that testosterone is important for maintenance of male sex drive and potency in humans (Davidson *et al.*, 1979) and that seasonal variations in testosterone level may influence the frequency of sexual activity in men (Reinberg and Lagoguey, 1978). Vermeulen (1979) has also published results suggesting that the decline in sexual activity in older men may be correlated with the decrease he observed in free serum testosterone index.

In order to further investigate this relationship, Tsitouras *et al.* (1982) examined testosterone and sexual activity levels in 180 additional men aged 60–80 years. They distributed men in each 5-year age interval into tertiles classified as high, medium, and low sexual activity. This was necessary because sexual activity changed so much between 60–80 years of age that a sexual frequency which would be low average in a 60–65-year-old man would be extremely high for a 75–80-year-old man. Thus, absolute numbers of sexual events were not simply comparable across the whole age range. Analysis of variance showed that the mean testosterone was significantly lower in the low activity group ($p < 0.05$) than in the other two groups (Fig. 7). Furthermore, χ^2 testing on the distribution of sexual activity groups into high (> 80th percentile), middle (20th–80th), and low (< 20th percentile) classes for serum testosterone showed significantly more men with high sexual activity in the high testosterone and with low sexual activity in the low testosterone classes ($p < 0.01$).

They next asked whether the correlation of testosterone with sexual activity might be specious or misleading in the sense of being due to some intervening variable related to both. For instance, heavy alcohol intake might lead independently to both low testosterone and low sexual activity levels. They compared body composition measurements made by the Metabolism Branch, Gerontology Research Center (GRC), and found that indices of obesity and muscularity did not differ among the sexual activity groups. There were also no differences in use of cigarettes or coffee, nor in the presence of detectable coronary vascular disease. Alcohol consumption was higher in the low sex group, but, although it is known that high levels of alcohol consumption can lower serum testosterone there was no apparent effect of alcohol on serum testosterone, at the levels consumed by these subjects. The correlation of sexual activity and serum testosterone in older men is open to several interpretations. It may be that sexual activity itself is a stimulus to increased testosterone secretion (although this has never been convincingly demonstrated in humans). It is also possible that the decreased sexual activity in older

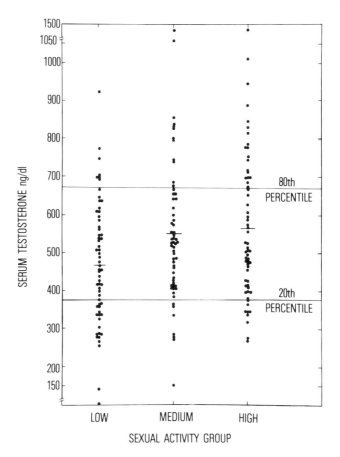

Fig. 7. Individual and mean serum testosterone concentrations in 180 BLS men aged 60–79 divided into tertiles by level of sexual activity in comparison with men in the same half-decade. (From Tsitouras *et al.*, 1982.)

men is, in part, a manifestation of decreasing sensitivity to testosterone of central nervous system structures pertinent to male erotic responsiveness (either through loss of androgen receptors or some other mechanism). This might explain why variation in testosterone in the normal range appears to be related to sexual activity in older, but not in younger men. Finally, it is possible that some third variable, perhaps as nonspecific as "general vigor" might be associated independently with higher testosterone levels and better maintenance of sexual activity in old age.

Further investigations into the effects of aging on hormones and hormone action should help to elucidate these issues.

6. References

Albert, A., 1956, Human urinary gonadotropins, *Rec. Prog. Horm. Res.* **12:**266.

Baker, H. W. G., Bremner, W. J., Burger, H. G., deKretser, D. M., Dulmanis, A., Eddie, L. W., Hudson, B., Keogh, E. J., Lee, V. W. K., and Rennie, G. C., 1976, Testicular control of follicle stimulating hormone secretion, *Rec. Prog. Horm. Res.*, **32:**429–476.

Bremner, W. J., and Prinz, P. N., 1981, The diurnal rhythm in testosterone levels is lost with aging in normal men, *Endocrine Soc. 63rd Annual Meeting* (Abst. 480), p. 202.

Carter, J. N., Tyson, J. G., Tolis, G., VanVliet, S., Faiman, C., and Friesen, H. G., 1978, Prolactin secreting tumors and hypogonadism in 22 men, *N. Engl. J. Med.* **299:**847–852.

Christiansen, P., 1972, Urinary follicle stimulating hormone and luteinizing hormone in normal adult men, *Acta Endocrinol. (Kbh.)* **71:**1–6.

Coppage, W. S., and Cooner, A. E., 1965, Testosterone in human plasma, *N. Engl. J. Med.* **273:**902–905.

Davidson, J. M., Camargo, C. A., and Smith, E. R., 1979, Effects of androgen on sexual behavior in hypogonadal men, *J. Clin. Endocrinol. Metabol.* **48:**955–958.

Desleypere, J. P., and Vermeulen, A., 1981, Aging and tissue androgens, *J. Clin. Endocrinol. Metabol.* **53:**430–434.

Dilman, V. M., and Anasimov, V. N., 1979, Hypothalamic mechanisms of aging and of specific age pathology I. On the sensitivity threshold of hypothalamic-pituitary complex to homeostatic stimuli in the reproductive system, *Exp. Gerontol.* **14:**161–174.

Forti, G., Pazzagli, M., Calabresi, E., Fiorelli, G., and Serio, M., 1974, Radioimmunoassay of plasma testosterone, *Clin. Endocrinol.* **3:**5–17.

Frick, J., 1969, Darstellung eine Methode (competitive protein binding) zur Bestimmung des Testosteronspiegels im Plasma und Studie uber den Testosteronmetabolismus beim Mann uber 60 Jahre, *Urol. Int.* **24:**481–501.

Gandy, H. M., and Peterson, R. E., 1968, Measurement of testosterone and 17 KS in plasma by the double isotope dilution derivative technique, *J. Clin. Endocrinol. Metabol.* **28:**949–956.

Giusti, G., Gonelli, P., Borreli, D., Fiorelli, G., Forti, G., Pazzagli, M., and Serio, M., 1975, Age related secretion of androstenedione, testosterone, and dihydrotestosterone by the human testis, *Exp. Gerontol.* **10:**241–245.

Harman, S. M., and Tsitouras, P. D., 1980, Reproductive hormones in aging men I: Measurement of sex steroids, basal LH, and Leydig cell response to hCG, *J. Clin. Endocrinol. Metabol.* **51:**35–40.

Harman, S. M., Martin, C. E., and Tsitouras, P. D., 1979, Aging, sex steroids and sexual function in healthy men, *Endocrine Soc. 61st Annual Meeting* (Abst. 132).

Harman, S. M., Tsitouras, P. D., Costa, P. T., and Blackman, M. R., 1982, Reproductive hormones in aging men II: Basal pituitary gonadotropins and gonadotropin responses to luteinizing hormone releasing hormone, *J. Clin. Endocrinol. Metabol.* **54:**547–551.

Hashimoto, T., Miyai, K., Izumi, K., and Kumahara, Y., 1973, Gonadotropin response to synthetic LHRH in normal subjects: Correlation between LH and FSH, *J. Clin. Endocrinol. Metabol.* **37:**910–916.

Haug, E. A., Aakvaag, A., Sand, T., and Torjesen, P. A., 1974, The gonadotropin response to synthetic LHRH in males in relation to age, dose, and basal levels of testosterone, estradiol-17-beta, and gonadotropins, *Acta Endocrinol. (Kbh.)* **77:**625–635.

Hollander, N., and Hollander, V. P., 1958, The microdetermination of testosterone in human spermatic vein blood, *J. Clin. Endocrinol. Metabol.* **38:**966–971.

Horst, H. J., Becker, H., and Voigt, K. D., 1974, The determination of specific testosterone and 5-α-dihydrotestosterone binding to sex hormone binding globulin by a differential dissociation technique, *Steroids* **23:**833–846.

Horton, R., Hsieh, P., Barberia, J., Pages, L., and Cosgrove, M., 1975, Altered blood androgens in elderly men with prostate hyperplasia, *J. Clin. Endocrinol. Metabol.* **41**:793–796.

Hossdorf, T., and Wagner, H., 1980, Secretion of prolactin in healthy men and women of different age, *Aktuel Gerontol.* **10**:119–126.

Kent, J. Z., and Acone, A. B., 1966, Plasma androgens and aging, in: *Androgens in Normal and Pathological Conditions*, ICS No. 101 (A. Vermeulen and D. Exley, eds.), Excerpta Medica, Amsterdam, pp. 31–40.

Kinsey, A. C., Pomeroy, W. B., and Martin, C. E., 1948, *Sexual Behavior in the Human Male*, W. B. Saunders, Philadelphia.

Kirschner, M. A., and Coffman, G. D., 1968, Measurement of plasma testosterone and delta-4-androstenedione using electron capture gas liquid chromatography, *J. Clin. Endocrinol. Metabol.* **28**:1347–1352.

Kley, H. K., Nieschlag, E., Bidlingmaier, F., and Kruskemper, H. L., 1974, Possible age dependent influence of estrogens on the binding of testosterone in plasma of adult men, *Horm. Metabol. Res.* **6**:213–215.

Kohler, P. O., Ross, G. T., and Odell, W. D., 1968, Metabolic clearance and production rates of human luteinizing hormone in pre- and postmenopausal women, *J. Clin. Invest.* **47**:38–47.

Lewis, J. G., Ghanadian, R., and Chisholm, G. D., 1976, Serum 5-α-dihydrotestosterone and testosterone, changes with age in man, *Acta Endocrinol. (Kbh.)* **82**:444–449.

Longcope, C., 1973, The effect of human chorionic gonadotropin on plasma steroid levels in young and old men, *Steroids* **21**:583–592.

Martin, C. E., 1977, *Sexual Activity in the Aging Male* (J. Money and H. Musaph, eds.), ASP Biol. Med. Press, Amsterdam.

Martin, C. E., 1981, Factors affecting sexual functioning in 60–79-year-old married males, *Arch. Sex. Behav.* **10**:399–420.

Mazzi, C., Riva, L. R., and Bernasconi, D., 1974, *Gonadotropins and Plasma Testosterone in Senescence* (V. H. T. James, M. Serio, and L. Martini, eds.), Academic Press, New York, pp. 51–62.

Murono, E. P., Nankin, H. R., Lin, T., and Osterman, J., 1982, The aging Leydig cell V. Diurnal rhythms in aged men, *Acta Endocrinol. (Kbh.)* **100**:455–461.

Murri, L., Barreca, T., Cerone, G., Massetani, R., Gallamini, A., and Baldassarre, M., 1980, The 24-hour pattern of human prolactin and growth hormone in healthy elderly subjects, *Chronobiologia* **7**:87–92.

Muta, K., Kato, K., Akamine, Y., and Ibayashi, H., 1981, Age-related changes in the feedback regulation of gonadotropin secretion by sex steroids in men, *Acta Endocrinol. (Kbh.)* **96**:154–162.

Nankin, H. R., Lin, T., Murono, E. R., Osterman, J., 1981, The aging Leydig cell III. Gonadotropin stimulation in men, *J. Androl.* **2**:181–189.

Natoli, A., Riondino, G., and Brancati, A., 1972, Studio della funzione gonadale ormonica e spermatogenica nel corso della senescenza maschile, *G. Gerontol.* **20**:1103–1119.

Newman, G., and Nichols, C. R., 1960, Sexual activities and attitudes in older persons, *J. Am. Med. Assoc.* **173**:33–35.

Nieschlag, E., Kley, K. H., and Wiegelmann W., 1973, Age dependence of the endocrine testicular function in adult men, *Acta Endocrinol. Scand. (Kbh.)* (Abst.) **177**(Suppl.):122.

Nieschlag, E., Lammers, U., Freischem, C. W., and Wickings, E. J., 1982, Reproductive function in young fathers and grandfathers, *J. Clin. Endocrinol. Metabol.* **55**:676–681.

Pazzagli, M., Forti, G., Cappellini, A., and Serio, M., 1975, Radioimmunoassay of plasma dihydrotestosterone in normal and hypogonadal men, *Clin. Endocrinol.* **4**:513–520.

Pedersen-Bjergaard, K., and Jonnesen, M., 1948, Sex hormone analysis: Excretion of sexual hormones by normal males, impotent males, polyarthritics, and prostatics, *Acta Med. Scand.* **213**(Suppl.):284–291.

Pepperell, R. J., deKretser, D. M., and Burger, H. G., 1975, Studies on the metabolic clearance rate and production rate of human luteinizing hormone and on the initial half-time of its subunits in man, *J. Clin. Invest.* **56**:118–126.

Pfeiffer, E., and Davis, G. C., 1972, Determinants of sexual behavior in middle and old age, *J. Am. Geriat. Soc.* **20**:151–158.

Pirke, K. M., and Doerr, P., 1973, Age related changes and interrelationships between plasma testosterone, estradiol, and testosterone binding globulin in normal adult male, *Acta Endocrinol. (Kbh.)* **74**:792–800.

Pirke, K. M., and Doerr, P., 1975a, Plasma DHT in normal adult males and its relation to T, *Acta Endocrinol. (Kbh.)* **79**:357–362.

Pirke, K. M., and Doerr, P., 1975b, Age related changes in free plasma testosterone, dihydrotestosterone, and oestradiol, *Acta Endocrinol. Scand. (Kbh.)* **80**:171–178.

Purifoy, F. E., Koopmans, L. H., and Mayes, D. M., 1981, Age differences in serum androgen levels in normal adult males, *Hum. Biol.* **53**:499–511.

Reinberg, A., and Lagoguey, M., 1978, Circadian and circannual rhythms in sexual activity and plasma hormones (FSH, LH, testosterone) of five human males, *Arch. Sex. Behav.* **7**:13–29.

Rubens, R., Dhont, M., and Vermeulen, A., 1974, Further studies on Leydig cell function in old age, *J. Clin. Endocrinol. Metabol.* **39**:40–45.

Ryan, R. J., 1962, The luteinizing hormone content of human pituitaries. I. Variations with sex and age, *J. Clin. Endocrinol. Metabol.* **22**:300–303.

Seymour, F. I., Duffy, C., and Koerner, A., 1935, A case of authenticated fertility in a man of 94, *J. Am. Med. Assoc.* **105**:1423–1425.

Snyder, P. J., Reitano, J. F., and Utiger, R. D., 1975, Serum LH and FSH responses to synthetic gonadotropin releasing hormone in normal men, *J. Clin. Endocrinol. Metabol.* **41**:938–945.

Sparrow, D., Bosse, R., and Rowe, J. W., 1980, The influence of age alcohol consumption, and body build on gonadal function in men, *J. Clin. Endocrinol. Metabol.* **51**:508–512.

Stearns, E. L., MacDonald, J. A., Kauffman, B. J., Lucman, T. S., Winters, J. S., and Faiman, C., 1974, Declining testis function with age: Hormonal and clinical correlates, *Am. J. Med.* **57**:761–766.

Tsitouras, P. D., Martin, C. E., and Harman, S. M., 1982, Relationship of serum testosterone to sexual activity in healthy elderly men, *J. Gerontol* **37**:288–293.

Vekemans, M., and Robyn, C., 1975, Influence of age on serum prolactin levels in women and men, *Brit. J. Med.* **4**:738–739.

Vermeulen, A., 1979, Decline in sexual activity in aging men: Correlation with sex hormone levels and testicular changes, *J. Biosoc. Sci.* **6**(Suppl.):5–18.

Vermeulen, A., and Verdonck, L., 1972, Some studies on the biological significance of free testosterone, *J. Steroid Biochem.* **3**:421–426.

Vermeulen, A., Rubens, R., and Verdonck, L., 1972, Testosterone secretion and metabolism in male senescence, *J. Clin. Endocrinol. Metabol.* **34**:730–735.

Zumoff, B., Strain, G. W., Kream, J., O'Connor, J., Rosenfeld, R. S., Levin, J., and Fukushima, D. K., 1982, Age variation of the 24-hour mean plasma concentration of androgens, estrogens, and gonadotropins in normal adult men, *J. Clin. Endocrinol. Metabol.* **54**:534–538.

CHAPTER 12

The Sexual Psychoendocrinology of Aging

JULIAN M. DAVIDSON, GARY D. GRAY, and ERLA R. SMITH

1. Introduction

If the need for sex changed with age in exact parallel to the capacity for sex, this chapter would be primarily an academic exercise instead of an attempt to explore the biological basis of a real human problem. This problem is well exemplified by the case of King David. *Prophets* 1:1 tells us: "Now King David was old and advanced in years and although they covered him with clothes, he could not get warm. Therefore his servants said to him, let a young maiden be sought for . . . and let her lie in your bosom . . . the maiden was very beautiful and she ministered to him; but the King knew her not." We may surmise that the aging David was not merely suffering from hypothermia. Rather, judging from the use of the biblical euphemism "knew," his problem was the discrepancy between libido and potency which is a common experience of aging men as has been substantiated in several studies (Verwoerdt *et al.*, 1969a,b; Kinsey *et al.*, 1948; Davidson *et al.*, 1983).

There is reason to believe that this gap, which is responsible for much unhappiness in the aging population, is even greater than might be expected from reading the (fairly sparse) modern literature on geriatric sexuality. This is related to the fact that the entity we term libido or sexual motivation is difficult to define, is not standardized among workers in the field and is often hard to separate from potency, the other "half" of sexuality (Davidson, 1980). If you ask a man whether he has sexual desire, he may answer "no" because he has given up the contest

JULIAN M. DAVIDSON, GARY D. GRAY, and ERLA R. SMITH • Department of Physiology, Stanford University, Stanford, California 94305.

after many failures, or because he thinks he shouldn't have those feelings at his age, or because he has learned to associate sexual desire with penile sensations which no longer seem to exist for him. As a result it is not clear that past studies (including our own) have asked the right questions. Even if one were to ask "Would you have sex if you could?" the answers might not be very helpful since moral or religious considerations can blind people to the appreciation of their own desires, or at least inhibit their expression.

The libido–potency gap is not limited to aged men. It is shared by a substantial population of younger psychogenically impotent men and sexually dysfunctional women,* as well as the much smaller population of dysfunctional individuals whose problems arise from demonstrable organic defects in the physiological sexual response. It is also a common experience among the large numbers of mild or heavy alcohol abusers in our society as described in the much celebrated quotation from Shakespeare "drink . . . provokes the desire and unprovokes the performance . . ." (*Macbeth,* Act II, Scene I). But in the course of aging, the libido–potency gap widens until sexual activity comes to a standstill in many men and in a much less determined number of women.

But while the libido–potency gap and associated phenomena provide the primary sociomedical relevance needed to motivate clinical research in this area, age-related changes in all aspects of sexuality undoubtedly occur and present an intriguing problem to the fundamental psychobiologist. The model of gradual, selective sexual deterioration presented by aging subjects lends itself to analysis of the component parts of sexuality and their collective or selective regulation by environmental and physiologic factors. This chapter is primarily concerned with the neuroendocrine mechanisms, which can be addressed directly in animals, since we have enough background information to discuss hormonal effects on neurally mediated behavioral phenomena. In humans, however, it is difficult, at this juncture, to separate such clearly defined biological factors from those loosely termed psychosocial or cultural. Nevertheless, the well-established neuroendocrine models derived from animal research are potentially applicable to humans, especially in the male (Davidson, 1977; Davidson *et al.,* 1978). We shall therefore first review the changes in sexual behavior which occur during aging in the

---

* Thanks in part to the wide publicity accorded to the work of Masters and Johnson (1966), it is widely recognized that male and female sexual responses are qualitatively very similar, subject only to anatomical differences. It is nonetheless not generally acknowledged, that "potency" (the vascular and muscular manifestations of the sexual response) may be just as relevant to achieving sexual satisfaction and orgasm in women as they are in men (see Davidson, 1980).

most studied animal species, briefly summarize the endocrine changes (dealt with in greater detail in other chapters), and then consider the relationship between hormonal and behavioral phenomena. This sequence will be applied to both males and females in turn.

Sexual behavior is the product of a combination of several more basic behavioral elements and a full understanding of age-related changes is not possible if we cannot specify the precise nature of the behavioral changes with age. In the male it is feasible to assess quantitatively sexual motivation or libido, and the "reflexes" of erection and ejaculation. In females, the comparable elements are sexual motivation or proceptive behavior (Beach, 1976), reflexes related to sexual receptivity (such as the common lordosis posture), and "sexual response" in the sense used by Masters and Johnson (1966), primarily vascular and muscular responses to sexual arousal/activity. A comprehensive description of sexual aging requires the differential evaluation of these behavioral elements rather than general statements about sexual behavior as a whole, which can be as misleading as they are inadequate. The various elements have different physiological, including neuroendocrine bases, and hence may be affected differentially during aging.

2. Male Animals

The dependence of masculine sexual behavior on testosterone (T) is perhaps the strongest known relationship in behavioral endocrinology, and it extends to all studied mammalian species, including the human (Davidson *et al.*, 1979; Skakkebaek *et al.*, 1980). Thus, there are substantial similarities in the neuroendocrine bases of sexual behavior across species, similarities which may extend to the aging process. Consideration of animal species may enhance our understanding of aging in general and may also provide experimental models applicable to problems of human dysfunction.

2.1. Endocrinology

As discussed elsewhere in this book, aging in the male rat involves a gradual decline in circulating T levels which is accompanied by a reduction in luteinizing hormone (LH) and follicle-stimulating hormone (FSH) levels (Meites *et al.*, 1976, 1978). The decline in LH and T is already apparent in the period we have described as early middle age, from about 1 year of age or before half of the average life span (Gray, 1978a). In aging mice, discrepant results have been reported regarding

decreases in LH and T in different strains of mice (Bronson and Desjardins, 1977; Eleftheriou and Lucas, 1975; Finch *et al.*, 1977). A recent
study using frequent blood sampling has clearly demonstrated reduced
T pulses related to decreased frequency and amplitude of LH pulses in
old CBF_1 mice (Coquelin and Desjardins, 1982).

The situation becomes somewhat more complicated in primates, in
part because of the role of sex hormone-binding globulin in regulating
androgen activity, a factor not present in laboratory rodents. Chambers
et al. (1981) failed to find significant differences in either total T level
or calculated free T between young and old (10 vs. 20 years) rhesus
monkeys, though a trend towards declining levels was clearly present.
Nevertheless, binding protein was elevated in the aged animals. In humans, most studies, with the exception of those on highly selected groups
of men (Sparrow *et al.*, 1980; Harman and Tsitouras, 1980; see below),
have shown decreases in total T and increases in binding protein activity,
generally leading to a greater decrease in calculated free T level than
in total T (Vermeulen, 1979; Stearns *et al.*, 1976; Baker *et al.*, 1976;
Davidson *et al.*, 1983).

A notable distinction between humans and laboratory rodents is that
gonadotropin levels rise in the former whereas they drop in the latter,
indicating that the hypogonadism of aging is primary in man and secondary in rats and mice. Nevertheless, it should be noted, without pre-
empting our later discussion on hormone–behavior relationships, that
the proximate cause of hypoandrogenicity in the aging male is probably
unimportant since T is the primary hormone relevant to the behavior.

2.2. Behavior in Rats

Not surprisingly, the most comprehensive data on aging and sexual
behavior are those dealing with laboratory rats and mice. With respect
to the nature of the changes, Larsson noted alterations in two elements
of the behavior of aged, sexually experienced individuals (Larsson, 1958a,b;
Larsson and Essberg, 1962). First, there was a decline in sexual motivation or arousal compared to young adults. Aged animals showed a
decrease in the number of tests with receptive females in which copulation was initiated and in the rate of copulation when it occurred, i.e.,
increased latencies for mounts, intromissions, and ejaculations (Larsson,
1958a; Larsson and Essberg, 1962). These differences were enhanced
in tests conducted during the light phase of the light-dark cycle, an
unfavorable condition for male copulation and one which therefore requires considerable motivation to overcome (Larsson, 1958b). This decline in sexual motivation contrasted with a second change in the be-

havior, namely an increase in number of ejaculations attained before satiety or "sexual exhaustion" (Larsson, 1958b; Larsson and Essberg, 1962). The increase was evident especially if arousal was maintained by the periodic introduction of new receptive females.

We have recently completed a series of studies directed at exploring the behavioral changes in aging male rats. Rather than examining animals of advanced age, we chose to focus on middle-aged rats (13–15 months) because it is at that stage that significant reductions in circulating T first develop (Gray, 1978a). Moreover, the general pathologies of murine senescence, e.g., tumors, lung disease, motor or sensory deficiencies, which may produce nonspecific effects on sexual behavior, are not yet prevalent in middle age. In order to evaluate the separate elements of sexual behavior, four different methods were employed:

1. Tests of mating or copulatory behavior in which the latency and frequency of mounts, intromissions, and ejaculation are recorded.

2. Tests of sexual motivation (or arousal) in which the rat's penis is anesthetized with tetracaine, eliminating the capacity to achieve intromission or ejaculation with a receptive female. The resulting mounting behavior, in the absence of sensory feedback, reflects only the male's attempts to initiate copulation and serves as a quantitative measure of motivation.

3. Tests of penile reflexes in which the male is lightly restrained in a supine position with the penis exposed. The frequency of resulting spontaneous reflex responses provides a quantitative measure of erection (and other reflex) potential independent of sexual stimulation and other aspects of sexual behavior.

4. Tests of spontaneous seminal emission, in which males are housed individually in wire-mesh cages for 72 hr after being fitted with a rigid corset which prevents grooming of the penis. Under these conditions, the ejaculatory plugs formed as a result of spontaneous ejaculation fall through a wire-mesh cage bottom and serve as a quantitative measure of ejaculatory potential, again independent of any other aspect of sexual behavior.

We compared the behavior of middle-aged rats with that of young adult rats and found differences in at least three components of sexual behavior. Middle-aged animals showed a significantly reduced probability of mating in copulatory behavior tests and longer latency measures (increased time to intromission and ejaculation) when mating occurred, suggestive of a decrease in sexual motivation (Fig. 1). This was confirmed in tests of sexual motivation during which middle-aged animals showed substantially fewer mounts than young adult animals (Gray et al., 1981). An aging decline in a second component of sexual behavior was evident

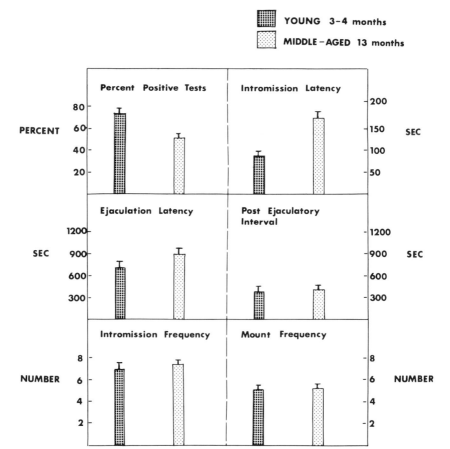

Fig. 1. The general pattern of behavior in middle-aged and young adult males in tests of copulatory behavior before testosterone treatment. Data represent mean ± SE. Data on latencies and frequencies include only rats which had positive copulatory tests. For percent positive, $n = 60$ (young) and 57 (middle–aged) rats. For the latency and frequency measures, $n = 49$ (young) and 36 (middle-aged) rats. (From Gray *et al.*, 1981.)

in the tests of penile erection (Gray, 1978b). The decrement in erections did not involve a complete failure of erectile ability in the middle-aged animals, but a quantitative reduction in erection frequency. The third difference involved ejaculatory mechanisms, but in this case, there was a slight *increase* in the number of ejaculatory plugs deposited by the middle-aged animals in tests of spontaneous ejaculation (Gray *et al.*, 1981). The decline in motivation, the reduction in erection potential, and the maintained or slight increase in ejaculation potential represent changes in separate distinct elements of sexual behavior, each of which surely affect the overall behavioral pattern of copulatory behavior in middle-aged male rats.

The changes in the first two components are undoubtedly limiting factors in mating as seen in the copulatory behavior tests. The significance of the third (and the only facilitatory) change is unclear, but is consistent with Larsson's finding, albeit differently assessed, of increased ejaculatory potential in considerably older rats during prolonged tests (see above). Together with this, however, the time required for ejaculation *in copula* was increased in our study, indicating a slower rate of ejaculatory responding in middle-aged rats (Gray *et al.,* 1981).

The major findings of our cross-sectional studies were recently confirmed in a newly completed longitudinal study on 89 sexually active male rats, the data from which are still being analyzed. Exposure to females commenced at 3 months and all animals received two recorded mating tests in 1 week, every 2 months from 7–27 months of age. The most striking change, beginning in early middle age, was the progressive decrease in probability of successful mating (Fig. 2). Among the 39% of

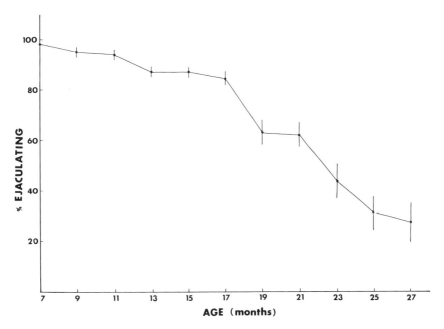

Fig. 2. Percentage of sexually experienced rats which showed complete copulatory behavior patterns, including ejaculation, from 7–27 months of age.

rats surviving to 27 months, 71% failed to mate in our usual copulatory test involving sequential exposure to different estrous females. Both in the cross-sectional and longitudinal studies, there was considerable overlap between behavioral scores of young and aged animals, and some 6% of the survivors maintained their behavior virtually unchanged through 27 months. Moreover, these animals who survived to 27 months showed an attenuated decline in sex behavior.

The longitudinal study confirmed and extended the specific and differential nature of age-related changes. Animals which failed to mate at 23 months did not show decreased erectile or ejaculatory reflexes as compared to their age matched cohorts (see Table 1). This situation resembles the loss of sexual behavior following lesions of the medial preoptic area, which is found in a variety of species (Hart, 1982); genital reflexes are maintained, according to the studies of Hart, in dogs and cats and probably in monkeys. Recently in this laboratory Stefanick (1982), has shown quantitative maintenance of normal erectile reflexes and of spontaneous emission patterns in lesioned rats following medial preoptic lesions. Thus, a possible mechanism of the aging decline could be a functional defect in medial preoptic function, as discussed below. At any rate, the pattern of failure of sexual motivation in the face of maintained reflex function is the converse of the libido–potency gap discussed in relation to humans at the beginning of this chapter. Another variable on which the longitudinal study provided information was the effect of sexual experience. In the cross-sectional experiments, minimal sexual experience at 3 months of age attenuated the decline in probability of copulation in middle-age, but not of erection potential, as assessed in reflex tests (Gray, 1978b). Thus, experience in young adulthood was

Table 1. The Relationship between Ejaculatory Behavior, Penile Reflexes, and Seminal Emission in 23-Month-Old Male Rats[a]

	N	No. erections[b]	% Positive	Plasma testosterone (ng/ml)	No. seminal plugs (per 3-day test)
Positive for ejaculation	26	11.06 + 1.92*	61.5	1.22 ± 0.11	2.8 ± 0.3
Negative for ejaculation	23	14.85 ± 1.31	87.0	1.13 ± 0.10	2.8 ± 0.4

[a] "Negative" animals showed apparently permanent loss of mating response.
[b] Data only from rats which showed *any* reflexes.
[c] Mean ± SE data.

sufficient to overcome aging deficits in specific elements of behavior including sexual motivation (initiation of mating) and erectile potency, given the stimulating conditions of the mating encounter as opposed to the nonarousing reflex test situation. In the longitudinal study, the rats showed a lower performance in general on the first of two tests performed within a week, every 2 months, than on the second of each series, indicating that repeated sexual experience after a period of deprivation attenuates the progressive decline in behavior noted as the animals age. A similar effect has been observed in mice (Huber and Bronson, 1980).

2.3. Hormone–Behavior Relationship in Rats

What is the cause of these changes in sexual behavior of aging rats? Given the tenuous nature of etiologic explanation in gerontology as a whole, this subject must be approached with great caution. Nevertheless, there is one rather compelling hypothesis which not only seems highly plausible, but has the additional advantage of great simplicity. Since adequate T titers are necessary for maintaining sexual activity in males and since T levels as well as sex behavior begin to decrease during middle-age, the decline in androgen may be responsible for the behavioral changes noted.

Previous attempts to address this issue in rats were made before the era of radioimmunoassay, and the investigators were unable to relate their treatments to hormone levels in the natural situation in young and old animals. This point is of particular relevance in view of the finding that Silastic capsules generating plasma T levels well below the naturally occurring range suffice for full maintenance of mating behavior. It follows that small decreases below the normal mean level are almost certainly irrelevant in rats (Damassa et al., 1977). The early, behaviorally unsophisticated report of Minnick and Warden (1946), on activation of sexual activity in very old rats, following adminstration of T propionate, adds little to our understanding of the problem. All sexual activity was virtually absent in the age-matched controls, and T levels may have dropped so far below the normal range that hormone administration might be expected to restore sexual activity to the usual middle-age level. The typical situation, in our experience with Long–Evans rats, is a gradual decline in T level and partial maintenance of behavior, even in 27-month-old animals. Unlike Minnick and Warden (1946), Larsson (1956) and Jakubczak (1964, 1967) argued that androgen could not be responsible for the aging changes since behavior declines before the accessory sexual tissues atrophy, an inconclusive argument which assumes equivalence in the dose-reponse curves of behavior and weights of these glands.

We have examined the behavior of young adult and middle-aged rats in which T levels were directly controlled by castration and implantation of T-filled Silastic capsules. In the first study, erectile capacity was investigated (Gray, 1978b). When T titers were equated at low and supraphysiological levels in the two age groups, differences in the responses were eliminated, indicating that the decline in the erectile reflex component of sexual behavior is due in large part to a decrease in T levels (Fig. 3). This was not the case, however, for sexual motivation assessed quantitatively by the mounting test; equating T levels did not eliminate the age differences in this component (Gray *et al.*, 1981; Fig. 4). In addition, the middle-aged rats continued to show a lower probability of mating and longer latency measures in tests of copulatory behavior. Even the administration of supraphysiological levels of T did

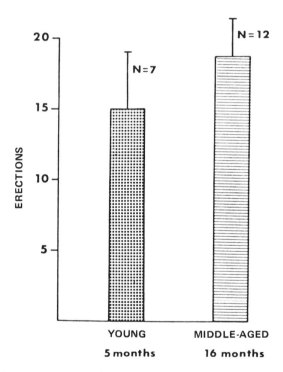

Fig. 3. Erection responses (test for reflexes) in castrated middle-aged and young rats with supraphysiological levels of testosterone. The results represent the mean ($\pm$ SE) number of erections in all tests, including the negative tests. n = number of animals per group. (From Gray, 1978b).

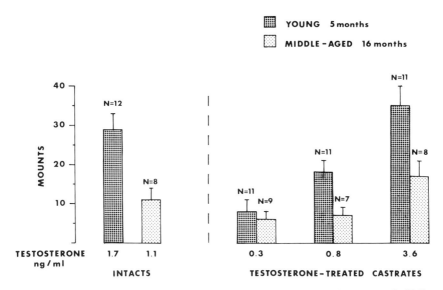

Fig. 4. Mounting behavior after genital anesthetization (mean ± SE) in groups of middle-aged and young adult males after T treatment. Groups include intacts that were sham castrated and implanted with empty capsules and castrates implanted with small, intermediate, or large T-filled capsules. Mean plasma T values for samples collected 3–5 days after the mounting tests are also presented for the various groups. n = number of rats. (From Gray *et al.*, 1981.)

not enhance the behavior of middle-aged males in these tests above that of untreated animals. Similarly, ejaculation latency was not restored to normal. Thus we concluded that the decrement in circulating T does not suffice to explain the decline of sexual motivation and ejaculatory behavior, and other factors will have to be considered (Gray *et al.*, 1981).

Since castration-replacement therapy is an artificial (albeit effective) approach, an important source of evidence in aging problems is correlational analysis in longitudinal experiments. From our recent study of this kind, preliminary data analysis shows no significant correlations between T levels (two samples taken every 2 months from 7–27 months of age) and parameters of copulatory behavior.

2.4. Other Species

The few studies on sexual aging in male guinea pigs originated from W. C. Young's laboratory in the 1950s and show slower rates of intromission and ejaculatory behavior in middle and old age with maintenance or increases in mounting frequency. Ejaculation latency was unaffected (reviewed in Jakubczak, 1967). Jakubczak (1964) could not improve intromission and ejaculation scores in 30-month-old animals with large doses of testosterone.

Systematic studies have recently been conducted in mice. Behavioral changes in laboratory mice (CBF_1 strain) are similar to those described for rats. There is a progressive decline in sexual activity beginning in middle age (Huber *et al.*, 1980). This is in large part the result of a decrease in sexual motivation or arousal, as evaluated separately in tests of copulatory behavior and in treadmill tests designed to assess a male's willingness to maintain contact with a receptive female (Craigen and Bronson, 1982). There is also a decrement in the capacity to achieve intromission (suggesting possible deficiencies in the erection response) and in ejaculatory capacity. Of the various parameters of copulation, only the decrement in ejaculatory capacity was associated with urogenital pathology (Huber *et al.*, 1980). In old (24 months) mice of this strain, sexual activity (as evaluated only by finding an ejaculatory plug in the vagina) and maintenance of pituitary-gonadal function (LH and T levels) were significantly related (Bronson and Desjardins, 1977). This correlation suggests, but does not prove, a functional relationship between the hormonal and behavioral changes, at least in very old mice. Whether such a relationship does exist, and whether it accounts entirely for the change in motivation, remains to be determined. It would be of particular interest in this regard to study the C57BL/6J strain of mice which does not show a decrement in T with increasing age (see Finch *et al.*, 1977).

The other nonhuman species for which there is a body of systematic data is rhesus macaques. Phoenix and co-workers have documented decrements in sexual behavior in older individuals of this species (Chambers and Phoenix, 1981; Phoenix and Chambers, 1982). In tests with receptive females, both the probability of mating to ejaculation and the rate of mating when it did occur were lower for male macaques over 20 years of age, than for those around 10 years of age. The authors suggest that this decline largely reflects a decrease in sexual motivation; older males are described as less persistent in pursuing females and more discriminating in the choice of partners. General disability is discounted as a major factor, but deficiencies in potency remain a possibility and need to be investigated.

In 1975, Robinson *et al.*, failed to find a relationship between total T level and sexual behavior in a small number of rhesus monkeys. The Phoenix group has recently examined the relationship of the behavioral changes to endocrine function in systematic fashion (Chambers *et al.*,

1981; Chambers and Phoenix, 1981). Circulating total T did not differ significantly between the young and old groups of male macaques, but sex steroid-binding globulin (SBP) was significantly higher in the old group. Calculated free T also did not quite differ significantly between young and old macaques, although the mean value of the older group was half that of the young group, a situation caused by a relatively small sample size (N = 9/group) and substantial variability in free T values. There was no correlation between behavior and free T in the old group, but surprisingly SBP showed high negative correlations with several behavioral measures, e.g., correlation coefficients were -0.68 for percent tests with ejaculation, -0.84 for intromissions/min, and -0.73 for contacts/min, a measure of sexual arousal. How SBP levels could affect behavior in the absence of free T effects is unknown. These correlations could of course simply mean that SBP levels reflect an aging deficiency in either pituitary–gonadal function or general physiology which develops concurrently with the behavioral deficiencies. It is of interest and perhaps of considerable relevance to this discussion that in many (all?) situations where androgen's effects are reduced, e.g., testicular feminization, SBP activity is increased (P. Siiteri, personal communication). Cortisol levels were also correlated with some behavioral measures in the older macaques, and levels of this hormone were significantly lower in the older groups. This may indicate a role for the ACTH-cortisol axis in the regulation of sexual behavior, though it is perhaps more likely that the lower cortisol titers represent a reduced level of arousal, sexual or otherwise. That attempts in the Phoenix laboratory to replicate the cortisol and SBP correlations with behavior have not been successful (C. Phoenix, personal communication) is indicative of the difficulty of establishing relationships by correlation analysis, unless large n's are available.

In addition to the correlational studies, Phoenix and Chambers (1982) administered T propionate to a group of old males at doses sufficient to maintain sexual behavior in young castrated macaques. They found no significant improvement in the males' behavior following treatment. This finding, along with the above-mentioned results, suggests that neither an alteration in T levels nor decreased sensitivity to T accounts for the behavioral changes reported in old macaques. Testosterone, along with other factors, may yet prove to play some partial role in the behavioral effects of aging, especially since all components of sexual behavior have not been examined in detail and the number of monkeys studied is small. Nevertheless the presently available data speak strongly against T being the predominant factor in the decline in sexual behavior of old rhesus monkeys.

3. Sexuality in Aging Men

The first step towards developing a neuroendocrinology of human sexual aging is to establish precisely the known age-related changes in sexuality. But since we are primarily concerned with those events which have a reasonable likelihood of showing a biological origin, we must scrutinize the data analytically to distinguish components which likely involve hormonal factors. Only then can we attempt to deal concretely with possible neuroendocrine mechanisms, within the constraints of the limited existing data.

On the basis of their extensive interview data Kinsey *et al.* (1948) maintained, in their classic study, that "from early and middle teens, the decline in sexual activity is remarkably steady, and there is no point at which old age suddenly enters the picture." While true for some of their measures (notably multiple orgasm and multiple forms of orgasmic activity), the data do not show any decline for others, including "total outlet," i.e., frequency of sexual activity, of any type, culminating in orgasm, until after 30 years. It should be noted that the numbers of aged individuals studied declined rapidly with age, from 3905 adolescents to two men over 80 (p. 220), which unfortunately limits the otherwise great reliability of their curves for the later years. A recent study

Table 2. Age and Erectile Impotence[a]

Age	Total population	% Impotent	Increment %
10	4108	0	
15	3948	0.05	0.05
20	3017	0.1	0.05
25	1627	0.4	0.3
30	1025	0.8	0.4
35	741	1.3	0.5
40	513	1.9	0.6
45	347	2.6	0.7
50	236	6.7	4.1
55	134	6.7	0.0
60	87	18.4	11.7
65	44	25.0	6.6
70	26	27.0	2.0
75	11	55.0	28.0
80	4	75.0	20.0

[a] An accumulative incidence curve, based on cases which are more or less totally and, to all appearances, permanently impotent. (From Kinsey *et al.*, 1948, p. 236.)

of men from 41–93 years shows that the major declines in sexual activity and capacity over this period occurred from the 7th decade of life on (Davidson *et al.*, 1983).

Kinsey's otherwise justifiable emphasis on frequency of sexual activity notwithstanding, the important point for the study of human aging is not minor (or even major) quantitative changes in frequency of sexual events but rather the onset of serious sexual dysfunction. Thus, if we look at frequency of "total impotence," the curve is not linear from adolescence on but exponential, with the first noticeable increase in slope occurring in the sixth decade (Table 2). Interestingly, the oldest men in several studies appear to show more sexual activity or interest than their next younger cohort (Pfeiffer *et al.*, 1972). This suggests that survival into advanced old age may correlate with a higher level of maintenance of sexual function, i.e., the oldest men include a sexually elite group of survivors. However, no systematic studies have been performed and the ages at which this phenomenon has been reported vary from late sixties (Pfeiffer *et al.*, 1972) to nineties! (Hegeler, 1981).

3.1. What Is Responsible for the Decrease in Sexual Activity?

A change in sexual activity can be due to decreases in (1) sexual interest or libido, (2) opportunity, or (3) capacity. In the recent cross-sectional questionnaire study on 220 aging men from 41–93 years of age conducted at Stanford University (Davidson *et al.*, 1983), self-reported sexual drive or interest did not significantly decrease with age, though significant decreases were found in measures of potency and another measure of libido, i.e., frequency of sexual fantasies/feelings (as well as in sexual activity; Table 3). From their data, Kinsey *et al.* (1948) felt unable to conclude anything about the extent to which the aging decline resulted from "psychologic situations, . . . availability of contacts . . . preoccupation with other social or business functions. . . ." Martin (1981) recently reported a retrospective interview study on several hundred highly selected white, upper middle-class, married, 60- to 70-year-old men from the Baltimore Longitudinal Study on Aging. He found that sexual frequency was not reportedly related to marital adjustment, husband's perception of sexual attractiveness of the wives, or sexual attitudes. Moreover, unlike the situation in aging women (see below) the availability or adequacy of sexual partners does not seem to be a major factor in reducing total sexual outlet. In fact, the men in the Duke studies (Pfeiffer *et al.*, 1972) overwhelmingly reported that their sexual decline had its origin from self rather than spouse (Table 4). In the Stanford study, there was no significant increase with age in attri-

Table 3. Sexuality Questionnaire Responses (Graded 1–5) of Men Aged 40–93

	Age Range				
Behavior	40–49 (n = 27)	50–59 (n = 70)	60–69 (n = 82)	70+ (n = 42)	$p <$ (Kruskall Wallis)
Frequency of sexual feelings/ fantasies	5.42 ±0.14	4.77 ±0.14	4.28 ±0.16	3.49 ±0.28	.01
Low sexual drive/interest[a]	3.74 ±0.19	3.55 ±0.15	3.70 ±0.16	3.29 ±0.27	.503(NS)
Frequency of sexual activity with orgasm	4.07 ±0.21	3.90 ±0.16	3.30 ±0.17	2.40 ±0.23	.01
Frequency of "morning" erections	4.07 ±0.26	3.73 ±0.15	3.28 ±0.17	2.61 ±0.22	.01
Frequency of spontaneous erections	3.93 ±0.35	3.97 ±0.19	3.58 ±0.18	2.63 ±0.27	.01
Failure to get erections[a]	4.12 ±0.21	3.64 ±0.16	3.50 ±0.16	2.73 ±0.23	.01
Failure to hold erections[a]	3.85 ±0.22	3.53 ±0.16	3.36 ±0.16	2.79 ±0.25	.02
Failure to have orgasm[a]	4.16 ±0.18	4.18 ±0.16	3.78 ±0.16	3.22 ±0.32	.01
Frequency of masturbation	2.44 ±0.27	2.26 ±0.16	1.89 ±0.14	1.64 ±0.17	.02
Enjoyment of sex	4.29 ±0.18	4.44 ±0.11	3.84 ±0.15	3.32 ±0.28	.001
Premature orgasm[a]	3.33 ±0.24	3.41 ±0.16	3.51 ±0.16	3.42 ±0.32	.92(NS)
Sexual dissatisfaction with partner[a]	4.00 ±0.19	3.98 ±0.14	3.90 ±0.15	3.67 ±0.26	.72(NS)
Lack of partner[a]	4.00 ±0.24	4.33 ±0.16	4.36 ±0.17	4.15 ±0.37	.25(NS)
Lack of opportunity for sex[a]	3.56 ±0.22	3.71 ±0.18	3.67 ±0.16	3.43 ±0.28	.74(NS)

[a] These questions were phrased "During the past six months, how frequently have each of the following problems prevented you from freely expressing or enjoying yourself in your sexual activity?" Higher scores, however, denote lower frequency of each problem.

bution of the limitation of sexual activity to lack of opportunity for sex or sexual partner-related variables (Table 3). There appears therefore to be no indication that psychosocial factors account for the behavioral changes of aging men. Rather, biological phenomena associated with aging should be considered the primary factors.

Though sexual interest declines with age in men, there is a growing discrepancy between this decrease and the greater decline in capacity, which is responsible for the libido–potency gap (Verwoerdt *et al.*, 1969a,b; Kinsey *et al.*, 1948; Table 3). Given then, that potency measures appear to be more robust indicators of the aging effect on sexuality than data

Table 4. Reasons for Cessation of Sexual Relations[a]

Reason	Men		Women	
	Number	Percent	Number	Percent
Death of spouse	0		35	36
Separation or divorce from spouse	0		12	12
Illness of spouse	5	14	19	20
Loss of interest by spouse	3	9	4	4
Spouse unable to perform sexually	2	6	17	18
Illness of self	6	17	2	2
Loss of interest by self	5	14	4	4
Self unable to perform sexually	14	40	4	4
Total	35		97	

[a] 261 men and 241 women aged 45–71 were surveyed. (From Pfeiffer *et al.*, 1972.)

related to libido, it seems more profitable to pursue the former in looking for correlations with hormonal factors. What are these changes in potency?

Among the elements of potency noted by Kinsey *et al.* (1948) to decline with age were erotic responsiveness, speed of attaining erection and its duration of maintenance with continuing stimuli, the amount of preorgasmic "mucus" secreted and capacity for multiple climax, nocturnal erections, and emissions. To these, Masters and Johnson (1966) added a generally decreased vasocongestive response affecting not only the penis but the testis and extragenital tissues such as the breasts. That these changes are not merely due to unresponsiveness to stimuli, i.e., libido factors, is suggested by the finding of Kahn and Fisher, (1969) and Karacan *et al.* (1972) that nocturnal penile tumescence also decreases with age, though to a limited extent. Quantitative laboratory measurements of specific elements of sexual physiology are needed to substantiate and extend data obtained from questionnaire/interview surveys and the sketchily described findings of Masters and Johnson (1966). A recent study (Solnick and Birren, 1977) assessed erection in response to erotic film using strain gauges measuring circumference change and thermistors measuring penile temperature. The rate of erection was approximately six times slower, and the circumference increase significantly smaller, in ten males aged 48–65 than in ten others aged 19–30 years; no data were given on maintenance of erection.

Changes in orgasmic function are described as involving an increase in the refractory period and decreased strength and frequency of contractions of the pelvic skeletal muscle (as measured for instance at the rectal sphincter), resulting in decreased force of expulsion of semen

(Masters and Johnson, 1966). Premature ejaculation in individuals with erectile capacity is as uncommon in the aged as it is common in young inexperienced males. In our sample, the frequency of premature ejaculation did not differ significantly between men in their 40's and those over 70 (Davidson et al., 1983). In fact, one of the few sexual bonuses the average aging man can expect is a reduction in what Masters and Johnson (1966) term "ejaculatory demand" (implying greater control over orgasm), a finding analogous to the increased ejaculation latency in aging rats.

The important variable of genital sensory function has not received due attention. Two investigations have concerned the decreased tactile sensitivity, usually measured as vibratory sense threshold. Newman (1970) demonstrated a gradual increase in vibrotactile threshold of the penis with advancing age, in 100 men, aged 17–88 years. The change became precipitous in the 65- to 74-year-old group, which showed an approximate tenfold increase over the 55- to 64-year-old group. The findings were corroborated in a smaller study by Edwards and Husted (1976).

But do these various changes in components of sex behavior importantly affect sexual function? Do they separately or collectively contribute to the aging decline? Undoubtedly the psychologically healthy individual can compensate for a large proportion of his relative inadequacy in sexual response by a variety of maneuvers, such as alterations of movement, pressure, and time taken during sexual activity. Nevertheless, it is a fair bet that the impotence which develops in increasing numbers of aging males is essentially an extension of the progressive changes described, to the point when satisfactory sexual activity becomes impossible in some men, no matter what adjustments are made. Since existing findings suggest that nocturnal penile tumescence normally continues into advanced age with only relatively small changes (Kahn and Fisher, 1969; Karacan et al., 1972), further studies are required on age-related impotence of otherwise unexplained origin. It will be important to determine the relative importance of the factors of responsivity to sexual stimuli vs. integrity of the erectile mechanism as expressed in its nocturnal reflex-like manifestation.

A fairly widespread concept (Masters and Johnson, 1966; Pfeiffer and Davis, 1972; Martin, 1981) is that sexual experience in presenescence contributes to the maintenance of sexual activity in old age (the idea that "if you use it, you don't lose it"). Pfeiffer and Davis (1972) showed by multiple regression analysis of interview data that past sexual interest, enjoyment, and frequency were highly correlated with continued sexual activity in old age in both men and women. This phenomenon might be related to the observation in male rats that prior sexual experience appears to reduce the aging decline in sexual behavior (Gray *et al.,* 1981). However, there is no evidence to indicate a causal relationship in humans between high sexual experience and sexuality in senescence, implying for instance, some kind of disuse atrophy. The data so far merely indicate that "high performers" in youth are more likely to remain high performers in old age.

3.2. Hormone–Behavior Relationships

The importance of testosterone (T) in male sexual function and the fact that T declines roughly in parallel with sexual function in aging men provide a strong basis for considering a direct hormone–behavior relationship in the aging process. As yet however, no systematic studies of the relationship between these two variables have been published. T has nevertheless been prescribed for the age-related decline in sexual function by some physicians, and some limited clinical data has been presented to support the effectiveness of this treatment (Greenblatt and Perez, 1974). Recent data from the Baltimore Longitudinal Study of Aging have relevance to this topic. In 19 men aged 70–89 there was a positive correlation between free-T index and sexual activity (Tsitouras *et al.,* 1982), though the subjects in their population, highly selected for optimal health, and education etc., did not show a significant aging decline in total or free-T levels (Harman and Tsitouras, 1980).

In our study on aging men (Davidson *et al.,* 1983) a single blood sample for hormone analysis and detailed questionnaire data were obtained. The subjects were recruited while entering an outpatient clinical laboratory to give a blood sample for a routine health check-up or other purposes. As described in the previous section, significant decreases were found in almost all aspects of sexual function examined when men over 70 were compared with others in early middle age (40–49). Moreover, this population (like most others studied) showed a significant drop in total T, a greater decline in calculated free T resulting from an elevation in sex hormone binding capacity, and a large increase in plasma LH and FSH with aging. No significant changes in estradiol and prolactin levels were found, which corresponds with some but not all other authors' conclusions (Davidson *et al.,* 1983).

A variety of correlations were obtained between questionnaire data and hormone levels in the population as a whole (Table 5). Significant correlations were more common with performance measures (sexual activity and potency) than with libido (self-perceived sex drive and frequency of sexual feelings). No correlations were found with total T and some weak but significant correlations with free T. Interestingly, LH

Table 5. Correlation Coefficients (Spearman): Hormones vs. Behavior[a]

	Libido			Performance						
	Gen. score[d]	Feels	Drive	Gen. score[d]	Org. frequ.	Noct. erect.	Spont. erect.	Get erect.	Hold erect.	Ejac. capac.
Free T		.13[b]		.15[b]	.19[c]					.16[b]
Total T										
LH	−.14[b]			−.29[c]	−.25[c]	−.27[c]	−.18[c]	−.18[c]	−.13[b]	
FT/E	.14[b]	.14[b]		.22[c]	.18[c]		.15[b]	.22[c]	.20[c]	.20[c]

[a] Only significant correlations shown.
[b] $p < .05$.
[c] $p < .005$.
[d] Gen. Score: general libido or performance scores for each man were constructed by averaging responses to the two libido and six performance questions, respectively.

and the ratio of free T to estradiol were more highly correlated than was T itself with a variety of measures, including frequency of orgasm and erectile capacity. However, in light of the finding that hormone levels decline along with sexual function in aging men, it is possible that the (low level) correlations between the two might be accounted for by colinear variation rather than by any true relationship between the two declining functions. Indeed, when hormone–behavior correlations were run within each decade rather than on the whole population, the effect was to reduce the incidence and extent of significant correlations (which could also be partly explained by the lower numbers of individuals in each group). Further analysis showed that partialling out disease and drug factors did not alter the correlations between free-T index and answers to specific questions (Davidson *et al.*, 1983). Finally the subjects were divide into tertiles (high, medium, and low) according to free T or LH levels and two-way analyses of variance were run to determine the effects of age and free T or LH on composite scores of libido or performance. In each of the four analyses, age was a significant variable and the hormonal variables were not significant, except for LH in the performance analysis (Table 6).

It was concluded that declining androgen levels (and the resulting increased LH levels) and reduced sexual activity and interest were separate and only partly related sequelae of the aging process in men. This finding is not contradictory to the well-established role of androgen in male sexuality, since T titer in aging men seldom falls to the level regarded clinically as being in the hypogonadal range. Similar to findings in male rat (see above), there seems to be no positive correlation between T levels and sexual function in a normal population of young men

Table 6. Sexual Performance: A Composite Score of Frequency of
Sexual Activities and Potency (Erection/Orgasm) in Men Grouped by
Age and by Tertiles of Free-T Index or LH[a]

	Free testosterone (pg/ml)			Luteinizing hormone (ng/ml)		
	<120	120–180	>180	<60	60–110	>110
40–49	4.5	3.9	3.7	3.9	3.8	4.7
50–59	3.3	3.5	4.0	3.8	3.9	3.1
60–69	3.5	3.2	3.2	3.6	3.0	3.0
70–93	2.2	2.3	3.0	3.1	2.2	2.3

[a] Tertile limits were based on approximate mean values for youngest and oldest age
groups. Two-way analysis of variance: Age, $p < 0.001$; Free T, $p > .05$; LH, $p < 0.03$.

(Brown *et al.,* 1978). Thus, the aging male presumably benefits from a
considerable redundancy of available androgen.

Our data therefore leaves unexplained much of the decline in sexual
function. Since this study was conducted in an outpatient clinic, it should
be noted that reported diseases (and alcohol consumption) contributed
virtually not at all to the variance in sexual behavior or in free-T index,
as determined by multiple regression analysis. The aging decline seems
unrelated to health factors; it was no less obvious in the Baltimore Study
of men who were exceptionally healthy (Martin, 1981; Tsitouras *et al.,*
1982), than in our population. Likewise, in an earlier study on 157
considerably less healthy men (60–74 years), impotence rose from 30%
to 60% with age but was independent of physical health, with particular
attention to present and past urologic disease (Bowers *et al.,* 1963).

There is an obligation to mention, before ending this section, that
the behavioral aspect of research in this field is still in a quite rudimentary
stage. Thus each study mentioned is flawed by inadequate or absent
statistical analysis or use of nonvalidated data-gathering techniques or
failure to take into account cohort vs. aging effects in cross-sectional
research. We believe, however, that the errors concern matters of detail
and that the major findings discussed are most likely valid.

4. The Male: Summary Statement and Discussion

The decline in sexual behavior in middle or advanced age is universal in all mammalian species studied, affecting most aspects of the
behavior, though not all to the same extent. While decreased circulating

T is a finding common to most studies, the origin of the change in androgenic status is different in different species. Thus, the primary change is testicular in humans, in the hypothalamo-hypophysial axis in laboratory rodents, and may (speculatively) be limited to target tissue insensitivity in rhesus. The search for causal relationships between the decline in androgenic status and sexual behavior is clearly motivated by our knowledge that a certain level of T is essential for maintaining sexual functioning in all species studied.

Yet the androgen hypothesis for the etiology of sexual aging is an inadequate explanation for various reasons. First, T level does not always decline. This has been found to be true for many individuals in all studied species, for group data in one mouse strain, in the only systematic study performed on rhesus monkeys, and in highly selected populations of men. Second, the level of sexual function associated with young adulthood could not be restored by administering T to older rats or monkeys. That the endocrine changes in aging can differentially affect different behavioral functions is indicated by the effective restoration of reflex erections in castrated, middle-aged rats with T treatment. Thirdly, statistical analyses on a reasonably large population of men showed that the decline in free T could account for only a small part of the decline in sexual function. Likewise, in a longitudinal study of aging rats, the behavioral changes were not correlated with the change in T level.

We conclude that sexual behavior as a whole and especially sexual motivation has not yet shown itself to be a simple function of the decline in T levels, free or total, in any species, and least of all in primates. However, the correlational studies in men suggest some relation between certain potency measures and testicular function, a finding reminiscent of the data on erection in rats.

Could there be another neuroendocrine factor or factors which is/ are responsible for these changes? Alterations in cerebral monoamine function, and particularly decreased dopaminergic transmission, have been documented in aging rodents and humans (Osterburg *et al.*, 1981) and such alterations have been implicated in sex hormone changes during the male's aging process (Riegle and Miller, 1978) and in sexual behavior of young adults (Beyer, 1979). Elucidation of the possible role of monoamines however, will not be easy, if only because of the multiplicity of their apparent functions in the central nervous system as mediators of endocrine action as well as regulators of hormone secretion and as direct neurobehavioral transmitters without endocrine involvement.

Various neuropeptides can also qualify as candidates for the role of mediators of the aging sexual decline. An interesting example is gonadotropin-releasing hormone (GnRH) which has a facilitatory effect on male sexual behavior in rats with low T levels (Moss *et al.*, 1975) and this could become limiting when T falls in aging. It is also capable of stimulating sexual arousal in rats by intraventricular injection of subliminal doses (Dorsa and Smith, 1980). Even more interesting, administration to castrated rats of a powerful GnRH analog, which antagonizes functions of the native peptide, facilitates the postoperative decline in sexual behavior (Dorsa *et al.*, 1981). A role of GnRH in aging is supported by data showing a decrease in GnRH content of the hypothalamus in aged rats (Riegle *et al.*, 1977), though there is no reliable method of assessing GnRH production rates except for the rigorous approach of portal vessel cannulation. If, however, the reduced LH level in aging rodents is of hypothalamic origin, decreased GnRH production may be assumed, at least in the hypophysiotropic areas of the hypothalamus.

Other neuropeptides which deserve consideration include the endogenous opiates which inhibit sexual behavior in various species. Steger *et al.* (1980) reported increased hypothalamic met-enkephalin content in old rats, but again production rate cannot be measured. Prolactin, which is also inhibitory to sexual behavior, may deserve some consideration since plasma levels are reportedly mildly elevated in aging rats (Meites *et al.*, 1980). However, in this laboratory no substantial increases in prolactin levels in aging men (Davidson *et al.*, 1983) or middle-aged Long–Evans rats (unpublished data) have been found. It should be noted that the levels of prolactin which have been related to sexual dysfunction in young adult subjects of both species are extremely high and well above those claimed to result from aging.

Finally, despite all that has been said, it may be premature to eliminate androgen as a major factor even in primates. The behavioral decline may be related less to blood T levels than to androgen receptor function or other factors affecting T sensitivity. Androgen receptors in prostate are reportedly reduced in old rats (Shain, 1973) and the foreskin of old men shows decreased 5α-reductase activity (Wilson, 1971) though not decreased androgen concentration (Desleypere and Vermeulen, 1981). There is, however, no predicting how long it will take to identify the relevant receptors in the CNS which could eventually prove to be substrates for aging changes in sexual behavior.

5. Female Animals

With increasing age, females of most mammalian species undergo dramatic alterations in reproductive function (Talbert, 1977) which are more substantial and abrupt than those of males. Aging effects on sexual behavior must therefore be considered in the light of these reproductive–endocrine transformations. For nonhuman species, sexual behavior in the female is closely tied to the reproductive cycle, and the dramatic endocrine alterations result in comparable disruptions in behavior. In the widely studied laboratory rat, most females cease regular cyclicity during middle age (9–13 months) and enter into a state of constant estrus or, less commonly, constant diestrus (reviewed in Schneider, 1978). Constant estrus denotes a state of continuous high levels of circulating estrogen, vaginal cornification, and the absence of ovulation. Sexual receptivity is also continuous as a result of the elevated estrogen titers. Constant diestrus is a state of continuous nonreceptivity as a result of repetitive periods of "pseudo-pregnancy" or pituitary hypofunction. In both cases, estrogen titers are low (Huang *et al.*, 1978). Central gonadotropin regulatory mechanisms are disrupted in the middle-aged rat. Both negative and positive feedback effects of ovarian steroids are severely attenuated (Meites *et al.*, 1978; Gray *et al.*, 1980a; Peng *et al.*, 1980). However, middle-aged (12–14 months) or older (18–20 months) female rats in constant vaginal estrus showed no change in sexual behavior as compared to 6-month-old controls. The older group showed a decline only in proceptive (female initiated) behavior (Borchardt *et al.*, 1980). Presumably those old rats which become acyclic without constant estrus ("pseudopregnant" or in "constant diestrus") are not sexually receptive. Their behavioral responsiveness to hormones has not been studied.

A report by Farrell *et al.* (1977) indicates a gradual decline in receptivity of spayed, steroid-treated hamsters, which becomes marked only in advanced old age. This probably reflects a decreased sensitivity to estrogen and/or progesterone.

Given the fact that alterations in circulating ovarian steroid levels account largely for the reported changes in female rat sexual behavior, we decided to examine whether changes also occur in the steroid sensitivity of neural mechanisms regulating receptivity. Since, as noted above, a pronounced reduction in steroid sensitivity occurs in brain–pituitary mechanisms regulating LH during middle age resulting in the loss of cyclicity, it was of interest to determine the generality of such a change in sensitivity with respect to other neural functions. Ovariectomized females of varying ages were treated with estrogen or estrogen plus progesterone and then their lordotic response to mating attempts by vigorous males was evaluated. Middle-aged females (14 months) did not differ from young adult females in their sexual receptivity, indicating no change in the steroid sensitivity with aging (Gray *et al.*, 1980a). Other investigators (Peng *et al.*, 1980) have similarly examined the sexual receptivity of spayed aging females, finding essentially no difference in the receptivity response (lordosis quotient) to high (supraphysiological) doses of estradiol benzoate among 5–8-, 15–23- and over 24-month-old groups. Although one report (Cooper, 1977) noted an increase in behavioral sensitivity to estrogen in old females, this remains an intriguing but not confirmed finding. The motivational (proceptive) component of female sexual behavior has not yet been studied in aging, in terms of hormone sensitivity.

The hormone–behavior relationships in female rats thus clearly contrast with those of the male, in that females seem to show no decline in sensitivity of the central nervous (Barfield and Chen, 1977) and/or peripheral (Komisaruk *et al.*, 1972) mechanisms subserving lordotic behavior. In both sexes the behavioral systems are clearly differentiated from the gonadotropin regulatory systems in the effects of aging on steroid sensitivity. Thus, aging female rats show reduced negative and positive feedback effectiveness of ovarian steroids (Gray *et al.*, 1980a) while aging males show increased negative feedback sensitivity (Gray *et al.*, 1980b).

6. Women

6.1. Sexual Decline and the Menopause

The questions to ask about sexuality in aging women are similar to those asked about men. Only the answers are different, though not as much as one might predict. In this section, we will examine available information regarding sexual aging in women and the sparse evidence on possible neuroendocrine mechanisms relating to it. The discussion will of necessity be dominated by menopause, which is second only to puberty as a dramatic natural transformation of the endocrine system.

The second Kinsey *et al.* (1953) study claimed that the peak frequency of sexual outlets occurred somewhat later in women than in men, i.e., in the 20's (but see comment Section 3). A marked decline was also noted in the 6th decade. Now, though 50 years is the approximate mean age at menopause, Kinsey *et al.* (1953, p. 735) interpreted the detailed data they collected on 173 females who had undergone natural menopause as indicating no effect of this phenomenon on the age-related decline of sexual response and activity. Rather the decline in the 6th decade was attributed to a reduction in sexual interest of the male partners. Yet a more objective interpretation of their data (39% and 42% of

127 orgasmic women reported no change in sexual response and total outlet, respectively, while 48% and 53% showed decreases) would be that menopause does result in a definite drop in these sexual functions, even if embedded in a more gradual overall age-related decline. Perhaps Kinsey's opposition to the influence of menopause is related to his down-grading of the importance of hormones in sexuality as a whole, expressed also in the case of the male, where he was clearly wrong (see above and Bermant and Davidson, 1974). This apparent bias against a role for menopausal hormone changes may be responsible for the suggestion that women might have "seized upon menopause . . . as an excuse for discontinuing sexual relationships in which they were never particularly interested" (Kinsey *et al.*, 1953). Interestingly, 13% of the respondents reported an *increase* in sexual function, which was ascribed by the authors to loss of fear of pregnancy. This explanation for enhanced sexuality, like that advanced for the more common decline, is certainly less applicable today than at the time of the Kinsey study.

Two prominent studies in the 1960's tended to support the conclusions of Kinsey. Thus, Masters and Johnson (1966) strongly supported the view that menopause was no necessary barrier to continued sexual life, but did not present data on the extent or frequency of change. The Duke University longitudinal and cross-sectional data on married couples also supported Kinsey's views and supplied data to show the powerful influence of the husband's aging on the wife. Unfortunately, these well-known studies (Verwoerdt *et al.*, 1969a,b; Pfeiffer *et al.*, 1972) did not pay direct attention to menopause. They did report that while only 7% of their women subjects aged 46–50 had totally lost sexual interest, this proportion had reached 51% by 61–65 years. Comparable figures in men were 0 to 11% respectively.

While men largely attributed responsibility for cessation of coitus to themselves, women attributed it to loss or incapacity of their husbands, to a very large extent (Table 4; Pfeiffer *et al.*, 1972).

The extent to which intercourse was replaced by other sexual activities was not assessed, though Christenson and Gagnon (1965) found that masturbation declines less after 50 than does intercourse. These workers and Van Keep and Kellerhalls (1974) were unable to substantiate the Kinsey and Masters and Johnson finding of a substantial number of women showing increased activity during the perimenopausal years. Various studies in addition to the Duke reports have demonstrated the sexual decline in coital activity in women during the 6th decade, but without specific focus on menopause (Christenson and Gagnon, 1965; Christenson and Johnson, 1973).

Hällström (1977) studied 800 women of 46–54 years of age living in the Swedish city of Göteborg and found a high incidence of decreased sexual activity, sexual interest, and orgasmic activity, while very few women reported increased sex drive. After comparing pre- and post-menopausal women of the same age they found by correlational analysis that the changes occurring in these years were due to menopause and not to aging *per se*. Moreover, they provided evidence that the changes did not result from the "husband effect." Thus, women who showed declining sexual interest more commonly did not have a greater age discrepancy with their husbands; their husbands had a greater sexual interest, and they were more sexually submissive to their husbands than those who did not decline. The findings of the Hällström study are more convincing and more applicable to present day conditions than the previous studies, in so far as specific focus on perimenopausal events is concerned. It is of interest that Hällström (1977) found declining sexual interest to be more common in lower socioeconomic groups. His interpretation was that education leads to greater freedom from cultural inhibitions and sexual stereotypes. Similar findings on socioeconomic factors on the impact of menopause on female sexuality were reported in another European study (Van Keep, 1975).

As discussed above for the male, it is also believed that maintained sexual behavior in aging women somehow protects against loss of sexual capacity. Any implication, however, that there is direct evidence for prevention of the sexual changes of senescence by a "treatment" with sexual activity would be unjustified. The data, in fact, may merely support what Pfeiffer and Davis (1972) term the "consistency of life style" throughout the aging process (Busse and Pfeiffer, 1969; Havighurst and DeVories, 1969).

We stated at the beginning of this chapter that libido and potency can be regarded as the major dimensions of sexuality in *both* sexes. That libido declines in an appreciable number of women from the 6th decade on is obvious from the data on "sexual interest," discussed above. Yet, there is still considerable lack of clarity or, at least agreement, as to whether this apparent loss of libido is the woman's "fault," i.e., derives from psychobiological changes in the woman or society or indeed from actual or potential sexual partners. It is hard to reconcile the conclusion that menopause is a major point of sexual decline with the belief that the cause is partner related. The problem cannot be resolved without further research, preferably by longitudinal study of menopause. But is failure of potency, i.e., physiological sexual response, an important element in the female sexual decline?

The cessation of ovarian cyclic activity at menopause has well-known consequences for the anatomy of the reproductive tract and some of these may be crucial for the declining sexual response. Masters and Johnson's (1966) list includes the following changes: decreased clitoral glans tumescence, thinning of the walls of the vagina and decreased vaginal vasocongestion and lubrication, changes in the labia related to reduction in its fatty tissue deposits, and absence of dilation of the cervical os and involution of the uterus, which ceases to elevate during arousal. Quantitative data on the extent and frequency of effects were not presented, nor were the changes related specifically to menopause. Semmens and Wagner (1982) present, in a "pilot study," a variety of measurements on vaginal functions in postmenopausal women, comparing the results to data collected separately under unspecified conditions on considerably younger premenopausal subjects. The authors interpreted the data as indicating that the postmenopausal women showed a lower volume of vaginal secretions and difference in electrical potential across the vaginal mucosa than younger cycling women. In addition, the vaginal pH was elevated in the postmenopausal group. The measurements were made under baseline conditions, i.e., subjects were presumably non-aroused.

The extent to which these changes in "potency" are limiting to the menopausal women's sexual function is not yet clear. Masters and Johnson (1966) concluded that a common problem in sexual activity of the postmenopausal female was failure of "lubrication" of the vagina because of reduced vasocongestive response and that this condition could be corrected by estrogen treatment or application of topical jellies. But despite Masters and Johnson's pioneering clinical data (1966) it remains an unfinished and important task to establish quantitatively the physiological response of the postmenopausal women *in sexual situations*. Studies are in progress in this laboratory, applying the photoplethysmographic method, to assess vaginal blood flow in response to erotic film and fantasy in young and postmenopausal women. The first study (Morrell *et al.,* 1983) shows significantly lower responses in the latter group. The two groups differed greatly in age as well as menopausal status but study of older premenopausal women indicated that the difference in response could be largely attributed to the menopause. However, the menopause is the crucial time of most rapid endocrine change, the influence of which will be considered next.

6.2. Hormones and Sexuality in Women

Because of the abruptness and extent of the gonadal endocrine change which occurs in middle-aged women, the prospect of identifying specific hormone–behavior relationships in sexual aging should be more promising in women than in men. This promise is yet unfulfilled, but with the recent increase in quantity and (more gradually) in quality of the research, a behavioral endocrinology of menopause is beginning to emerge.

One approach used is correlational. It is an attempt to demonstrate specific relationships between incidence/degree of sexual dysfunction and extent of change in blood estrogen or androgen levels. Although various studies have skirted this issue, none have approached it head-long. Studd *et al.* (1977) could find no correlation between "the presenting symptom of loss of libido" and plasma androgen level in post-menopausal women visiting a menopause clinic. Later, the same group (Chakravarti *et al.*, 1979) found that perimenopausal women attending the clinic and presenting with vasomotor symptoms (hot flushes) had significantly lower estradiol levels (but no difference in testosterone) and a considerably lower incidence of loss of libido (9/40) than those without hot flushes and with normal estrogen (19/42). The latter group also had a high incidence of depression (36/42). A much higher percent of patients in the former group had their symptoms relieved by estrogen.

There are, however, difficulties with these studies; their validity in terms of hormone–behavior relationships is limited for reasons related to subject selection, demand characteristics, and lack of proper control procedures in this clinical population. Also deficient in this area of research are appropriate measures of behavior change, and careful sampling and validation procedures, as pointed out by Zussman *et al.* (1981). An example of the previous generation of superficial investigations is the well publicized conclusion of Utian (1975) that loss of libido is not related to estrogen deprivation. This was based on the suggestive, but certainly not conclusive evidence that hysterectomy resulted in loss of libido in a high percentage of patients which did not differ whether or not ovariectomy was also performed.

There are a large number of studies on estrogen replacement therapy in postmenopausal women, but very few have paid more than nominal attention to the analysis of sexuality. One double-blind study (Campbell, 1976) reported a significantly decreased incidence of vaginal dryness, but no change in coital frequency or satisfaction, nor in masturbation or orgasms. Another double-blind study (Fedor-Freybergh, 1977) utilized a number of measures related to libido as well as sexual activity and found that estrogen significantly improved both, as well as orgasmic capacity. The most thorough work relevant to this question dealt with ovarian hormone replacement therapy in "artificial menopause." Using a double-blind crossover design, Dennerstein *et al.* (1980) gave women who had undergone hysterectomy–ovariectomy for benign disorders, 3 months each of treatment with a synthetic estrogen, a synthetic progestin, a combination of the two and a placebo. Estrogen had the most beneficial effects on reported sexual desire, enjoyment, and orgasmic frequency. No significant differences were observed in coital rate or in daily-scored analog rating scales for depression, anxiety, and sexual response, although the authors expressed doubt about the validity of analog scales. The synthetic progestin norgestrel produced a clear inhibitory trend, though no statistical significance was reported. If menopause is said to be roughly equivalent to functional ovariectomy, these results suggest that adverse effects of the menopause can logically be ascribed to estrogen deficiency, affecting various aspects of sexuality, at least in part.

From a maze of discrepant and often inadequate reports as to what exactly is/are the relevant changes in female aging, two conclusions emerge. Decreased vaginal response is a not infrequent result of menopause and there is enough evidence to relate this phenomenon to hypoestrogenemia, regardless of its still unclear interactions with libido factors. Laboratory studies are still greatly needed to specify quantitatively the nature and extent of the estrogen-related defects in sexual response. Semmens and Wagner (1982) have developed several methods applicable to this objective. Their preliminary study suggests that estrogen replacement can be effective in restoring several baseline measurements of vaginal function in postmenopausal women, particularly pH.

What is still completely undetermined is whether the hormonal decline produces changes in the brain or other branches of the nervous system(s) affecting sexuality, or only in genitopelvic structures, such as the vascular bed, sensory receptors, etc. If topical administration of estrogen is more effective than systemic treatment, we might postulate a largely direct effect of estrogen on the vagina. Unfortunately, estrogen in vaginal creams is more efficiently absorbed into the circulation than the common oral preparations (Studd and Thom, 1981). If and when vaginal dryness in a subject can be effectively treated, from the sexual point of view, by local application of nonhormonal lubricating jelly, it is hard to argue that an *important* dimension of estrogen-mediated sexuality is involved, rather than a relatively trivial mechanical problem.

The other major structure which undergoes atrophy in menopausal women and can be restimulated with estrogen, is the uterus. Its possible role in sexual experience is unclear but persistent suggestions have been made that it contributes importantly to orgasm, in some women at least, due perhaps to direct stimulation of the cervix in coitus (reviewed by Zussman *et al.*, 1981). The role of the uterus during sexual arousal and activity remains to be adequately studied. It has implications apart from menopause for other questions such as the effects of hysterectomy, probably the most common (and often controversial) operation on women at present (Dennerstein *et al.*, 1980; Zussman *et al.*, 1981).

The role of androgen remains elusive. It has been much less studied then estrogen and progestin because the clinical indications for its use are not nearly as clear as those of the ovarian steroids. Moreover, despite persistent clinical claims and some inadequate research, its importance as a natural regulator of sexuality in women is still not established (Bancroft, 1980; Davidson, 1978; McCauley and Ehrhardt, 1976). Several clinical researchers have nevertheless used androgen alone, or more often in combination with estrogen, and report successful treatment of sexual dysfunction in the menopausal woman (Greenblatt and Perez, 1974; Studd *et al.*, 1977; Studd and Thom, 1981). The requisite double-blind studies have not yet been published, nor has the possibility been considered that effects of androgen could be mediated by its aromatization to estrogen. It should be noted that because of the adrenal contribution and production of androgen by the ovarian stroma, androgen level is less affected by menopause than estrogen.

This review has not treated the question of hormone release resulting from coital activity, mostly because the subject seems only marginally germane to aging. Two observations, however, deserve mention. In rats, a spontaneously ovulating species in which coitus nevertheless can release a large surge of LH, (Brown-Grant *et al.*, 1973; Davidson *et al.*, 1973), mating-induced LH release is one of the first to decline in early middle-aged females (Gray *et al.*, 1980a). And to end on what may seem to be a bizarre note, we have observed that regular weekly coitus is clearly associated with low incidence or severity of hot flushes in perimenopausal women (Table 7). A credible interpretation of this finding,

Table 7. Incidence of Hot Flushes in Relation to Frequency of Coitus in Perimenopausal Volunteers[a]

Hot flushes	Coital frequency	
	Sporadic	Weekly
Present	25	3
Absent	9	7

[a] Behavioral data were collected prospectively by daily calendars over a period of ten weeks. Weekly = coitus at least once each week; Sporadic = less than once weekly. (From Cutler, McCoy, and Davidson, unpublished.)

though not the only one, is that regular sexual activity maintains estrogen levels *via* enhanced gonadotropin release.

7. Concluding Discussion

The lesser amount of attention given to females than to males in this review is not due to any bias on our part, but to the smaller corpus of data of possible relevance to the reproductive psychoneuroendocrinology of aging. Age-related deterioration of sexual behavior has not been reported in female animals, except for one study showing the reduction of proceptive behavior only in old rats and one showing declining receptivity in hamsters. In women, even the involvement of hormones in the CNS regulation of sexual behavior is far from established, unlike the situation in men and female mammals. Nevertheless, this situation could change overnight if definitive research were to show that androgen has a major role to play in women's sexual functioning.

The barely explored frontier which faces us is the mechanism of the action of aging on the hormone sensitivity of sexually relevant central or peripheral tissues in either sex. This could involve changes in receptors or other mechanisms of hormonal action, including membrane alterations or enzymatic transformations such as the aromatization of androgen likely involved in the sexual differentiation of perinatal rat brains (see MacLusky and Naftolin, 1981). If mechanisms of this type were to be established in explanation of the aging decline, they could be potentially applicable to all species and sexes in which there is such a decline. An appropriate neuroendocrine model for these phenomena could be the aging changes in the putative feedback receptors for gonadal steroids involved in the regulation of gonadotropin secretion. The age-related alterations in feedback sensitivity differ between sexes and species, and the direction of effects on feedback sensitivity differ from those on behavioral sensitivity. Thus, in experimental rodents, negative and positive feedback sensitivity declines in middle-aged females (Gray *et al.*, 1980a) while negative feedback sensitivity in the male actually increases (Gray *et al.*, 1980b). In humans, the situation differs in that reproductive aging entails a primary gonadal decline in both sexes. In addition, postmenopausal women are reported to show a significant decline in negative (but not positive) feedback sensitivity to estrogen (Mills and Mahesh, 1978), and old men show a similar decline in negative feedback response to androgen (Muta *et al.*, 1981). Investigation of the central mechanisms underlying these changes, and similar ones in the reproductive tissues, could provide a powerful impetus for work on the mechanisms of steroid–behavioral interactions in aging.

In closing this chapter, we return to the phenomenon presented at its outset, the libido–potency gap. Assuming the equivalence of this dichotomous characterization of sexual behavior across sexes and species, how general is the gap? We may conclude that it does indeed exist in men and in part is due to androgen deficiency, but in small part only. In male rodents, it does not seem to exist. All measures of sexual behavior decline with age, with no obvious major discrepancy in rate except for ejaculatory potency. In female animals, no very prominent sexual decline with aging has been demonstrated, certainly no clear decrease in steroid sensitivity of the behavior. In women, it is hard to discern with clarity a libido–potency gap as we peer through the obscuring mists of culture-bound expectations, male-originated influences, and our ignorance of the nature and physiologic bases of female sexuality. There certainly seem to be hormonal effects on behavior in women, but their precise definition and degree of importance for women's sexuality elude us at this present time.

ACKNOWLEDGMENTS. The authors' work was supported by NIH grants AG01437, AG01312, and MH21178. The technical assistance of Brenda Siddall, Dorothy Tallentire, Rich Humbert, and Diane Szumowski is gratefully acknowledged, as is the secretarial support of Cathy Spruck and Jean Caldwell.

8. References

Baker, H. W. G., Burger, H. G., de Kretser, D. M., Hudson, B., O'Connor, S., Wang, C., Mirovics, A., Court, J., Dunlop, M., and Rennie, G. C., 1976, Changes in the pituitary-testicular system with age, *Clin. Endocrinol.* **5**:349–372.

Bancroft, J., 1980, Endocrinology of sexual function, *Clin. Obstet. Gynecol.* **7**:253–281.

Barfield, R. J., and Chen, J., 1977, Activation of estrous behavior in ovariectomized rats by intracerebral implants of estradiol benzoate, *Endocrinology* **101**:1716–1725.

Beach, F. A., 1976, Sexual attractivity, proceptivity and receptivity in female mammals, *Horm. Behav.* **7**:105–138.

Bermant, G., and Davidson, J. M., 1974, *Biological Bases of Sexual Behavior*, Harper and Row, New York.

Beyer, C., 1979, *Endocrine Control of Sexual Behavior*, Raven Press, New York.

Borchardt, C. M., Lehman, J. R., and Hendricks, S. E., 1980, Sexual behavior and some of its physiological consequences in persistent estrous aging female rats, *J. Aging* **3**:59–63.

Bowers, L. M., Cross, R. R., and Lloyd, F. A., 1963, Sexual function and urologic disease in the elderly male, *J. Am. Geriat. Soc.* **11:**643–652.

Bronson, F. H., and Desjardins, C., 1977, Reproductive failure in aged CBF, male mice: Interrelationships between pituitary gonadotropic hormones, testicular function and mating success, *Endocrinology* **1:**939–945.

Brown, W. A., Monti, P. M., and Corriveau, D. P., 1978, Serum testosterone and sexual activity and interest in men, *Arch. Sex. Behav.* **7:**97–103.

Brown-Grant, K., Davidson, J. M., and Greig, F., 1973, Induced ovulation in albino rats exposed to constant light, *J. Endocrinol.* **57:**7–22.

Busse, E. W., and Pfeiffer, E. F., 1969, Functional psychiatric disorders in old age, in: *Behavior and Adaptation in Late Life* (E. W. Busse and E. F. Pfeiffer, eds.) Little Brown, Boston.

Campbell, S., 1976, Double blind psychometric studies on the effects of natural estrogens on postmenopausal women, in: *The Management of the Menopause and Post-Menopausal Years* (S. Campbell, ed.), University Park Press, Baltimore, pp. 149–158.

Chakravarti, S., Collins, W. P., Thom, M. H., and Studd, J. W. W., 1979, Relation between plasma hormone profiles, symptoms, and response to oestrogen treatment in women approaching the menopause, *Brit. Med. J.* **1:**983–985.

Chambers, K. C., and Phoenix, C. H., 1981, Diurnal patterns of testosterone, dihydro-testosterone, estradiol and cortisol in serum of rhesus males: Relationship to sexual behavior in aging males, *Hor. Behav.* **15:**416–426.

Chambers, K. C., Hell, D. L., and Phoenix, C. H., 1981, Relationship of free and bound testosterone to sexual behavior in old rhesus males, *Physiol Behav.* **27:**615–620.

Christenson, C. V., and Gagnon, J. H., 1965, Sexual behavior in a group of older women, *J. Gerontol.* **20:**351–356.

Christenson, C. V., and Johnson, A. B., 1973, Sexual patterns in a group of older, never married women, *J. Geriat. Psychiat.* **6:**80–98.

Cooper, R. L., 1977, Sexual receptivity in aged female rats. Behavioral evidence for increased sensitivity to estrogen, *Horm. Behav.* **9:**321–333.

Coquelin, A., and Desjardins, C., 1982, Luteinizing hormone and testosterone secretion in young and old male mice, *Am. J. Physiol.* E257–E263.

Craigen, W., and Bronson, F. H., 1982, Deterioration of the capacity for sexual arousal in aged male mice, *Biol. Reprod.* **26:**869–874.

Cutler, W., McCoy, N., and Davidson, J. M., Relationships between estrogen level, hot flashes, and sexual behavior in premenopausal women (unpublished).

Damassa, D. A., Smith, E. R., and Davidson, J. M., 1977, The relationship between circulating testosterone levels and sexual behavior, *Horm. Behav.* **8:**275–286.

Davidson, J. M., 1977, Neuro-hormonal bases of male sexual behavior, in: *Reproductive Physiology II, International Review of Physiology,* Vol. 13 (R. O. Greep, ed.), University Park Press, Baltimore, pp. 225–254.

Davidson, J. M., 1978, Gonadal hormones and human behavior, in: *Hormonal Contraceptives, Estrogen and Human Welfare,* Chap. 12 (M. C. Diamond and C. C. Korenbrot, eds.), Academic Press, New York, pp. 123–131.

Davidson, J. M., 1980, The psychobiology of sexual experience, in: *The Psychobiology of Consciousness* (J. M. Davidson and R. J. Davidson, ed.), Plenum Press, New York, pp. 271–332.

Davidson, J. M., Smith, E. R., and Bowers, C. Y., 1973, Effects of mating on gonadotropin release in the female rat, *Endocrinology* **93:**1185–1192.

Davidson, J. M., Gray, G. D., and Smith, E. R., 1978, Animal models in the endocrinology of reproductive behavior, in: *Animal Models for Research on Contraception and Fertility*, Harper and Row, New York, p. 61.

Davidson, J. M., Camargo, C. A., and Smith, E. R., 1979, Effects of androgen on sexual behavior in hypogonadal men, *J. Clin. Endocrinol. Metabol.* **48:**955–958.

Davidson, J. M., Chen, J. J., Crapo, L., Gray, G. D., Greenleaf, W. J., Catania, J. A., 1983, Hormonal changes and sexual function in aging men, *J. Clin. Endocrinol. Metab.* (in press).

Dennerstein, L., Burrows, G. D., Wood, C., and Hyman, G., 1980, Hormones and Sexuality: Effect of Estrogen and Progestogen, *Obstet. Gynecol.* **56:**316–322.

Desleypere, J. P., and Vermeulen, A., 1981, Aging and tissue androgens, *J. Clin. Endocrinol. Metabol.* **53:**430–434.

Dorsa, D. M., and Smith, E. R., 1980, Facilitation of mounting behavior in male rats by intracranial injection of luteinizing hormone-releasing hormone, *Regul. Pep.* **1:**147–155.

Dorsa, D. M., Smith, E. R., and Davidson, J. M., 1981, Endocrine and behavioral effects of continuous exposure of male rats to a potent LHRH agonist: Evidence for CNS actions of LHRH, *Endocrinology* **109:**729–735.

Edwards, A. E., and Husted, J. R., 1976, Penile Sensitivity, Age and Sexual Behavior, *J. Clin. Psychol.* **32:**697–700.

Eleftheriou, B. E., and Lucas, L. A., 1975, Age-related changes in testes, seminal vesciles and plasma testosterone levels in male mice, *Gerontologia,* **20:**231–238.

Farrell, A., Gerall, A. A., and Alexander, M. J., 1977, Age-related decline in receptivity in normal, neonatally androgenized female and male hamsters. *Exp. Aging Res.* **3:**117–128.

Fedor-Freybergh, P., 1977, The influence of oestrogens on the well-being and mental performance in climacteric and Post-menopausal women, *Acta Obstet. Gynecol. Scand.* (Suppl.) **64:**1.

Finch, C. E., Jones, V., Wisner, J. R., Jr., Sinha, Y. N., de Vellis, G. S., and Swerdloff, R. S., 1977, Hormone production by the pituitary and testes of male, C57BL/6J mice during aging, *Endocrinology* **101:**1310–1317.

Gray, G. D., 1978a, Changes in the levels of luteinizing hormone and testosterone in the circulation of aging male rats, *J. Endocrinol.* **76:**551–552.

Gray, G. D., 1978b, Age-related changes in penile erections and circulating testosterone in middle-aged male rats, in: *Aging and Neuroendocrine relationships* (A. D., Kenny, D. E. Potter, and C. E. Finch, eds.), Plenum Press, New York.

Gray, G. D., Tennent, B., Smith, E. R., and Davidson, J. M., 1980a, Luteinizing hormone regulation and sexual behavior in middle-aged female rats, *Endocrinology* **107:**187–194.

Gray, G. D., Smith, E. R., and Davidson, J. M., 1980b, Gonadotropin regulation in middle-aged male rats, *Endocrinology* **107:**2021–2026.

Gray, G. D., Smith, E. R., Dorsa, D. M., and Davidson, J. M., 1981, Sexual behavior and testosterone in middle-aged male rats, *Endocrinolgy* **109:**1597–1604.

Greenblatt, R. B., and Perez, D. H., 1974, Problems of libido in the elderly, in: *The Menopausal Syndrome* (R. B. Greenblatt, V. B. Mahesh, and P. G. McDonough, eds.), Medcom Press, New York, pp. 95–101.

Hällström, T., 1977, Sexuality in the climacteric, *Clin. Obstet. Gynecol.* **4:**227–239.

Harman, S. M., and Tsitouras, P. D., 1980, Reproductive hormones in aging men. I. Measurement of sex steroids, basal luteinizing hormone, and Leydig cell response to human chorionic gonadotropin, *J. Clin. Endocrinol. Metabol.* **51:**35–40.

Hart, B., 1982, Neural bases of sexual behavior: A comparative analysis, in: *Handbook of Behavioral Neurobiology* (R. W. Goy, and D. W. Pfaff, eds), Plenum Press, New York (in press).

Havighurst, R. J., and DeVories, A., 1969, Life styles and free time activities of retired men, *Hum. Dev.* **12:**34–54.

Hegeler, S., 1981, The sexual function of 1161 elderly danish males, *5th World Congress of Sexology*, Jerusalem.

Huang, H. H., Steger, R. W., and Meites, J., 1978, Patterns of sex steroid and gonadotropin secretion in aging female rats, *Endocrinology* **103:**1855–1859.

Huber, M. H. R., and Bronson, F. H., 1980, Recovery of sexual activity with experience in aged male mice, *Exp. Aging Res.* **6:**385–391.

Huber, M. H. R., Bronson, F. H., and Desjardins, C., 1980, Sexual activity of aged male mice: Correlation with level of arousal, physical endurance, pathological status and ejaculatory capacity, *Biol. Reprod.* **23:**305–316.

Jakubczak, L. F., 1964, Effects of testosterone propionate on age difference in mating behavior, *J. Gerontol.* **19:**458–461.

Jakubczak, L. F., 1967, Age, Endocrines and Behavior, in: *Endocrines and Behavior* (L. Gitman, ed.), C. C. Thomas, Springfield, Illinois, pp. 231–245.

Kahn, E., and Fisher, C., 1969, The sleep characteristics of the normal aged male, *J. Nerv. Ment. Dis.* **148:**477–494.

Karacan, I., Hursch, C. J., and Williams, R. L., 1972, Some characteristics of nocturnal penile tumescence in elderly males, *J. Gerontol.* **27:**39–45.

Kinsey, A. C., Pomeroy, W. B., and Martin, C. E., 1948, *Sexual Behavior in the Human Male*, W. B. Saunders, Philadelphia.

Kinsey, A. C., Pomeroy, W. B., Martin, C. E., and Gebhard, P. H., 1953, *Sexual Behavior in the Human Female*, W. B. Saunders, Philadelphia.

Komisaruk, B., Adler, N., and Hutchinson, J., 1972, Genital sensory field: Enlargement by estrogen treatment in female rats, *Science* **178:**1295–1298.

Larsson, K., 1956, *Conditioning and Sexual Behavior in the Male Albino Rat*, Almkvist and Wiksell, Stockholm.

Larsson, K., 1958a, Sexual activity in senile male rats. *J. Gerontol.* **13:**136–139.

Larsson, K., 1958b, Age Differences in the diurnal periodicity of male sexual behavior, *Gerontologia* **2:**64–72.

Larsson, K., and Essberg, L., 1962, Effect of age on the sexual behavior of the male rat, *Gerontologia* **6:**133–143.

MacLusky, N. J., and Naftolin F., 1981, Sexual differentiation of the central nervous system, *Science* **211:**1294–1306.

Martin, C. E., 1981, Factors affecting sexual functioning in 60–79-year-old married males, *Arch. Sex. Behav.* **10:**399–420.

Masters, W. H., and Johnson, V. E., 1966, *Human Sexual Response*, Little Brown, Boston.

McCauley, E., and Ehrhardt, A. A., 1976, Female sexual response: Hormonal and behavioral interactions, *Prim. Care* **3:**455–476.

Meites, J., Huang, H. H., and Riegle, G. D., 1976, Relation of the hypothalamo-pituitary-gonadal system to decline of reproductive functions in aging female rats, in: *Hypothalamus and Endocrine Functions* (F. Labrie, J. Meites, and G. Pelletier, (eds.), Plenum Press, New York, pp. 3–20.

Meites, J., Huang, H. H., and Simpkins, J. W., 1978, Recent studies on neuroendocrine control of reproductive senescence in rats, in: *The Aging Reproductive System* (E. Schneider, ed.), Raven Press, New York, pp. 213–236.

Meites, J., Steger, R. W., and Huang, H. H. H., 1980, Relation of neuroendocrine system to the reproductive decline in aging rats and human subjects, *Fed. Proc.* **39:**3168–3172.

Mills, T. M., and Mahesh, V. B., 1978, Pituitary function in the aged. in: *Geriatric Endocrinology* (R. B. Greenblatt, ed.), Raven Press, New York, pp. 1–11.

Minnick, R. S., and Warden, C. J., 1946, The effects of sex hormones on the copulatory behavior of white rats, *Science* **103**:749–751.

Morrell, M., Dixen, J., Carter, S., and Davidson, J. M., 1983, *Am J. Ob. Gynec.* (submitted).

Moss, R. L., Dudley, C. A., Foreman, M. M., and McCann, S. M., 1975, Synthetic LRF: Potentiator of Sexual Behavior in the Rat, in: *Hypothalamic Hormones* (M. Motta, P. G. Crosignonni, and L. Martini, eds.), Academic Press, New York, p. 269.

Muta, K., Kato, K., Akamine, Y., and Ibayishi, H., 1981, Age related changes in the feedback regulation of gonadotropin secretion by sex steroids in men, *Acta Endocrinol. (Copenhagen)* **96**:154.

Newman, H. F., 1970, Vibratory sensitivity of the penis, *Fertil. Steril.* **21**:791–793.

Osterburg, H. H., Donahue, H. G., Severson, J. A., and Finch, C. E., 1981, Catecholamine level and turnover during aging in brain regions of male C57BL/6J Mice, *Brain Res.* **224**:337–352.

Peng, M. T., Yao, C. T., and Wan, W. C. M., 1980, Dissociation between female sexual behavior and luteinizing hormone release in old female rats, *Phsiol. Behav.* **25**:633–636.

Pfeiffer, E., and Davis, G. C., 1972, Determinants of sexual behavior in middle and old age, *J. Am. Geriat. Soc.* **4**:151–158.

Pfeiffer, E., Verwoerdt, A., and Davis, G., 1972, Sexual behavior in middle life, *Am. J. Psychiat.* **128**:1262–1267.

Phoenix, C. H., and Chambers, K. C., 1982, Sexual behavior in aging male rhesus monkeys, in: *Advanced Views in Primate Biology* (B. Chiarelli and R. S. Corruccini, eds.), Springer Verlag, Heidelberg, pp. 95–104.

Riegle, G. D., and Miller, A. E., 1978, Aging effects on the hypothalamic-hypophyseal-gonadal control system in the rat, in: *The Aging Reproductive System* (E. L. Schneider, ed.), Raven Press, New York, p. 159–191.

Riegle, G. D., Meites, L., Miller, A. E., and Wood, S. M., 1977, Effects of aging on hypothalamic LH-releasing and prolactin inhibiting activity and pituitary responsiveness to LH-RH in the male laboratory rat, *J. Gerontol.* **32**:13–18.

Robinson, J. A., Scheffler, G., Eisele, S. G., and Goy, R. W., 1975, Effects of age and season on sexual behavior and plasma testosterone and dihydrotestosterone concentrations of laboratory-housed male rhesus monkeys (Macca Mulatta), *Biol. Reprod.* **13**:203–210.

Schneider, E. L. (ed.), 1978, *The Aging Reproductive System*, Raven Press, New York.

Semmens, J. P., and Wagner, G., 1982, Estrogen deprivation and vaginal function in postmenopausal women, *J. Am. Med. Assoc.* (in press).

Shain, S. A., 1973, Prostatic receptors and the aging phenomenon, in: *Symposium on the Normal and Abnormal Problems of the Prostate* (M. Goland, ed.), C. C. Thomas, Springfield, Illinois, pp. 712–730.

Skakkeback, N. E., Bancroft, J., Davidson, D. W., and Warner, P., 1980, Androgen replacement with oral testosterone undecanoate in hypogonadal men: A double-blind controlled study, *Clin. Endocrinol.* **14**:49–61.

Solnick, R. L., and Birren, J. E., 1977, Age and male erectile responsiveness, *Arch. Sex. Behav.* **6**:1–9.

Sparrow, D., Bosse, R., and Rowe, J. W., 1980, The influence of age, alcohol consumption and body build on gonadal function in men, *J. Clin. Endocrinol. Metabol* **51**:508–512.

Stearns, E. L., MacDonnell, J. A., Kaufman, B. J., Lucman, T. S., Winter, J. S., and Faiman, C., 1976, Declining testicular function with age, *Am. J. Med.* **57**:761–766.

Stefanick, M. L., 1982, Ph.D. Dissertation, Stanford University, Palo Alto, California.

Steger, R. W., Sonntag, W. E., Van Vugt, D. A., Forman, L. J. and Meites, J., 1980, Reduced ability of naloxone to stimulate LH and testosterone release in aging male rats; possible relation to increase in hypothalamic met-enkephalin. *Life Sci.* **27**:747–753.

Studd, J. W. W., and Thom, M. H., 1981, Ovarian failure and aging, *Clin. Endocrinol. Metabol.* **10**:1.

Studd, J., Chakravarti, S., and Oram, D., 1977, Climacteric, *Clin. Obstet. Gynecol.* **4**:3–29.

Talbert, G. B., 1977, Aging of the reproductive system, in: *Handbook of the Biology of Aging* (C. E. Finch and L. Hayflicks, eds.), New York, p. 318.

Tsitouras, P. D., Martin, C. E., Harman, S. M., 1982, Relationship of serum testosterone to sexual activity in healthy elderly men, *J. Gerontol.* **37**: 288–293.

Utian, W. H., 1975, Effect of hysterectomy, oophorectomy and estrogen therapy on libido, *Int. J. Gynecol. Obstet.* **13**:97.

Van Keep, P. A., and Kellerhalls, J. M., 1974, The aging woman, *Acta Obstet. Gynecol. Scand.* (Suppl. **51**) 19–27.

Van Keep, P. A., and Kellerhalls, J. M., 1974, Die alterwerdende frau., *Therapiewoch* **45**:5170–5194.

Vermeulen, A., 1979, Decline in sexual activity in ageing men: Correlation with sex hormone levels and testicular changes, *J. Biosoc. Sci.* (Suppl.) **6**:5–18.

Verwoerdt, A., Pfeiffer, E., and Wang, H. S., 1969a, Changes in sexual activity and interest of aging men and women, *J. Geriat. Psychiat.* **2**:163–180.

Verwoerdt, A., Pfeiffer, E., and Wang, H. S., 1969b, Sexual behavior in senescence, *Geriatrics,* **24**:137–154.

Wilson, J. D., 1971, *Testosterone Metabolism in Skin,* 17th Symposium Dtsch. Ges. Endokrinol., Springer Verlag, Berlin, pp. 11–18.

Zussman, L., Zussman, S., Sunley, R., and Bjornson, E., 1981, Sexual response after hysterectomy-oophorectomy: Recent studies and reconsideration of psychogensis, *Am. J. Obstet Gynecol.* **140**:725–729.

CHAPTER 13

Regulation of Thyrotropin Physiology during Aging

ROBERT I. GREGERMAN

1. Introduction

The relationship of age to the functional state of the hypothalamic-pituitary-thyroid axis has been studied in a variety of ways to both animals and man. Basal concentrations of pituitary and of blood thyrotropin (TSH) have been measured and attempts made to relate these to circulating concentrations of the thyroid hormones. Thyrotropin-releasing hormone (TRH) has been administered to provoke pituitary secretion of TSH. The immunologic and functional characteristics of pituitary and blood TSH have been examined. Intact animals have been subjected to maneuvers (stress) which affect the secretion of TSH. It is safe to conclude from all of these observations that age certainly has an influence on the parameters studied, but the information that has thus far emerged from studies in animals and man is incomplete and does not fall into a single pattern.

2. Methodological Considerations

Assays for the thyroid hormones thyroxine (T_4) and triiodothyronine (T_3) in plasma are well developed and standardized for use with human plasma. Most of the methods in current use are radioimmunoassays. Many laboratories use "kits," packaged reagents which include antibody, labeled iodothyronine, standards, etc. These immunoassays

ROBERT I. GREGERMAN • Gerontology Research Center, National Institute on Aging, NIH, Baltimore City Hospital, Baltimore, Maryland 21224.

are frequently affected by nonspecific protein effects, so that their application to assays of thyroid hormone in rat or other animal sera sometimes produces inaccurate results. Any report which does not specify that the methodology has been appropriately validated is suspect. Unfortunately, many reports in the gerontology literature fail to provide this information. The interpretation of studies which attempt to approximate thyroid hormone binding for estimation of "free" (non-protein-bound) hormones are even more difficult to interpret. Many of these methods are not quantitative in any case. Moreover, when kits that are devised for use with human sera are used for rat serum, only gross approximation of the thyroid hormone binding may result. Even the best studied technique, equilibrium dialysis, yields results which are difficult to interpret. When a study uses a commercial kit and reports values in arbitrary units, even comparative data may be of little value.

The assay of TSH in serum (or pituitary) is perhaps even more complex. The fact that antibody specificity is not absolute is too often ignored. Instead of considering assays to represent "immunoassayable material" or "TSH-like immunoreactivity," the material at hand is considered to be TSH itself. In the absence of meticulous examination of immunologic reactivity and/or concurrent bioassay of the "TSH" being assayed, grossly erroneous conclusions may be reached concerning age-related alterations of TSH content.

Beyond these rather obvious, if frequently ignored considerations, studies of both animals and man too often fail to appreciate the characteristics of the populations being studied. For example, different investigators may report widely differing values for T_4 in plasma. Are these differences methodological (see above), due to differences of strain, i.e., genetically determined, or are the animals in different states of health? Investigators who work with experimental animals are often loathe to consider this last variable, but clinically oriented investigators have for some time been well aware of the influence of illness on plasma thyroid hormone levels and have recently recognized the effect of illness on pituitary responsiveness to thyrotropin. Even capable physician/clinical investigators may have trouble sorting out the difference between age and illness. Do we have any reason to believe that "basic" scientists, working with rats, are better able to recognize illness and its possible consequences in their animals? If, for no other reason than the increasing probability of death in the old animals, their state of health must be considered. The older the animal, the greater must be the suspicion that "age" may not be the proximate cause of the observed effect and that inapparent illness may be contributing in a major way.

Studies in animals may yield different results as a consequence of genetic influences with different rat strains showing different responses. Clinical investigations have also pointed to population differences (see below). These studies strongly suggest, for example, that genetic factors may be important determinants of age-related alterations of pituitary responsiveness to TRH, although factors of health status are by no means excluded.

Another consideration in the evaluation of age effects in animals is the precise ages of the animals compared. Frequently, comparison of young, still growing rats (2–4 months) is made with old but not necessarily senescent animals (18 months). Such comparisons are very likely to reveal effects of "aging," since many metabolic parameters differ between such groups of animals. But does this constitute "aging" or maturation? Would the same conclusion have been drawn had animals of 2–3 months been compared with others of 6 or 12 months?

Although many investigators are understandably eager to generalize from their work, numerous comparisons of results of endocrine studies in man and animals clealy reveal major species differences. Studies in animals can and should serve as models for those in man (or vice versa), but attempts to extrapolate observations made in one species to what "must" be found in another are completely unwarranted. When valid but different observations are made in different species, the results are not best interpreted as being "in conflict." Rather, the manifestations of age-related processes are simply likely to differ between unrelated species! Examples of these considerations will become apparent in the ensuing discussion.

3. Assessment of the Status of the Feedback System in the Basal State

3.1. Circulating Levels of Thyroid Hormones

Interpretation of the plasma concentrations of TSH must be made in the context of the simultaneous concentrations of the thyroid hormones. Accordingly, the available literature on the concentration of thyroid hormones will be reviewed here.

3.2. Studies in Animals

Studies of aging and plasma T_4 and T_3 in animals are interesting but are not appropriate model systems for the situation in man, since the plasma binding of thyroid hormones is quite different in animals than in man. It is of interest that a study of two strains of mice showed that plasma T_4 (measured as protein-bound iodine) decreased 30% and 65%, respectively, at advanced age (Eleftheriou, 1975). These observations cannot be simply interpreted in terms of TSH control of thyroid function, since no information was available on protein binding in plasma. However, the importance of genetic determinants is made obvious by such determinations. Other workers have presented data suggesting that changes of T_4 occurring in the rat during aging might well relate to alterations of changes of protein binding rather than to altered TSH regulation of thyroid function. For example, recent studies of the regulation of TSH during aging in rats have included data on T_4 and free T_4 (determined by equilibrium dialysis). A modest but significant decrease of plasma T_4 was seen between young and middle-aged male animals. The small further change of T_4 that was seen during senescence could be related to decreased protein binding (Klug and Adelman, 1979). In the relatively small number of animals studied, no significant decrease of free T_4 could be demonstrated between any of the groups. In another study of male rats, young (3–5 months) and old (22–24 months) animals were compared (Chen and Walfish, 1979). A rather striking difference of total T_4 could also be attributed to altered T_4 binding, since free hormone concentrations were the same in both groups. Others have also reported a similar pattern of T_4 and free T_4 in male rats (Valueva and Verzhikovskaya, 1977). Young animals (1–2 months) had the highest T_4 which fell with maturation (8–10 months) and fell even slightly more in the old and senescent animals (18–24 months). Similarly, estimates of free T_4 indicated that T_4 binding was altered, so that free T_4 remained essentially unchanged or decreased only slightly in comparing old and senescent animals with the mature. Similar observations using equilibrium dialysis had shown an identical pattern (Frolkis, et al., 1973).

The data for old male rats are in striking constrast to those reported for females (Chen and Walfish, 1978). In females, total T_4 was less in the old group, but, in contrast to the males, no major difference of protein binding was evident. As a result, in the females, decreased T_4 *was* accompanied by decreased free T_4. This study has a major limitation. Plasma T_4 was compared only between young (3–4 months) and old (18 months) rats. Since no comparison was made of mature vs. old (senescent) animals, the data are not to be interpreted as representative of aging in anything but the broadest sense.

Plasma T_3 and free T_3 in the male rat were considerably less in old than in young animals (Chen and Walfish, 1979; Klug and Adelman, 1979). In female rats, free but not total T_3 was decreased in the older animals studied (Chen and Walfish, 1978; Table 1).

Table 1. Thyroid Hormone Levels in
Blood of Old Rats Relative to Those in
Younger Animals[a]

	T_4	Free T_4	T_3	Free T_3
Old ♀	↓	↓	↔	↓
Old ♂	↓	↔	↓	↓

[a] See text for details and qualifications. ↓ = decrease; ↔ = no change.

3.3. Studies in Man

Until recently, in most studies of normal healthy adults, plasma (T_4) showed no change or decreased only slightly. Recent studies of large numbers of subjects do suggest that, even excluding subjects who may be ill, a modest decrease of T_4 may be seen at advanced age. This change does not exceed about 15% (Gregerman and Davis, 1978). In one report on several hundred apparently healthy elderly men and women (ages greater than 60 years) there was no significant decrease of T_4. However, a significant number (about 20% of individuals) had modest but clear elevations of TSH. In this group the mean T_4 was reduced (Sawin *et al.*, 1979). Another large survey reported similar results (Tunbridge, *et al.*, 1977). The implications of these findings will be discussed below. Suffice it to say at this point that aging in normal human populations reveals subgroups of persons with lowered T_4 and raised TSH, findings compatible with the simplest possible explanation, viz., age-related increase in the occurence of *hypothyroidism* due to thyroid gland failure. Most of these cases would have to be considered subclinical. However, other explanations are possible (see below).

The relationship of age to plasma triiodothyronine (T_3) concentrations in the human appears finally to have been resolved. Numerous early reports *seemed* to establish a substantial decrease of T_3 with aging. Later work suggested only a modest decrease in plasma T_3 (about 20% over the adult age span. However, a reexamination of the issue has firmly denied any decrease of T_3 with aging when the elderly were carefully screened for illness (Olsen et al., 1978). Plasma T_3 is now well-known to be affected by clinical status (especially the state of nutrition). The results of the early studies clearly reflect failure to select appropriate subjects for study. The entire saga presents a compelling argument for the need for careful clinical screening of subject populations and determination of the influence of illness on plasma hormone levels before attributing changes to aging *per se*.

Interpretation of plasma concentrations of T_4 (and to a lesser extent of T_3) must be made in relationship to the concentrations in plasma of the iodothyronine-binding proteins. A number of reports have suggested that the major T_4 carrier of man, thyroxine-binding globulin (TBG), increases while the lesser carrier, thyroxine-binding prealbumin (TBPA) falls at advancing age. However, neither plasma free T_4 concentration nor the free T_4 index appears to be affected at advanced age, although a single report suggests a significant fall of free T_4 (Gregerman and Davis, 1978). In evaluating these reports one should bear in mind again that the influence of illness may not have been appreciated. For example, in one report elderly healthy subjects were said to have shown a substantial increase of TBG and decreases of T_4 and T_3 (Hesch et al., 1977). The change in T_3 suggests, however, that the population may have included more ill persons than was appreciated; one can only speculate whether the TBG and T_4 results were similarly affected. Acute and chronic illnesses can certainly affect the plasma T_4, the concentrations of both TBG and TBPA, and the free T_4 (Lutz et al., 1972). Since such illnesses are, of course, common in the elderly, changes of these parameters are not readily attributable to age alone (Jefferys et al., 1972).

3.4. Regulation of Thyrotropin

In conventional considerations of the feedback control of TSH, decreased plasma levels of T_4 and T_3 should result in increased basal levels of TSH and increased responsiveness of the pituitary to exogenous TRH. It is clear from the preceding evaluation of plasma T_4 and T_3 (and free T_4 and T_3) during aging that some evidence for decreased plasma levels of thyroid hormones does exist, although the picture is incomplete and inconstant.

However, it will be obvious from the following discussion that no single pattern of TSH levels or responsiveness to TRH can be related to the levels of thyroid hormone in plasma and their changes with age. Nonetheless, age-related phenomena clearly influence basal levels of TSH, responsiveness to TRH, and other aspects of the regulation of TSH.

3.5. Thyrotropin under Basal Conditions and after TRH

Interpretation of TSH levels during aging in rats must be made in terms of the following considerations: differences between females and males, dissociation between biological and immunological activity, and the effect of circadian rhythms. These variables are discussed below and summarized in Table 2.

Table 2. Thyrotropin (TSH) in Blood of Old Rats and Responses of TSH to Thyrotropin-Releasing Hormone (TRH). Values are Relative to Young Animals[a]

	Basal TSH	TSH increase after TRH	Effect of castration on TRH response
Old ♀[b]	↔	↔	↓
Old ♂[c,d]	↑ or ↔	↑ or ↔	↔

[a] ↓ = decrease; ↑ = increase; ↔ = no change.
[b] Old ♀ rats were only 18 months.
[c] In one study in which basal TSH of old male rats was unchanged, circadian rhythm was obtained (see text).
[d] Castration decreased responsiveness to TRH in young but not old male animals.

Basal levels of TSH in young vs. old female rats were not increased, as one might have expected, despite the decrease of plasma T_4, free T_4, and free T_3. Moreover, the TSH increment after TRH was not different (Chen and Walfish, 1978). An influence of age could not be shown after ovariectomy and/or estradiol treatment. Ovariectomy of old rats decreased the response to TRH from six- to sevenfold before to three- to fourfold after castration. Comparing maximum levels of TSH *increment* after TRH, the change was reduced by nearly one-half for the older animals and remained the same for the younger animals. Treatment of ovariectomized rats with estradiol increased the response to TRH in both young and old animals, but the increase was much smaller in the old. These results clearly indicate that age is in an important determinant of pituitary responsiveness to *pharmacologic* doses of TRH under certain experimental conditions (castration, estrogen treatment) but do little to explain the age-related decrease of thyroid hormones in this group of older female rats. The failure of basal levels of TSH to rise in the face of lowered circulating levels of thyroid hormones does suggest an acquired derangement of hypothalamic-pituitary function, while the pharmacologic manipulations support this notion. Interpretation of TSH levels in rats is, however, complicated by the demonstration (see below) that immunologic and biologic activities are dissociated. Incidentally, the possibility of thyroid gland hyporesponsiveness to endogenous TSH was also raised by failure of T_3 to rise after administration of TRH to intact old rats.

In contrast to the findings in old female rats, several reports indicated modest but significant *increases* of basal TSH in old male rats (Chen and Walfish, 1979; Valueva and Verzhikovskaya, 1977; but see below). On the other hand, still different results and a more complicated effect of age was revealed by studies of the circadian rhythmn of TSH secretion (Klug and Adelman, 1979). Maximal levels of TSH were seen at 1000 hours at all ages. One-half of the mature (12 months) and none of the old (24 months) animals showed a clear drop at later hours, but young (2 months) animals showed a clear nadir at 2200 hours.

3.6. Response to TRH

The response of the male rat to TRH has not been uniform. A comparison of 3- to 5-month-old rats with others at 22–25 months found a significant decrease of responsiveness to TRH (Chen and Walfish, 1979). Castration decreased the response to TRH in young animals but had no effect on the old. Testosterone reversed the effect of orchidectomy in the young and significantly increased the response in the old. In contrast, in another study, there was no difference of responsiveness to TRH between mature (12 months) and senescent (24 months) animals (Klug and Adelman, 1979). In this study, young animals (2 months) exhibited the least responsiveness at low doses of TRH whether the TRH was injected into the pituitary or was given intravenously.

In a study of TSH in blood and pituitaries of male rats at various ages, progressively higher blood TSH values were reported in young (1–2 months) vs. middle-aged (8–10 months) vs. old animals (18–24 months); the old group had nearly twice the concentrations of the young (Valueva and Verzhikovskaya, 1977). A senescent group (28–32 months) showed a marked decrease of TSH responsiveness to TRH to less than one-half that of the old. Unfortunately, it is difficult to evaluate this report. The TSH values are stated to be in the range of 3–9 ng/ml, values far lower than those reported by several other groups (0.5–2.0 µg/ml or 500–2000 ng/ml). Whether this discrepancy represents a reporting error or some standardization problem in the immunoassay is unclear. If the changes can at least be thought of as relative, the pattern is still grossly different from the reports cited earlier. The corresponding pituitary concentrations, measured by bioassay, are in the range given in the literature. Whether expressed as total TSH in the pituitary or as TSH content/mg pituitary, the amount of TSH increased as animals matured, fell modestly in the old, and decreased in senescence to one-half the values seen at maturity. A parallelism was therefore observed between blood TSH and that in the pituitary. The plasma T_4 in these animals has been commented upon earlier. It is clear that TSH fell in the oldest animals despite maintenance of plasma-free T_4.

An attempt has been made to relate the pituitary's deiodinating capacity for T_4 to changes of pituitary TSH content (Valueva and Verzhikovskaya, 1977). Enhanced deiodination of T_4 was observed in old rats. This phenomenon was postulated to result in greater intrapituitary generation of T_3, and consequently more efficient suppression of pituitary TSH synthesis in the old animals. This postulate, while interesting, must be considered speculative. Disturbances of hypothalamic/pituitary regulation and impaired intrapituitary synthetic mechanisms have not been excluded as causes of the observed decrease of pituitary TSH content.

3.7. Molecular Aspects of TSH during Aging

Interpretation of blood and pituitary TSH concentrations and hence of the interpretation of experiments which alter TSH concentration are complicated by the demonstration that immunologically reactive TSH exists in large molecular forms (Klug and Adelman, 1977). The total immunoassayable TSH of serum was unchanged with age in the rats studied. However, when rat serum was subjected to gel filtration and the fractions assayed for TSH, several molecular species with apparent molecular weights much larger than that of TSH were measurable. The serum of old rats contained a much greater amount of this material. When serum from old rats was subjected to bioassay, much less bioassayable material was present in the sera of the old as compared to the young rats. Moreover, when gel filtered the fractions containing large molecular weight species also contained an inhibitor of TSH bioactivity. The implication of this observation is that circulating TSH may not exert its full biological effect in old rats, but such an interpretation should be made with caution. It remains to be shown that the inhibitor material, as assayable in a bioassay in the mouse, is also an effective inhibitor *in vivo* in the rat.

When the TSH of pituitaries was labeled with [^{3}H]leucine, heterogeneity of TSH-like immunoprecipitable materials was also demonstrable. The nature of these materials, whether precursors of TSH or unrelated materials, is not known. This pituitary TSH-like immunoreactivity was quantitatively much less than the material found in the serum.

3.8. Effect of Age on Stress-Induced TSH Secretion

The responsiveness of the hypothalamo-pituitary system to several stimuli is decreased in old rats. Thus, gonadotropin (FSH, LH) secretion is decreased in response to ovariectomy in old rats. Other stimuli such as progesterone treatment of estrogen-primed ovariectomized rats and ether stress also induce less release of FSH and LH in old rats. TSH secretion in rats is also known to be inhibited by several stress situations. Comparing young (2–3 months) and old (18–20 months) male rats, the stress of serial bleeding, ether exposure, and physical restraint inhibited serum TSH in the young animals but had a much smaller effect in the old (Simpkins *et al.*, 1978). Conversely, the augmented release of TSH that occurs with cold exposure was less in old than in young rats. Thus, the regulation of TSH secretion, like that of the gonadotropins, is age-related. In the case of TSH, the limited data to this point do not permit a differentiation between effects of maturation and those of senescence. Furthermore, the conflicting information on whether or not pituitary responsiveness to TRH is altered (Chen and Walfish, 1979; Klug and Adelman, 1979) does not permit assignment of a functional level at which the age-effect is manifest.

3.9. Thyrotropin Secretion during Aging in the Human

Aging in the human is well-known to be associated with an increasing incidence of hypothyroidism due to autoimmune disease of the thyroid that leads to gland failure. This phenomenon must be distinguished from alterations of thyroid function due to aging, *per se* (Gregerman and Bierman, 1981). However, since hypothyroidism is clearly increasingly frequent in the elderly, it is not surprising that surveys of older individuals should show elevation of TSH. Early studies of this issue from the U.S. assessed only small numbers of subjects and failed to note such age-related changes of TSH (Azizi *et al.*, 1975; Snyder and Utiger, 1972a). However, a number of European reports noted increased TSH levels in the elderly (see Gregerman and Davis, 1978). The most recent survey of several hundred relatively healthy men and women in the U.S. showed that about 20% had elevated TSH. Of these, 6% (3% of elderly men and 8% of elderly women) had clearly elevated (>10 μU/ml) basal levels of TSH (Sawin *et al.*, 1979). Minor but definite elevations were seen in an additional 14% (>5 ≤ 10 μU/ml). Similar results were reported in a community survey in Great Britain (Tunbridge *et al.*, 1977). On average, those older persons with *clearly elevated* TSH had lower levels of T_4 than those with a normal serum TSH. Those persons with *slightly elevated* TSH had no decrease of T_4 compared with the normal values for their age.

The issue of thyroid gland failure in the elderly was approached many years ago by studies of the responsiveness of the thyroid to exogenous TSH. One extensive and carefully conducted study of this type was made using supraphysiologic amounts of heterologous (bovine) TSH. No evidence of diminished thyroidal responsiveness was seen (Einhorn,

1958). On the other hand, two other smaller studies did report decreases (Lederer and Bataille, 1969; Scazziga and Lemarchand-Béraud, 1968). Until such time as similar studies of responsiveness to TSH are repeated in a sizeable number of elderly persons with elevated blood levels of TSH, and possibly until the issue of dose-response to exogenous TSH is settled, no firm conclusions will be possible from this approach.

The results available from studies showing frequent elevation of TSH might seem to be indicative of widespread latent hypothyroidism in the elderly. Such a view does not seem justified at this time. It should not be forgotten that T_4 and T_3 levels in the elderly human are well maintained (Gregerman and Bierman, 1981). Without doubt, a small but definite proportion of the elderly have hypothyroidism due to some degree of thyroid failure. In such persons, TSH is clearly elevated and T_4, while possibly still within the usual rather wide and normal range is, on average, low.

What then of that sizeable group with minimal elevations of TSH whose mean T_4 levels, like those of most elderly persons, are not decreased? Several obvious possibilites remain. The first may be that the elderly human, like the old rat, has elevated serum levels of *TSH-like*, immunoassayable material which may bear no functional relationship to TSH. Another possibility is that thyroidal responsiveness to TSH may decrease. In this case, the minimal increases of TSH seen in the elderly are homeostatic and necessary to maintain serum T_4 levels within the range seen in the young.

3.10. Response to Thyrotropin-Releasing Hormone

Highly variable results have been reported. Early findings from U.S. studies were a clear decrease with age of responsiveness in elderly men (Snyder and Utiger, 1972a) but no effect of age in elderly women (Snyder and Utiger, 1972b; Azizi, *et al.*, 1975). Another report on a large group of individuals from Europe indicated no effect of age in men but a clear decrease of responsiveness in women (Wenzel *et al.*, 1974). The reason for these variable results are not apparent, but characteristics of the populations must be considered in view of still another study of a Japanese population. In these apparently normal individuals, responses to TRH were unequivocably *increased* in the elderly (Ohara *et al.*, 1974). Moreover, doses of TRH that produced suboptimal responses in young adults were already maximal in the elderly. Thus, in this population of apparently normal elderly subjects, also characterized by unchanged levels of T_4 but frequently showing elevated levels of basal TSH, aging was accompanied by both increased sensitivity to TRH and hyperresponsiveness with maximal doses. Such results suggest that genetic or subtle environmental factors may strongly influence endocrine responses during aging in man and call for caution in drawing generalized conclusions from single populations.

3.11. The Hypothalamo-Pituitary-Thyroid Axis during Stress in the Elderly

Severe, life-threatening illness (often associated with septicemia, overwhelming pneumonia, or similar diseases) may be associated with development of a low T_4 in serum. Values for T_4 may be very low and into the hypothyroid range. Free T_4 is normal, low, or high. The TSH is "normal." The phenomenon has been termed the "euthyroid sick syndrome." The majority of such individuals do not survive, presumably because of the nature of their underlying illness. Most often, but not invariably, the affected individual is elderly. Although stress is associated with inhibition of TSH secretion in animals, no evidence exists to date that a similar phenomenon occurs in man, let alone under clinical circumstances of the type described. A major obstacle is the difficulty of measuring in the human values of TSH *within the normal range.** Thus, TSH secretion could conceivably fall during such illness. Since T_4 metabolism is accelerated during stressful illness (Gregerman and Solomon, 1967; Lutz *et al.*, 1972), the serum T_4 would be expected to fall to very low levels as the result of impairment of TSH-driven T_4 release *plus* accelerated T_4 disposal. Although response to TRH under these conditions of stress is often reported as "normal," recent work suggests that response to TRH is in fact grossly blunted, thus providing a possible mechanism for the suspected failure of TSH secretion that we postulate here. In the recovery phase, preliminary evidence is already at hand that "rebound" TSH oversecretion occurs.

The usual interpretion that has been given for the phenomenon of the euthyroid sick syndrome is that normal levels of free T_4 are maintained and that TSH secretion is normal and appropriate to the free T_4. In fact, the evidence suggests an alternative sequence. Free T_4 is often low in these cases (Slag, *et al.*, 1981) and thus the low T_4 may contribute to the morbidity and mortality of the syndrome. Since the serum TSH, as mentioned, has not heretofore been accurately assessed, stress-related failure of TSH secretion may well contribute to the pathogenesis of the

* TSH values by conventional immunoassays are reported as 0–6 µU/ml. In reality, many persons have undetectable values while the immunochemical significance of the "normal" values observed is unknown and may not pertain to the TSH molecule.

syndrome. Further work to define the role of TSH is clearly necessary and is underway in our laboratory using a TSH assay of improved sensitivity. Whether aging will also be found to play a dominant role in the development of the euthyroid sick syndrome remains to be determined.

4. Summary

Studies in animals and man of the basal and stress-related secretion of thyrotropin (TSH) have been reviewed in relation to the influence of age. Although it is now apparent from studies in man that illness may have a profound effect on function of the hypothalamic-pituitary-thyroid axis, most studies in animals have paid little or no attention to the possibility that "effects of age" may in fact be the consequences of inapparent disease in the old animals. Methodologic problems in the assays of TSH and even the thyroid hormones continue to receive inadequate attention with the result that the conclusions of many available studies are open to question. Failure to recognize possible genetic differences between animal strains continues to result in unwarranted generalizations, as do extrapolations from one species to another. A continuing problem is the lack of a generally accepted definition of aging, which is often coupled with failure of investigators to distinguish effects of maturation from those of senescence. Interpretation of the physiology of TSH during aging must also be considered in terms of already demonstrated differences between female and male animals, dissociation between biological and immunological activity of TSH, and age-related alterations of circadian rhythms.

Studies of TSH secretion in old animals are available only for the rat. In this species, basal levels of TSH have been reported not to increase in old females, despite reported decreases of plasma T_4, free T_4, and free T_3 in the old animals. Such evidence suggests an age-related derangement of hypothalamic-pituitary function, since basal levels of TSH fail to increase in the face of lowered levels of circulating thyroid hormones. In old males, basal levels of TSH have been reported to increase as expected from the concomitant age-related decrease of circulating thyroid hormones. However, the additional very important finding of immunologic heterogeneity of TSH during aging in the rat makes the increase of TSH difficult to evaluate.

Responsiveness of the pituitary to stimulation with thyrotropin-releasing hormone (TRH) has been reported to remain intact in old female rats. Responsiveness of old males has been reported to decrease in one study but not in two others. Old male rats fail to show the clear circadian rhythm of TSH secretion that is apparent in young and many mature animals.

In the rat, most forms of stress inhibit secretion of TSH. A variety of experimental stress-induced situations have a much smaller effect, i.e., suppress TSH secretion less, in old animals than in young. Conversely, the augmented release of TSH that occurs with cold exposure is less in old animals than in young.

Studies of thyrotropin secretion during aging in man are limited to observations in intact persons. These studies are, moreover, complicated by an increasing incidence of age-related but clinically inapparent thyroid disease. A significant proportion of elderly persons (up to 20%) have elevations of basal TSH. It seems probable, but is not established, that many or all of these individuals have autoimmune (Hashimoto's) thyroiditis and that the increase of TSH is a consequence of reduced thyroid gland secretion of thyroxine. The possibility that the elevations of TSH in the elderly human, like the old rat, may relate to elevated levels of TSH-like, immunoassayable material which is not biologically active remains to be examined.

The responsiveness of the pituitary of the aging human to TRH has been highly variable in different reports from around the world. The importance of genetic or subtle environmental factors seems inescapable from these reports.

Serious, life-threatening illness in the human results in a syndrome of low circulating thyroid hormones ("euthyroid sick syndrome"). The plasma T_4 may be well into the range seen in hypothyroidism and the plasma T_3 is invariably very low. TSH does not increase as would be expected from the low plasma T_4 and T_3, and responsiveness to TRH is blunted. The possibility that failure of TSH secretion may occur in these very ill individuals is currently under investigation. This situation is most often seen in elderly patients, perhaps because it is the elderly who most often become ill, and the phenomenon is not confined to the old. Whether advanced age is a major predisposing factor in the development of this syndrome remains to be established.

5. References

Azizi, F., Vagenakis, A. G., Portnay, G. I., Rapoport, B., Ingbar, S. H., and Braverman, L. E., 1975, Pituitary-thyroid responsiveness to intramuscular thyrotropin-releasing hormone based on analyses of serum thyroxine, tri-iodothyronine and thyrotropin concentrations, *N. Engl. J. Med.* **292**:273–277.

Chen, H. J., and Walfish, P. G., 1978, Effects of age and ovarian function on the pituitary–thyroid system in female rats, *J. Endocrinol.* **78**:225–232.

Chen, H. J., and Walfish, P. G., 1979, Effects of age and testicular function on the pi-tuitary–thyroid system in male rats, *J. Endocrinol.* **82**:53–59.

Einhorn, J., 1958, Studies on the effect of thyrotropic hormone on thyroid function in man, *Acta Radiol.* (Suppl. 160), 1–107.

Eleftheriou, B. E., 1957, Changes with age in protein-bound iodine (PBI) and body tem-perature in the mouse, *J. Gerontol.* **30**:417–421.

Frolkis, V. V., Verzhikovskaya, N. V., and Valueva, G. V., 1973, The thyroid and age, *Exp. Gerontol.* **8**:285–296.

Gregerman, R. I., and Bierman, E. L., 1981, Hormones and aging, in: *Textbook of Endo-crinology*, Chap. 29 (R. H. Williams, ed.), W. B. Saunders, Philadelphia, pp. 1192–1212.

Gregerman, R. I., and Davis, P. J., 1978, Effects of intrinsic and extrinsic variables on thyroid hormone economy. Intrinsic physiologic variables and nonthyroidal illness, in: *The Thyroid* (S. C. Werner, and S. H. Ingbar, eds.), Harper and Row, New York, pp. 223–246.

Gregerman, R. I., and Solomon, N., 1967, Acceleration of thyroxine and triiodothyronine turnover during infections and fever. Implications for the functional state of the thyroid during stress and in senescence, *J. Clin. Endocrinol.* **27**:93–105.

Hesch, R. D., Gatz, J., Jüppner, H., and Stubbe, P., 1977, TBG-dependency of age related variations of thyroxine and triiodothyronine, *Horm. Metab. Res.* **9**:141–146.

Jefferys, P. M., Farran, H. E. A., Hoffenberg, R., Fraser, P. M., and Hodkinson, H. M., 1972, Thyroid-function tests in the elderly, *Lancet* **1**:924–927.

Klug, T. L., and Adelman, R. C., 1977, Evidence for a large thyrotropin and its ac-cumulation during aging in rats, *Biochem. Biophys. Res. Commun.* **77**:1431–1437.

Klug, T. L., and Adelman, R. C., 1979, Altered hypothalamic-pituitary regulation of thyrotropin in male rats during aging, *Endocrinology* **104**:1136–1142.

Lederer, J., and Bataille, J. P., 1969, Senescence et fonction thyroidienne, *Ann. Endocrol. (Paris)* **30**:598–603.

Lutz, J. H., Gregerman, R. I., Spaulding, S. W., Hornick, R. B., and Dawkins, A. T., Jr., 1972, Thyroxine binding proteins, free thyroxine and thyroxine turnover interrela-tionships during acute infectious illness in man, *J. Clin. Endocrinol. Metabol.* **35**:230–249.

Ohara, H., Kobayashi, T., Shiraishi, M., and Wada, T., 1974, Thyroid function of the aged as viewed from the pituitary-thyroid system, *Endocrinol. Jap.* **21**:377–386.

Olsen, T., Laurberg, P., and Weeke, J., 1978, Low serum triiodothyronine and high serum reverse triiodothyronine in old age: An effect of disease not age, *J. Clin. Endocrinol. Metabol.* **47**:1111–1115.

Sawin, C. T., Chopra, D., Azizi, F., Mannix, J. E., and Bacharach, P., 1979, The aging thyroid. Increased prevalence of elevated serum thyrotropin levels in the elderly, *J. Am. Med. Assoc.* **242**:247–250.

Scazziga, B., and Lemarchand-Béraud, T., 1968, *Problèmes de Gériatrie*, Sandoz, Paris, p. 15.

Simpkins, J. W., Hodson, C. A., and Meites, J., 1978, Differential effects of stress on release of thyroid-stimulating hormone in young and old male rats, *Proc. Soc. Exp. Biol. Med.* **157**:144–147.

Slag, M. F., Morley, J. E., Elson, M. K., Labrosse, K. R., Crowson, T. W., Nuttal, F. Q., and Shafter, R. B., 1981, Free thyroxine levels in critically ill patients, *J. Am. Med. Assoc.* **246**:2702–2706.

Snyder, P. J., and Utiger, R. D., 1972a, Response to thyrotropin releasing hormone (TRH) in normal man, *J. Clin. Endocrinol.* **34**:380–385.

Snyder, P. J., and Utiger, R. D., 1972b, Thyrotropin response to thyrotropin releasing hormone in normal females over forty, *J. Clin. Endocrinol.* **34**:1096–1098.

Tunbridge, W. M. G., Evered, D. C., Hall, R., Appleton, D., Brewis, M., Clark, F., Grimley Evans, J., Young, E., Bird, T., and Smith, P. A., 1977, The spectrum of thyroid disease in a community: The Wickham survey, *Clin. Endocrinol.* **7**:481–493.

Valueva, G. V., and Verzhikovskaya, N. V., 1977, Thyrotropic activity of hypophysis during aging, *Exp. Gerontol.* **12**:97–105.

Wenzel, K. W., Meinhold, H., Herpich, M., Adkofer, F., and Schleusener, H., 1974, TRH-Stimulationstest mit Alters- und Geschlechtsabhängigem TSH-Anstieg bei Normalpersonen, *Klin. Wochenschr.* **52**:722–727.

CHAPTER 14

Changes in Growth Hormone Secretion in Aging Rats and Man, and Possible Relation to Diminished Physiological Functions

WILLIAM E. SONNTAG, LLOYD J. FORMAN, and JOSEPH MEITES

1. Introduction

Growth hormone (GH) is the most important protein-anabolic agent in the body and is essential for protein synthesis in body tissues throughout life. Growth hormone promotes body growth, bone growth, and liver, kidney, and hematopoietic functions. It stimulates the thymus gland that produces T cells and the hormone thymosin, which stimulates antibody production. Growth hormone also affects other physiological processes, including carbohydrate, lipid, vitamin, and mineral metabolism. The actions of GH appear to be mediated by direct action on tissues, and also through a family of hormones secreted by the liver, the somatomedins.

In general, aging in mammalian species is characterized by decreases in protein synthesis in many tissues and organs, a reduction in immunological vigor, diminished kidney and liver function, a decrease in bone mass, and other changes in metabolic processes. Growth stasis occurs in mature female rats and administration of GH has been shown to reinitiate body growth in these animals (Greenspan *et al.*, 1950). A decrease in GH secretion may be partially responsible for these aging events

WILLIAM E. SONNTAG and JOSEPH MEITES ● Department of Physiology, Neuroendocrine Research Laboratory, Michigan State University, East Lansing, Michigan 48824. **LLOYD J. FORMAN** ● Department of Medicine, University of Medicine and Dentistry of New Jersey, Camden, New Jersey 08103.

(Everitt and Burgess, 1976; Sonntag *et al.*, 1980, 1981). This suggests that there may be a deficiency in hypothalamic stimulation of GH secretion during aging.

It has been established that a correlation exists between some aspects of body growth and longevity. In many species, a positive correlation has been demonstrated between length of the growth period and lifespan (Asdell, 1946; Hammond and Marshall, 1952; Rockstein *et al.*, 1977). Food restriction, which increases the length of the growth period (albeit at a slower rate), has been reported to increase longevity in rats and mice (Northrop, 1917; McCay *et al.*, 1935; Saxton, 1945; Lansing, 1948; Everitt, 1959; Berg and Simms, 1960, 1961; Comfort, 1963, 1964; Miller and Payne, 1968). Food restriction in rats reduces secretion of GH and other hormones. However, administration of GH in attempts to maintain body growth and possibly reverse some of the age-related changes in metabolism due to aging have met with only limited success. Several investigators claimed to have restored some components of metabolic functions by injections of GH, but others found no effects (Asling *et al.*, 1952; Emerson, 1955; Everitt, 1959; Beck *et al.*, 1960; Jelinkova and Hrúza, 1954; Marelli, 1968; Root and Oski, 1969). These early studies concluded that one aspect of aging is a decline in tissue responsiveness to GH, which in the light of present knowledge, could involve a decrease in GH receptors in some body tissues.

In the last decade, many advances have been made in the understanding of the hypothalamic regulation of GH release from the pituitary. It is now known that GH secretion is episodic and is controlled by at least two hypothalamic hormones, GH release inhibiting factor or hormone (GHRIF or somatostatin) and a GH releasing factor (GHRF). The synthesis, release, and degradation of these hypothalamic hormones are believed to be regulated by a number of hypothalamic neuropeptides and neurotransmitters. In addition, other factors such as thyroid, gonadal, adrenal cortical, and pancreatic hormones, as well as physiological stimuli, such as stress, exercise, sleep, and diet have been reported to influence GH secretion either by acting directly on the pituitary, or acting via the hypothalamus. Earlier workers who investigated GH secretion during aging were unaware of the pulsatile nature of GH secretion, and of its intricate hypothalamic control. Also, radioimmunoassays for analysis of GH in the systemic blood were not available. Most of the early investigators concluded that there were no significant changes in GH secretion during aging.

The purpose of this chapter is to review what is presently known about age-related changes in the regulation of GH secretion, and to speculate on the significance of diminished GH secretion in relation to decreased functions of some body tissues and organs.

2. Alterations in Episodic Growth Hormone Secretion with Age

Early studies on GH secretion in both animals and man were compromised by the absence of sensitive assays and by lack of knowledge of the pulsatile nature of GH release. We are now aware that frequency and amplitude of GH pulses are specific for animals of different species, ages, and sex. In young adult male rats, for example, immunoreactive GH pulses range from trough values of 10 ng/ml to peak values greater than 600 ng/ml, with a period of approximately 3 hr (Tannenbaum and Martin, 1976; Sonntag et al., 1980). In the adult female rat, the amplitudes of the pulses are smaller and the secretory episodes occur at approximately hourly intervals (Saunders et al., 1976). It has been reported that GH pulses are entrained to the light-dark cycle in rats, but there is much variation in the onset, amplitude, and duration of these pulses. This inherent variation between GH pulses makes comparisons unreliable without frequent blood sampling. Furthermore, pulsatile secretion of GH is known to be influenced by stress and anesthetics. These difficulties in measuring GH release have been resolved by obtaining serial samples of blood via an atrial cannula from unanesthetized, unrestrained animals at frequent intervals for several hours. The frequency, amplitude, and duration of GH pulses can then be compared, and estimates made on the total amount of GH secreted from the pituitary.

Early investigators of pituitary and plasma values of GH in old animals reported levels to be increased, decreased, or unchanged with age. It is now known that at least part of the causes for these discrepancies were due to assaying single rather than multiple samples of blood, and collecting blood from anesthetized animals. More recently, studies which assessed pulsatile release of GH in old male rats revealed a significant decrease in amplitude of these pulses as compared to those in young animals (Sonntag et al., 1980). Greater than 57% of the young rats (3- to 4-months old) exhibited high amplitude pulses of GH (greater than 300 ng/ml), whereas only 7% of the old animals (18–20 months old) exhibited pulses of this amplitude (Fig. 1). There was no apparent change in the periodicity of these pulses or entrainment to the light-dark cycle. Moreover, trough GH levels were not different, but mean GH concentrations were approximately three times greater in young than in old

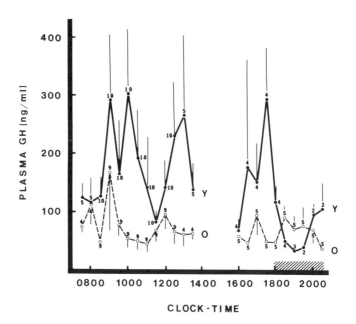

Fig. 1. Mean plasma GH concentrations in young (Y) and old (O) male Sprague–Dawley rats. Each point represents the mean for the number of observations indicated. Vertical bars represent the SEM. Shaded area is the dark phase of the light-dark cycle. (From Sonntag *et al.*, 1980, with permission of the publisher.)

animals. In the female rat, GH pulses occur at hourly intervals with individual values ranging from 10 to 180 ng/ml. As in the male rat, old constant estrous females exhibited a reduction in the amplitude of GH pulses (Forman *et al.*, 1982). However, as a result of increased trough GH concentrations in the old female rats, mean values were similar to those of young animals.

In humans, age-related changes in pulsatile GH secretion have been found. In young adults, small GH pulses occur throughout the day, and a marked surge of GH occurs approximately 2 hr after the onset of sleep (Takahashi *et al.*, 1968; Sassin *et al.*, 1969; Carlson *et al.*, 1972; Finkelstein *et al.*, 1972). The sleep related increase in GH accounts for the major portion of GH secreted during a 24-hr period. Age-related changes in basal GH levels in humans have been controversial, with reports of increases (Sandburg *et al.*, 1973; Blichert-Toft, 1975), decreases (Danowski *et al.*, 1969; Vidalon *et al.*, 1973), or no changes with age (Kalk *et al.*, 1973). Although differences in basal levels of GH between young and old individuals may be the result of differences in body weight or alterations in levels of other hormones that contribute to GH release, analysis of the sleep-related increase in GH has revealed a consistent reduction in the amplitude of these pulses with age (Carlson *et al.*, 1972; Finkelstein *et al.*, 1972; Thompson *et al.*, 1972; Blichert-Toft, 1975; Bazarre *et al.*, 1976; Prinz *et al.*, 1981). The reduction of GH pulse amplitude contributes to, or may be primarily responsible for, the age-related decrease in integrated concentrations of human GH during a 24-hr period.

Since evidence for attenuation of the pulsatile release of GH during aging in rats and man has only recently been demonstrated, its possible relation to decrements in the function of many body tissues and organs is unknown at present. It seems probable that diminished GH secretion is directly related to some of the changes observed in GH target tissues and organs during aging such as loss of muscle mass and bone, and the decline in immunological vigor, kidney, liver, and possibly other functions. It will be of interest to determine whether the return in old male rats of high amplitude pulsatile GH secretion by administration of L-dopa (Sonntag *et al.*, 1982a), also can reverse some of the decrements in body functions seen in these old animals.

3. Mechanisms Responsible for Alterations in Growth Hormone Secretion with Age

3.1. Pituitary

The hypothesis that age-related changes within the hypothalamus are responsible for many of the deficits in the secretion of anterior pituitary hormones is well documented (Meites *et al.*, 1978). However, evidence for age-related changes which are intrinsic to the pituitary gland is only beginning to be recognized. There are two lines of evidence to support this hypothesis: (1) there is a reduction in the capacity of synthetic hypothalamic hormones to stimulate anterior pituitary hormone release, possibly due to alterations in the mechanism of hypothalamic hormone action, and (2) there are qualitative changes in the hormone synthesized and released by the anterior pituitary.

Both synthetic luteinizing hormone-releasing hormone (LHRH) and thyrotropin-releasing hormone (TRH) administration have been reported to increase LH, follicle-stimulating hormone (FSH), and thyrotropin (TSH) secretion, respectively, more in young than in old animals (Bruni *et al.*, 1977a; Meites *et al.*, 1978; Sonntag *et al.*, 1982b). Also, as early as 1965, investigators reported that partially purified hypothalamic extracts increased GH release more in young than in old animals (Pecile *et al.*, 1965). However, the assay method used by Pecile *et al.* (1965) can be considered questionable, and the hypothalamic extract used undoubtedly contained somatostatin as well as GHRF. The reduced capacity of the pituitary of old rats to respond normally to hypothalamic hormones may be the result of (1) a reduced ability of the pituitary to produce receptors for hypothalamic hormones, (2) an increase in enzymatic degradation of hypothalamic hormones, (3) a diminished capacity of the pituitary to synthesize hormones, or (4) changes in the capacity of hypothalamic hormones to initiate mechanisms involved in the release of pituitary hormones. There is also the possibility that hypersecretion of somatostatin may contribute to diminished GH release (refer to Section 3.3). Some of these possibilities are currently being investigated in our laboratory.

There is also evidence that qualitative changes in pituitary hormones occur with age. For example, there is evidence that immunoreactive TSH (Klug and Adelman, 1977) LH (Conn *et al.*, 1980), and β-endorphin (Forman *et al.*, 1981) circulate in higher molecular weight forms in old animals. The higher molecular weight variants of TSH and LH have been reported to exhibit diminished biological activity when compared to the lower molecular weight forms normally found in the plasma of young rats. Although the biological activity of circulating GH has not been compared between young and old animals, we have preliminary evidence that immunoreactive GH in old male and female rats also circulates as a higher molecular weight species (Sonntag *et al.*, unpublished). If these qualitative changes in GH result in diminished biological activity, it may be a significant factor in the altered metabolic functions of old animals.

3.2. GHRF

Although its structure is unknown, there is considerable physiological evidence for the existence of a hypothalamic GHRF (Deuben and Meites, 1964; Martin, 1979; Meites and Sonntag, 1981). Bioassayable GHRF is believed to be present in the ventromedial nucleus (VMN) of the rat hypothalamus, since electrical stimulation of the VMN produces an increase in GH release, whereas lesions of this area reduce GH release and result in growth retardation (Frohman *et al.*, 1968; Frohman and Bernardis, 1968). In the original work by Deuben and Meites (1964), dose–response effects of hypothalamic extract on GH release *in vitro* were demonstrated. Also, boiling of the hypothalamic acid extract did not destroy its biological activity, indicating it is probably a peptide. A recent private communication by R. Guillemin to J. Meites (June 1982) indicates that structural determination of the GHRF peptide is close at hand.

3.3. Somatostatin

There is a substantial body of evidence which suggests that somatostatin participates in the control of pulsatile GH secretion (Martin, 1979). Electrical stimulation of the preoptic area (which contains somatostatin perikarya) increased somatostatin release into the hypothalamic hypophysial portal circulation (Chihara et al., 1979), and decreased GH release from the pituitary (Martin, 1974). Lesions of the preoptic area decreased hypothalamic somatostatin content and resulted in increased GH secretion (Rice and Critchlow, 1976; Critchlow et al., 1978), whereas episodic GH release appears to continue (Martin, 1979). Recently, in vivo measurement of somatostatin secretion in the median eminence, using a push-pull cannula system, revealed that somatostatin was released in discrete pulses which were inversely correlated with GH secretory episodes (Kasting et al., 1981). Together, these results suggest that somatostatin is released in discrete pulses which may contribute to or regulate episodic GH release. To date, there have been no studies of pulsatile release of hypothalamic hormones in old animals.

In old animals, somatostatin content measured by radioimmunoassay (RIA) was decreased in rostral (associated with somatostatin synthesis) and caudal (associated with somatostatin release) hypothalamic areas (Sonntag et al., 1980). Immunocytochemical studies found decreased staining of somatostatin fibers in the hypothalami of old animals, in agreement with our results (Sladek and Hoffman, 1980). Since hypothalamic somatostatin content is the result of synthesis, degradation, and release of the peptide, age-related changes in content fail to give significant information on the relationship between somatostatin and diminished amplitude of GH release.

We have attempted to assess the importance of somatostatin in old animals by passive immunization with somatostatin antiserum. When old and young animals were injected with 5 ml/kg antiserum, there was a similar rise in GH in both age groups (Fig. 2). However, a higher dose of the antiserum (8 ml/kg) increased GH more in old than in young rats. This suggested that aging rats retain the capacity to secrete as much GH as young animals when the inhibitory effects of somatostatin are removed. Somatostatin release from the hypothalamus of old animals may

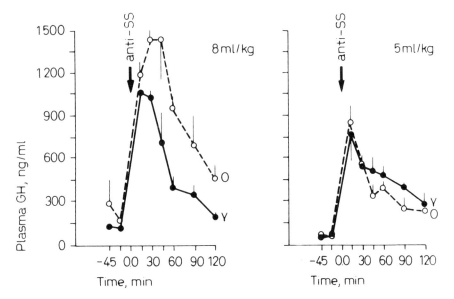

Fig. 2. Plasma GH in young (Y) and old (O) male rats after passive immunization with somatostatin antiserum (anti-SS number 774: courtesy of Dr. Akira Arimura). Vertical bars represent SEM. (From Sonntag *et al.*, 1981, with permission from the publisher.)

be increased or the pituitaries of old animals may be more sensitive to the inhibitory effects of the hormone. There is also recent evidence that higher molecular weight forms of somatostatin exist which can be secreted into the hypothalamic hypophysial portal circulation (Chihara *et al.*, 1979). Higher molecular weight species of somatostatin (somatostatin-28, somatostatin-25) have been reported to exhibit increased biological activity as compared to somatostatin-14 (Tannenbaum *et al.*, 1981). There are no studies of higher molecular weight species of somatostatin in the hypothalamus of old rats, but if these forms are increased in old animals, they could participate in the decline in pulsatile GH release.

There is no direct evidence at present that hypothalamic somatostatin or GHRF secretion is altered with age. The decrease that was observed in somatostatin content in old rats together with studies of passive immunization with somatostatin antiserum, suggest that regulation of somatostatin secretion by the hypothalamus or pituitary sensitivity to somatostatin is altered with age.

3.4. Neurotransmitters

Growth hormone release can be stimulated by neurotransmitters which act to increase GHRF secretion or inhibit somatostatin release (Meites and Sonntag, 1981). For example, dopamine and dopaminergic drugs such as apomorphine and piribedil have generally been shown to increase plasma levels of GH in mature male and female rats (Mueller *et al.*, 1976; Vijayan *et al.*, 1978), whereas some antidopaminergic drugs and catecholamine synthesis inhibitors decreased GH release (Kato *et al.*, 1973). In man, the release of GH is clearly stimulated by L-dopa, dopamine, bromoergocryptine, or subemitic doses of apomorphine (Boyd *et al.*, 1970; Mims *et al.*, 1973; Lal *et al.*, 1975), whereas the dopamine receptor blocker, pimozide, attenuated the GH rise produced by arginine infusion or exercise (Martin, 1976).

There is also evidence for an α-adrenergic component in the regulation of GH secretion. In the male rat, both α-methyl-para-tyrosine, a catecholamine synthesis inhibitor, and phenoxybenzamine, an α-adrenergic receptor antagonist, abolished the episodic release of GH, whereas clonidine, an α-adrenergic receptor agonist, increased GH release (Durand *et al.*, 1977). Clonidine has also been reported to increase plasma GH in man (Lal *et al.*, 1975). Phentolamine, an α-adrenergic receptor blocker, inhibited GH release induced by insulin hypoglycemia, arginine, vasopressin, L-dopa, exercise, or stress (Martin, 1976). It is unclear if these putative neurotransmitters increase GH by stimulating release of GHRF or by inhibiting release of somatostatin.

The role of serotonin in the physiological regulation of GH secretion in rats and humans is uncertain. In the rat, some investigators reported that the serotonin antagonist, parachlorophenylalanine (PCPA) did not affect the pulsatile release of GH (Eden *et al.*, 1979), whereas others observed that PCPA administration abolished pulsatile release of GH (Arnold and Fernstrom, 1978). However, intraventricular injections of serotonin were reported to increase plasma levels of GH in the rat (Collu *et al.*, 1972), and this effect was blocked by the serotonin antagonist, cyproheptadine (Smythe *et al.*, 1975). Similarly, in humans, some laboratories reported that serotonin increased GH secretion (Bivens *et al.*, 1973; Imura *et al.*, 1973; Nakai *et al.*, 1974), whereas others found no effect (Benkert *et al.*, 1973; Müller *et al.*, 1974). Cyproheptadine also decreased or abolished the sleep-related increase in plasma GH levels (Chihara *et al.*, 1976), and diminished the rise in serum GH associated with exercise (Smythe and Lazarus, 1974), arginine infusion (Nakai *et al.*, 1974), and insulin-induced hypoglycemia (Bivens *et al.*, 1973; Smythe and Lazarus, 1974). In general, it appears that serotonin can influence GH secretion in rats and humans, but the exact nature of its physiological role remains to be determined.

The presence of endogenous opiate peptides in the brain and pituitary, and the observed increase in GH secretion produced by opiates, suggest that endogenous opiates may participate in the regulation of anterior pituitary function, including secretion of GH. In the rat, administration of the opioid peptides, β-endorphin or met[5]-enkephalin, produced a rapid elevation in plasma GH (Dupont *et al.*, 1977; Rivier *et al.*, 1977; Bruni *et al.*, 1977b), which was antagonized by the opiate receptor antagonist, naloxone (Rivier *et al.*, 1977; Bruni *et al.*, 1977b; Shaar *et al.*, 1977). However, the role of endogenous opioid peptides in the physiological regulation of GH secretion in the rat is controversial, since opiate antagonists appear to have no effect on basal pulsatile secretion of GH in the rat (Martin *et al.*, 1979; Tannenbaum *et al.*, 1979). In humans, enkephalin analogs were reported to increase GH secretion (Stubbs *et al.*, 1978; Delitala *et al.*, 1981; Grossman *et al.*, 1981). However, naloxone administration alone decreased GH release induced by arginine infusion or exercise stress, but failed to reduce basal levels of GH or to abolish the rise in GH produced by apomorphine, L-dopa, insulin hypoglycemia, or sleep (Lal *et al.*, 1979; Martin *et al.*, 1979; Morley *et al.*, 1980; Spiler and Molitch, 1980; Wakabayashi *et al.*, 1980). These observations suggest that under some circumstances, endogenous opiate peptides may participate in the regulation of GH secretion.

We have tested the capacity of several potent CNS active drugs to increase GH release in young and old animals (Sonntag *et al.*, 1981). The α-adrenergic receptor agonist, clonidine (Fig. 3), the dopamine receptor agonist, piribedil (Fig. 4), and morphine (Fig. 5) produced a smaller increase in GH release in old than in young male rats. Similar results were found in old female rats after administration of clonidine and morphine (Forman *et al.*, 1982). There also are reports of diminished release of GH in man after L-dopa (Bazarre *et al.*, 1976), exercise (Bazarre *et al.*, 1976), or insulin-induced hypoglycemia (Laron *et al.*, 1970). The capacity to increase GH in response to pharmacological stimuli with age may be the result of an inadequate release of GHRF, a failure of these drugs to reduce somatostatin secretion, or altered pituitary responsiveness to these hormones. It is also possible that these differences are the result of a deficiency in postsynaptic neurotransmitter receptors that have been reported to occur with aging (Govoni *et al.*, 1978; Greenberg and Weiss, 1978; Maggi *et al.*, 1979).

Many of the neuroendocrine changes that develop with aging may be related to changes in synthesis or release of neurotransmitters (refer

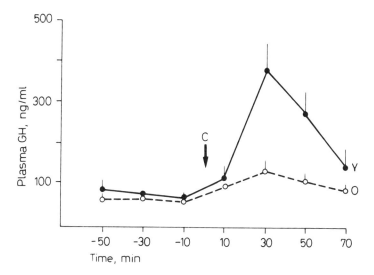

Fig. 3. Effect of an intravenous injection of clonidine hydrochloride (150 μg/kg) on plasma GH levels in young (Y) and old (O) male rats. α-methyl-p-tyrosine (250 mg/kg, i.p.) was injected 1 hr prior to the experiment. Vertical bars represent SEM. (From Sonntag *et al.*, 1981, with permission of the publisher.)

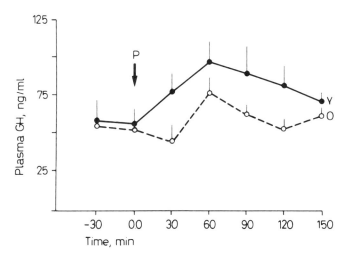

Fig. 4. Effect of piribedil methane sulfonate (1 mg/kg, s.c.) on plasma GH concentrations in young (Y) and old (O) male rats. Vertical bars represent SEM. (From Sonntag *et al.*, 1981, with permission of the publisher.)

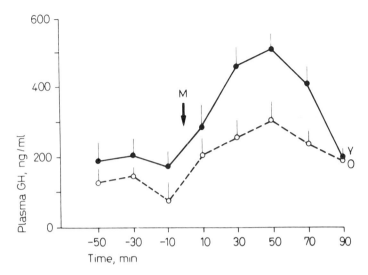

Fig. 5. Effect of an intravenous injection of morphine sulphate (5 mg/kg) on plasma GH in young (Y) and old (O) male rats. Vertical bars represent SEM.(From Sonntag *et al.*, 1981, with permission of the publisher.)

to Chapter 6 by Simpkins, this text). It appears to be well established that the content and turnover of the hypothalamic catecholamines, dopamine, and norepinephrine, are reduced in old rats, whereas, the turnover of hypothalamic serotonin is increased (Huang *et al.*, 1979; Simpkins *et al.*, 1977). Similar decreases in hypothalamic catecholamines may occur in elderly humans (Robinson *et al.*, 1972). Administration of the catecholamine precursor, L-dopa, which increases brain catecholamine levels in young animals, may increase brain catecholamine levels in old animals as well. Treatment of old male rats with L-dopa (100 mg/kg) for 8 days increased high-amplitude GH secretion (Fig. 6) and mean GH levels to those observed in young male rats (Sonntag *et al.*, 1982a). L-dopa treated old rats appeared to show no significant changes in pituitary GH concentration or hypothalamic somatostatin content, as compared to vehicle-treated animals. Preliminary evidence from our laboratory also suggests that L-dopa administration to old rats may not reverse the diminished response to clonidine or morphine observed in old animals. The mechanism(s) responsible for the L-dopa induced increase in high amplitude pulsatile release of GH in old animals is currently under investigation.

Neurotransmitters are important in the control of GH release, and the decline in hypothalamic content and turnover of some of these substances in old animals, particularly the catecholamines, suggest that they

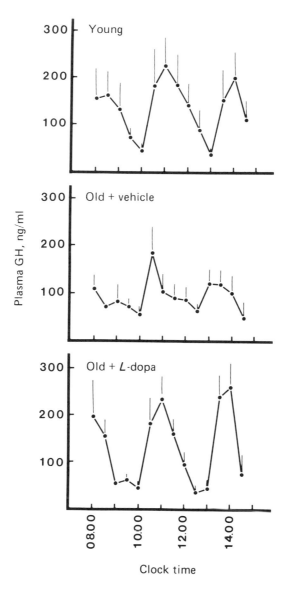

Fig. 6.   Pulsatile release of GH in young (Y) and old (O) male rats, and old rats chronically injected with the catecholamine precursor, L-dopa (100 mg/kg twice daily for 8 days). Vertical bars represent SEM. (From Sonntag *et al.*, 1982a, with permission of the publisher.)

may contribute to the decline in high amplitude GH pulses. The attenuated rise in GH in old animals after clonidine, piribedil, and morphine, and the finding that L-dopa restores pulsatile GH release without affecting the response to these drugs, suggests that other deficiencies in the neuroendocrine system of old rats may contribute to the decrease in GH pulses.

3.5. Autoregulation of Growth Hormone Secretion

There are many indications that GH participates in the regulation of its own secretion, via a short-loop feedback mechanism (Berelowitz et al., 1981; Richman et al., 1981). Intraventricular injection of GH was shown to stimulate release of somatostatin into hypophysial portal blood (Chihara et al., 1981) and to abolish pulsatile release of GH (Tannenbaum, 1980). In addition, somatomedin C, a hormone which is regulated by GH and is responsible for some of the effects of GH at the tissue level, promoted the release of somatostatin by the hypothalamus in vitro (Berelowitz et al., 1981). These observations suggest that the somatomedins and GH itself may regulate GH secretion by stimulating the release of somatostatin.

There are no direct studies on the regulation of GH feedback in aging animals or man. However, it seems reasonable to suggest that the decrease in GH in aging animals may be partially attributable to the inability of the hypothalamus to recognize diminished levels of GH in plasma and to respond by stimulating GHRF release or by inhibiting release of somatostatin.

3.6. Other Hormones

3.6.1. Thyroid Hormone

The thyroid hormones, thyroxine and triiodothyronine, appear to be involved in the regulation of GH synthesis and release by the anterior pituitary. In the rat, thyroidectomy reduces both serum and pituitary GH (Reichlin, 1966; Peake et al., 1973; Hervas et al., 1975), and abolishes the pulsatile release of GH (Takuchi et al., 1978). Thyroid hormone replacement in these animals increases plasma and pituitary GH within 24 hr (Hervas et al., 1975; Coiro et al., 1979).

In humans, the GH response to insulin-induced hypoglycemia or arginine infusion was impaired in the absence of normal thyroid hormone secretion. In addition, hypothyroid children exhibited a reduction of normal body growth (Iwatsubo *et al.*, 1967; MacGillivray *et al.*, 1968; Kato *et al.*, 1969). Administration of thyroid hormone restored body growth and promoted the release of GH in response to various stimuli. The mechanism by which thyroid hormones influence GH secretion is not established, but one report suggests that they may increase the activity of hypothalamic enzymes which metabolize somatostatin (Dupont *et al.*, 1978).

Age-related changes in the secretion of thyroid hormones appear to be controversial in man and less so in rats. There is evidence for an age-related decline in thyroid function in the rat (Huang *et al.*, 1980; see Gregerman, Chapter 14, this volume). It is possible that other aspects of thyroid hormone physiology may change with age and ultimately influence GH secretion. These include possible changes in uptake of thyroid hormones into tissues by receptors and diminished responsiveness of tissue to the effects of thyroid hormones. The interactions between thyroid hormones and GH secretion during aging remain to be investigated.

3.6.2. Steroid Hormones

Various steroid hormones are known to influence the secretion of GH. The gonadal steroids, estrogen and testosterone, appear to potentiate GH secretion in both the rat and human. In the rat, early studies suggested that estrogen stimulated GH release (Dickerman *et al.*, 1971), but more recent data suggest that estrogen does not have a major role in regulating the pulsatile secretion of GH (Saunders *et al.*, 1976). In humans, the GH response to arginine infusion was positively correlated with circulating estrogen levels in women, and in children and men given estrogen (Frantz and Rabkin, 1965; Merimee *et al.*, 1969). The pulsatile release of GH is initiated at puberty, a time when circulating levels of estrogen and testoterone are increasing (Finkelstein *et al.*, 1972).

Progesterone and glucocorticoids appear to inhibit GH release. In humans, medroxyprogesterone diminished the GH responses to insulin hypoglycemia and arginine infusion (Simon *et al.*, 1967), and inhibited the normally occurring nocturnal surge of GH (Lucke and Glick, 1971). Children suffering from hypercortisolemia (Cushing's Disease), or receiving glucocorticoid therapy, routinely demonstrated patterns of impaired body growth which may be associated in part with decreased secretion of GH (Frantz and Rabkin, 1964; Hartog *et al.*, 1964; Krieger and Glick, 1972).

The secretion of steroid hormones has been reported to be altered in aged animals and man. As female rats age, estrous cycles become lengthened and irregular (at approximately 10–12 months), followed by constant vaginal estrus, characterized by chronically high estrogen levels, or by long recurrent pseudopregnancies with high progesterone levels, and in the oldest animals an anestrous state is reached characterized by low estrogen and progesterone secretion (Huang and Meites, 1975). In male rats, testosterone concentrations decline with age (Riegle and Miller, 1978). In humans, circulating estrogen levels in females (Pincus *et al.*, 1954; Furuhjelm, 1966) and testosterone levels in males (Vermeulen *et al.*, 1972; Longscope, 1973; Pirke and Doerr, 1973) also decrease significantly with age. These aging alterations in gonadal steroid hormone levels may influence GH secretion in both rats and man, but their effects, as well as their mechanisms of action on GH secretion, remain to be investigated.

4. Possible Implications of Attenuated Growth Hormone Pulses in Old Animals and Humans

4.1. Somatomedins

Many of the effects of GH are the result of its direct action on target tissues. These effects include stimulation of protein synthesis, RNA synthesis, amino acid transport, and incorporation into liver, muscle (including heart), fat, and hematopoietic tissues. However, all of the effects of GH cannot be attributed to a direct action on tissues. One of the most potent actions of GH *in vivo* is stimulation of bone growth as measured by enlargement of the epiphysial plate cartilage or stimulation of chondroitin sulphate synthesis in cartilage. However, *in vitro* GH administration or serum from hypophysectomized rats was unable to stimulate chondroitin sulphate synthesis, whereas serum from normal or hypophysectomized rats treated with GH produced a significant increase in chondroitin sulphate synthesis (Salmon and Daughaday, 1957). These observations led to the hypothesis that some of the actions of GH were mediated by other factor(s). Recently, several of these factors have been isolated and termed somatomedins (Daughaday *et al.*, 1972; Van Wyk *et al.*, 1974; Rinderknecht and Humbel, 1978a,b). It appears that the somatomedins represent a family of peptide hormones, including somatomedin A and C, insulinlike growth factors (IGF-1 and IGF-2), and multiplication-stimulating activity. These hormones compete for the same receptors on many cell types, and exhibit common properties such as potent mitogenic actions *in vitro*, stimulation of sulphate uptake into cartilage, and weak insulinlike effects. Somatomedins generally are synthesized in the liver and released in response to GH stimulation (McConaghey and Sledge, 1970; Hintz *et al.*, 1972; Phillips *et al.*, 1976; Moses *et al.*, 1979; Schalch *et al.*, 1979).

Although there are few studies of age-related changes in the secretion of somatomedins, somatomedin concentrations in rat plasma measured by bioassay or radioreceptor assay were reported to decrease with age (Florini and Roberts, 1980; Florini *et al.*, 1981). Similarly, somatomedin C levels in aging men were reported to be approximately 1/2 to 1/3 of values in young men, and administration of GH restored somatomedin-C levels in older men to levels in young men (Johanson and Blizzard, 1981). In the rat, the ability of a somatomedin analog to stimulate amino acid uptake into isolated omohyoideus muscle did not appear to vary as a function of age, indicating that tissue responsiveness of this muscle did not decline with age (Florini and Roberts, 1980). These results suggest that decreases in GH may contribute to decreases in somatomedin levels, and to the reductions in protein synthesis and metabolic functions that occur with age in some, but not necessarily all tissues in both rats and man.

Little meaningful work has yet been done to determine the effects of exogenous administration of GH on organ function and protein synthesis during aging. Preliminary observations from our laboratory indicate that GH administration can increase weight of the heart, kidneys, liver, and spleen in old rats (Sonntag *et al.*, unpublished data). The biological significance of these changes in organ weights of old animals in response to GH injections is currently being investigated.

4.2. Metabolic Function

4.2.1. Protein Metabolism

One of the primary effects of GH is the ability to stimulate protein synthesis. Hypophysectomy, which eliminates GH secretion, was reported to decrease amino acid transport and protein synthesis in diaphragm muscle (Riggs and Walker, 1960). Growth hormone replacement returned both amino acid transport and protein synthesis to levels observed in intact animals. Similar findings have been reported *in vitro* (Kostyo *et al.*, 1959; Kipnis and Reiss, 1960). The effects of GH on protein synthesis may be the result of increasing amino acid transport into cells (Noall *et al.*, 1957; Riggs and Walker, 1960), stimulating the synthesis or activity of amino acid-transporting proteins (Kostyo, 1968;

Hjalmarson, 1968), or possibly by increasing mRNA translation (Kostyo and Rillema, 1971).

It is generally accepted that with progressive aging, there is a decrease in lean body mass which may be indicative of decreased protein content and reduction in mass of individual muscles. However, recent data suggest that not all muscles or other tissues lose mass with age, and these may be age- and strain-specific. In the rat, a decrease in protein synthesis with age has been reported in the liver, hind limb musculature, heart, brain, and testes (Richardson, 1981). These observations, however, tend to be quite variable and may be subject to methodological errors.

Determinations of "total body protein synthesis" in human subjects revealed a 37% decrease in individuals 69–91 years of age, as compared to individuals 20–23 years of age (Young *et al.*, 1976; Winterer *et al.*, 1976). The decline in protein synthesis appears to be greater in elderly female than in male subjects.

4.2.2. Carbohydrate Metabolism

In man, postprandial GH levels decline, whereas insulin secretion is increased. The interactions between GH and insulin promote glucose uptake and formation of glycogen and triglycerides (Rabinowitz *et al.*, 1966; 1968). Chronic administration of GH appears to produce a diabetogenic effect. Blood glucose increases significantly, whereas tissue sensitivity to insulin is reduced (Engel and Kostyo, 1964; Weil, 1965). The diabetogenic effect of GH may be the result of increased fatty acid metabolism, which inhibits glycolysis and glycogenesis (Weil, 1965). In elderly humans, fasting blood glucose is significantly elevated (Albanese *et al.*, 1954; Streeten *et al.*, 1965; Balodimos *et al.*, 1967; O'Sullivan *et al.*, 1971; O'Sullivan, 1974). Aged individuals demonstrate a decrease in glucose tolerance (Silverstone *et al.*, 1957) and reduced sensitivity to insulin (Himsworth and Kerr, 1939; Silverstone *et al.*, 1957; Dyck and Moorhouse, 1966), which increases the possibility of these individuals being labeled as diabetic, when in fact they show none of the other symptoms of this disease (Levine, 1980).

4.2.3. Lipid Metabolism

Acute GH treatment decreases fatty acid synthesis (Knobil and Hotchkiss, 1964), whereas chronic administration of GH inhibits glyceride synthesis and decreases body fat accumulation (Goodman, 1963). The reduction in fat formation attributed to GH is partly the result of a decrease in glucose utilization and its subsequent conversion to fatty acids (Goodman, 1969). Growth hormone also may act by mobilizing fatty acids (inhibiting re-esterification) and accelerating lipolysis (Goodman, 1969; Winkler *et al.*, 1969).

In the rat, plasma cholesterol and phospholipids increase with age, whereas plasma triglycerides do not change (Carlson *et al.*, 1968). Liver cholesterol content increased from 1–18 months of age (Carlson *et al.*, 1968), but the phospholipid content of the kidney and liver microsomal fractions derived from 24-month-old rats was diminished as compared to rats 6 months of age (Grinna and Barber, 1972).

In humans, plasma cholesterol (primarily cholesterol esters) increases between the second and sixth decades of life and then remains unchanged or decreases slightly. A similar pattern was observed for plasma triglycerides and cholesterol associated with low-density protein (Kritchevsky, 1978; Nicholson *et al.*, 1979). With age, there is also a decreased lipolytic response to adrenalin (Stuchlikova *et al.*, 1966) and an increase in total brain phospholipid as a percentage of total brain lipids (Rouser and Yamamoto, 1968).

4.2.4. Bone Metabolism

Growth hormone has a major influence on bone growth, especially growth of the epiphysial plate and articular cartilage (Becks *et al.*, 1949). Growth hormone also participates in the remodeling of bone, favoring an increase in cortical thickness and a decrease in accumulation of cancellous bone (Rasmussen, 1974). It has been shown that the promotion of chondrogenesis in bone involves the somatomedins secreted by the liver (Van Wyk and Underwood, 1975). Administration of GH produces hypercalcemia and hyperphosphatemia by increasing calcium and phosphate absorption from the intestine (Knobil and Hotchkiss, 1964; Root, 1972), and by promoting tubular resorption of calcium and phosphate by the kidney (Corvilain and Abramow, 1962). It is unknown if some of these effects are mediated through parathyroid hormone.

In the aging rat, there is a decrease in periosteal osteoblasts and conversion of osteoblasts to osteocytes. In addition, the number of mitochondria and their enzymatic activity are reduced (Tonna and Pillsbury, 1959). These changes produce a decrease in periosteal thickness and bone mass (Tonna and Cronkite, 1961).

It is well known that as humans age, degenerative changes occur in skeletal integrity leading to an increased incidence of vertebral atrophy, compression fractures, and long bone fractures (Tonna, 1977). Bone resorption is part of the normal remodeling process which occurs continuously in adult human bone, but with age the number of resorption sites per unit bone increases significantly (Sedlin *et al.*, 1963). The occurrence of osteoporosis (increased bone resorption) is greater in human females than in males, and there is a marked increase in osteoclastic activity after the menopause (Sedlin *et al.*, 1963). Reduced estrogen levels in postmenopausal women appear to contribute to osteoporosis, since estrogen administration has been shown to diminish the occurrence of osteoporosis (Henneman and Wallach, 1957). Growth hormone appears to have a major role in bone growth and osteogenesis, and dimished secretion of GH may contribute to the fragility of the aging skeleton.

4.2.5. Liver Function

Growth hormone significantly influences the metabolic functions of the liver. Liver protein synthesis is stimulated by GH both *in vivo* (Kostyo and Nutting, 1974) and *in vitro* (Jefferson and Korner, 1967; Clemens and Korner, 1970), which may be due to an increase in both transcriptional and translational events (Daughaday, 1974; Kostyo and Reagan, 1976). Growth hormone promotes glucose production by influencing gluconeogenesis, and stimulates ketone-body formation by increasing lipid metabolism (Altszuler *et al.*, 1968). The synthesis of fatty acids by the liver is decreased by GH (Altszuler *et al.*, 1968). The rat liver exhibits a decrease in weight as a percentage of total body weight with age (Calloway *et al.*, 1965), and shows an impaired ability to demonstrate enzyme adaptation in response to glucose and adrenocorticotrophic hormone (ACTH) (Adelman, 1970a,b,c). Glucose-6-phosphate (Kritchevsky, 1978) and α-glycerophosphate dehydrogenase (Bulos *et al.*, 1971) activity are reduced in the livers of old animals, as is the activity of microsomal-linked NADPH-linked electron transport systems (Kato and Takanaka, 1968a,b). The oxidation and reduction of drugs by the liver is also impaired in old male rats (Kato and Takanaka, 1968a,b). Several investigators have reported that in man, there is a progressive diminution in liver weight with age (Calloway *et al.*, 1965; Thompson and Williams, 1965). However, there appears to be no major reduction of hepatic functions in human males or females with age (Cohen *et al.*, 1960).

4.2.6. Renal Function

Renal function can be significantly influenced by GH. Glomerular filtration rate and renal plasma flow of the kidney are increased by GH administration, as is tubular reabsorption of calcium and phosphorous (Tonna and Pillsbury, 1959; Knobil and Hotchkiss, 1964). A role for GH in renal function is also suggested by the report that hypophysectomy reduces the capacity for renal compensatory hypertrophy, and that GH administration can restore this capacity (Knobil and Hotchkiss, 1964).

In both animals (Dunnill and Halley, 1973) and humans (Lungquist and Lagergren, 1962), the size of the kidneys decreases with age. In man, there is a decrease in the number of glomeruli (Arataki, 1926; Takazakura *et al.*, 1972) and a reduction in the length and volume of the proximal tubules (Darmady *et al.*, 1973). The human kidney also demonstrates numerous age-related physiological alterations. Glomerular filtration rate (Davies and Shock, 1950), creatinine clearance (Roe *et al.*, 1976), and renal blood flow (Lindeman *et al.*, 1966) are markedly diminished with age. Tubular function also declines. There are decreases in free water clearance (Adler *et al.*, 1968), total acid excretion (Adler *et al.*, 1968), maximum concentrating ability (Lindeman *et al.*, 1960), the capacity to reabsorb glucose (Miller *et al.*, 1952), and the response to acid load (Adler *et al.*, 1968). The tubular cells of the kidney show fewer mitochondria (Barrows *et al.*, 1960), lower enzyme concentration (Burich, 1975), and a reduced transport capacity (Beauchene *et al.*, 1965). The capacity to exhibit renal compensatory hypertrophy is also reduced in aged humans (Boner *et al.*, 1973) and rats (Barrows *et al.*, 1962).

4.2.7. Immune Function

There are sufficient data to implicate an important role for GH in immune function. Administration of antiserum against GH resulted in atrophy of the thymus and a wasting syndrome (Pierpaoli and Sorkin, 1968). In addition, GH increased immune function in immune-deficient dwarf mice (Pierpaoli *et al.*, 1969), and was reported to increase DNA synthesis by the thymus and spleen of both hypophysectomized and intact rats (Pandian and Talwar, 1971). Growth hormone also stimulated *in vitro* incorporation of [³H]uridine into RNA in thymocytes (Pandian and Talwar, 1971).

With age there is atrophy of the thymic cortex and a decrease in thymic lymphatic mass in both rats and man (Boyd, 1932). In addition, there is an increase in reticular structures (Chino *et al.*, 1971; Peter, 1973) and in the occurrence of aneuploid lymphocytes (Jacobs *et al.*, 1964), and a decrease in the number of germinal centers (Chino *et al.*, 1971; Peter, 1973). With aging, the capacity of T cells to proliferate in response to challenge is reduced in both rats and humans (Alder *et al.*, 1971; Hallgren *et al.*, 1973; Hori *et al.*, 1973; Roberts-Thomson *et al.*, 1974). In the rat, both *in vivo* and *in vitro* studies suggest that T cell regulatory function is altered with age (Price and Makinodan, 1972; Heidrick and Makinodan, 1973; Hardin *et al.*, 1973). A similar decline has also been observed (Makinodan and Peterson, 1964). The relation of GH to these changes in immune function remain to be studied.

5. Conclusions

Recent studies have indicated that high-amplitude GH pulses are diminished during aging in both rats and humans. These changes in pulsatile release of GH are associated with diminished mean blood GH secretion in rats and decreased integrated GH values in humans. The mechanisms responsible for the decreased high-amplitude GH pulses are unclear at present. It is possible that these changes are due to (1) alterations in the release of GHRF or somatostatin from the hypothalamus, (2) decreases in activity of neurotransmitters that modulate GHRF and somatostatin release into the portal vessels, (3) reductions in thyroid and gonadal hormone secretion, (4) changes in the sensitivity of the pituitary to GHRF or somatostatin, or (5) other causes. It has been shown that administration of L-dopa can restore GH secretion in old male rats to levels found in young male rats. Other neurotransmitters, as well as thyroid or gonadal hormones may also favorably influence GH secretion during aging. There is evidence for decreases in thyroid function in rats, and for decreased gonadal function in both rats and humans.

Growth hormone influences many physiological processes, but it remains to be determined to what extent the decline in GH secretion during aging is responsible for decrements in protein synthesis, bone loss, decline in immunologic functions, decreases in kidney and liver functions, and other metabolic changes. It would be of interest to determine whether administration of GH, hormones, or drugs that increase GH secretion can inhibit or reverse some of these deficiencies in old rats. The decreases with age of somatomedin levels in humans and rats also appear to be associated with decreased GH secretion, since GH administration has been shown to raise somatomedin C levels in the plasma of elderly human individuals. Therefore, somatomedins also may be involved in the decline in many body functions during aging. With the recent advances in knowledge of hypothalamic control of GH secretion, there are possibilities for improving some body functions in aging individuals by use of central-acting drugs that increase GH secretion, and by use of human GH (clonal) or GHRH (when commercially available).

ACKNOWLEDGMENTS. The authors' work was supported by NIH post-doctoral fellowships AG-5147, AG05208, and AG00416 from the National Institute on Aging, CA10771 from the National Cancer Institute, and AM04784 from the National Institute of Arthritis, Diabetes, and Digestive and Kidney Diseases.

6. References

Adelman, R. C., 1970a, Reappraisal of biological aging, *Nature* **228:**1095–1096.

Adelman, R. C., 1970b, An age-dependent modification of enzyme regulation, *J. Biol. Chem.* **245:**1032–1035.

Adelman, R. C., 1970c, The independence of cell division and age-dependent modification of enzyme induction, *Biochem. Biophys, Res. Commun.* **38:**1149–1153.

Adler, S., Lindeman, R. D., Yiengst, M. J., Beard, E., and Shock, N. W., 1968, Effect of acute acid loading on urinary acid secretion by the aging human kidney, *J. Lab. Clin. Med.* **72:**278–289.

Adler, W. H., Takiguchi, T., and Smith R. T., 1971, Effect of age upon primary alloantigen recognition by mouse spleen cells *J. Immunol.* **107:**1357–1362.

Albanese, A. A., Higgons, R. A., Orto, L., Belmont, A., and DiLallo, R., 1954, Effect of age on the utilization of various carbohydrates by man, *Metabolism* **3:**154–159.

Altszuler, N., Steele, R., Rathgeb, I., and De Bodo, R. C., 1968, Influence of growth hormone on glucose metabolism and plasma insulin levels in the dog, in: *Growth Hormone, Proc. 1st Int. Symp. on Growth Hormone, 1967, Milan* (A. Pecile and E. E. Müller, eds.), North Holland, Amsterdam, pp. 309–318.

Arataki, M., 1926, On the postnatal growth of the kidney, with special reference to the number and size of the glomeruli (albino rat). *Am. J. Anat.* **36:**399–450.

Arnold, M. A., and Fernstrom, J. D., 1978, Serotonin receptor antagonists block a natural, short-term surge in serum growth hormone levels, *Endocrinology* **103:**1159–1163.

Asdell, S., 1946, *Patterns of Mammalian Reproduction*, Comstock, Ithaca, New York.

Asling, C. W., Moon, H. D., Bennett, L. L., and Evans, H. M., 1952, Relation of the anterior hypophysis to problems of aging, *J. Gerontol.* **7:**292.

Balodimos, M. C., Balodimos, P. M., and Davis, C. B., 1967, Abnormal carbohydrate tolerance and diabetes in elderly patients, *Geriatrics* **22:**159–166.

Barrows, S. H., Jr., Falzone, J. A., Jr., and Shock, N. W., 1960, Age differences in the succinoxidase activity of homogenates and mitochondria from the livers and kidneys of rats, *J. Gerontol.* **15:**130–133.

Barrows, C. H., Jr., Roeder, L. M., and Olewine, D. A., 1962, Effect of age on renal compensatory hypertrophy following unilateral nephrectomy in the rat, *J. Gerontol.* **17:**148.

Bazarre, T. L., Johanson, S. J., Huseman, C. A., Varma, M. M., and Blizzard, R. M., 1976, Human growth hormone changes with age, *Proc. 3rd Int. Symp. on Growth Hormone, 1975, Milan*, North Holland, Amsterdam.

Beauchene, R. E., Fanestil, D. D., and Barrows, C. H., 1965, The effect of age on active transport and sodium-potassium activated ATPase activity in renal tissues of rats, *J. Gerontol.* **20:**306–310.

Beck, J. C., McGarry, E. E., Dyrenfurth, I., Morgen, R. O., Bird, E. D., and Venning, E. H., 1960, Primate growth hormone studies in man, *Metabolism* **9:**699.

Becks, H., Asling, C. W., Simpson, M. E., Li, C. H., and Evans, H. M., 1949, The growth of hypophysectomized female rats following treatment with pure pituitary growth hormone. III. Skeletal changes: tibia, metacarpal, costochondral junction, and caudal vertebrae, *Growth* **13:**175–189.

Benkert, O., Laakman, G., Souvatzoglou, A., and Von Werder, K., 1973, Missing indicator function of growth hormone and luteinizing hormone blood levels for dopamine and serotonin concentration in the human brain, *J. Neural Trans.* **34**:291–299.

Berelowitz, M., Szabo, M., Frohman, L.A., Fierstone, S., and Chu, L., 1981, Somatomedin-C mediates growth hormone negative feedback by effects on both the hypothalamus and the pituitary, *Science* **212**:1279–1281.

Berg, B., and Simms, H., 1960, Nutrition and longevity in the rat. II. Longevity and onset of disease with different levels of food intake, *J. Nutrition* **71**:255.

Berg, B., and Simms, H., 1961, Nutrition and longevity in the rat. III. Food restriction beyond 800 days. *J. Nutrition* **74**:23.

Bivens, C. H., Lebovitz, H. E., and Feldman, J. M., 1973, Inhibition of hypoglycemia-induced growth hormone secretion by the serotonin antagonists cyproheptadine and methysergide, *N. Engl. J. Med.* **289**:236–239.

Blichert-Toft, M., 1975, Secretion of corticotrophin and somatotrophin by the senescent adenohypophysis in man, *Acta Endocrinol.* **195**(Suppl.): 78.

Boner, G., Shelp, W. D., Neton, M., and Rieselbach, R. E., 1973, Factors influencing the increase in glomerular filtration rate in the remaining kidney of transplant donors, *Am. J. Med.* **55**:169–174.

Boyd, E., 1932, The weight of the thymus gland in health and in disease, *Am. J. Dis. Child,* **43**:1162–1214.

Boyd, A. E., Lebovitz, H. E., and Pfeiffer, J. B., 1970, Stimulation of human growth hormone secretion by L-dopa, *N. Engl. J. Med.* **283**:1425.

Bruni, J. F., Huang, H. H., Marshall S., and Meites, J., 1977a, Effects of single and multiple injections of synthetic GnRH onserum LH, FSH and testosterone in young and old male rats, *Biol. Reprod.* **17**:309–312.

Bruni, J. F., Van Vugt, D. A., Marshall, S., and Meites, J., 1977b, Effects of naloxone, morphine and methionine enkephalin on serum prolactin, luteinizing hormone, follicle stimulating hormone, thyroid stimulating hormone and growth hormone, *Life Sci.* **21**:461–466.

Bulos, B., Sacktor, B., Grossman, I. W., and Altman N., 1971, Thyroid control of mitochondrial α-glycerolphosphate dehydrogenase in rat liver as a function of age, *J. Gerontol.* **26**:13–19.

Burich, R. L., 1975, Effects of age on renal function and enzyme activity in male C57BL/6 mice, *J. Gerontol.* **30**:539–545.

Calloway, N. O., Foley, C. F., and Lagerbloom, P., 1965, Uncertainties in geriatric data. II. Organ size, *J. Am. Geriat. Soc.* **13**:20–29.

Carlson, L. A., Forberg, S. O., and Nye, E. R., 1968, Effect of age on the blood and tissue lipid levels in the male rat, *Gerontologia* **14**:65–79.

Carlson, H. E., Gillin, J. C., Gorden, P., and Snyder, F., 1972, Absence of sleep-related growth hormone peaks in aged normal subjects and in acromegaly, *J. Clin. Endocrinol. Metabol.* **34**:1102.

Chihara, K., Kato, Y., Maeda, K., Matsukura, S., and Imura, H., 1976, Suppression by cyproheptidine of human growth hormone and cortisol secretion during sleep, *J. Clin. Invest.* **57**:1392–1402.

Chihara, K., Arimura, A., and Schally, A. V., 1979, Immunoreactive somatostatin in rat hypophysial portal blood: Effects of anesthetics, *Endocrinology* **104**:1434.

Chihara, K., Minamitani, N., Kaji, H., Arimura, A., and Jufita, T., 1981, Intraventricularly injected growth hormone stimulates somatostatin release into rat hypophysial portal blood, *Endocrinology* **109**:2279–2281.

Chino, F., Makinodan, T., Lever, W. H., and Peterson, W. J., 1971, The immune systems of mice reared in clean and dirty conventional laboratory farms. I. Life expectancy and pathology of mice with long life-spans, *J. Gerontol.* **26:**497–507.

Clemens, M.J., and Korner, A., 1970, Amino acid requirement for the growth hormone stimulation of incorporation of precursors into protein and nucleic acids of liver slices, *Biochem. J.* **119:**629–634.

Cohen, T., Giltman, L., and Lipshutz, E., 1960, Liver function studies in the aged, *Geriatrics* **15:**824–236.

Coiro, V., Braverman, L. E., Christianson, D., Fang, S., and Goodman, H. M., 1979, Effect of hypothyroidism and thyroxine replacement on growth hormone in the rat, *Endocrinology* **105:**641.

Collu, R., Fraschini, F., Visconti, P., and Martini, L., 1972, Adrenergic and serotonergic control of growth hormone secretion in adult male rats, *Endocrinology* **90:**1231–1237.

Comfort, A., 1963, Effect of delayed and resumed growth on the longevity of a fish (Lebistes Reticulatus) in captivity, *Gerontolgia* **8:**150.

Comfort, A., 1964, Growth and senescence, in: *Aging—The Biology of Senescence* (A. Comfort, ed.), Holt, Rinehart and Winston, New York, p. 206.

Conn, P. J., Cooper, R., McNamara, C., Rogers, D. C., and Shoenbardt, L., 1980, Qualitative change in gonadotropin during normal aging in the male rat, *Endocrinology* **106:**1549.

Corvilain, J., and Abramow, M., 1962, Some effects of human growth hormone on renal hemodynamics and on tubular phosphate transport in man, *J. Clin. Invest.* **41:**1230–1235.

Critchlow, V., Rice, R., and Vale, W., 1978, Somatostatin content of the median eminence in female rats with lesion-induced disruption of the inhibitory control of growth hormone secretion, *Endocrinology* **103:**817.

Danowski, T., Tsai, T., Morgan, C., Sieracki, J., Alley, R., Robbins, T., Sabeh, G., and Sunder, J., 1969, Serum growth hormone and insulin in females without glucose tolerance, *Metabolism* **18:**811.

Darmady, E. M., Offer, J., and Woodhouse, M. A., 1973, The parameters of the aging kidney, *J. Pathol.* **109:**195–207.

Daughaday, W. H., 1974, The adenohypophysis, in: *Textbook of Endocrinology* (R. H. Williams, ed.), W. B. Saunders, Philadelphia, pp. 31–79.

Daughaday, W. H., Hall, K., Raben, M. S., Salmon, W. D., Vanden Brande, L. L., and Van Wyk, J. J., 1972, Somatomedin: Proposed designation for sulfation factor, *Nature* **235:**107.

Davies, D. F., and Shock, N. W., 1950, Age changes in glomerular filtration rate, effective renal plasma flow, and tubular excretory capacity in adult males, *J. Clin. Invest.* **29:**496–507.

Delitala, G., Grossman, A., and Besser, G. M., 1981, Changes in pituitary hormone levels induced by met-enkephalin in man—the role of dopamine, *Life Sci.* **29:**1537–1544.

Deuben, R. R., and Meites, J., 1964, Stimulation of pituitary growth hormone release by a hypothalamic extract *in vitro*, *Endocrinology* **74:**408.

Dickerman, E., Dickerman, S., and Meites, J., 1971, Influence of age, sex, and estrous cycle on pituitary and plasma growth hormone levels in rats, in: *Growth Hormone, Proc. 2nd Int. Symp. on Growth Hormone, 1971, Milan* North Holland, Amsterdam, p. 252.

Dunnill, M. S., and Halley, W., 1973, Some observations of the quantitative anatomy of the kidney, *J. Pathol.* **110:**113–121.

Dupont, A., Cusan, L., Garon, M., Labrie, F., and Li, C. H., 1977, β-endorphin: Stimulation of growth hormone release *in vivo*, *Proc. Natl. Acad. Sci.* **74:**358–359.

Dupont, A., Merand, Y., and Barden, N., 1978, Effect of propylthiouracil and thyrozine on the inactivation of somatostatin by rat hypothalamus, *Life Sci.* **23:**2007.

Durand, D., Martin, J. B., and Brazeau, P., 1977, Evidence for a role of α-adrenergic mechanisms in regulation of episodic growth hormone secretion in the rat, *Endocrinology* **100:**722.

Dyck, D. R., and Moorhouse, J. A., 1966, A high dose intravenous glucose tolerance test, *J. Clin. Endocrinol. Metabol.* **26:**1032–1037.

Eden, S., Bolle, P., and Modegh, K., 1979, Monoaminergic control of episodic growth hormone secretion in the rat: Effects of reserpine, α-methyl-p-tyrosine, p-chlorophenylalanine, and haloperidol, *Endocrinology* **105:**523.

Emerson, J. D., 1955, Development of resistance to growth promoting action of pituitary growth hormone, *Am. J. Physiol.* **181:**390.

Engel, F. L., and Kostyo, J. L., 1964, Metabolic actions of pituitary hormones, in: *The Hormones*, Vol. 5 (G. Pincus, K. V. Thimann, and E. B. Astwood, eds.) Academic Press, New York, pp. 69–158.

Everitt, A. V., 1979, The effect of pituitary growth hormone on the aging male rat, *J. Gerontol.* **14:**415.

Everitt, A. V., and Burgess, J. A., 1976, Growth hormone and aging, in: *Hypothalamus, Pituitary and Aging* (A. V. Everitt and J. A. Burgess, eds.), C. C. Thomas, Springfield, Illinois, p. 464.

Finkelstein, J. W., Roffwarg, H. P., Boyar, R. M., Kream, J., and Hellman, L., 1972, Age-related changes in the twenty-four hour spontaneous secretion of growth hormone, *J. Clin. Endocrinol. Metabol.* **35:**665–670.

Florini, J. R., and Roberts, S. B., 1980, Effect of rat age on blood levels of somatomedin-like growth factors, *J. Gerontol.* **35:**23.

Florini, J. R., Harned, J. A., Richman, R. A., and Weiss, J. P., 1981, Effect of rat age on serum levels of growth hormone and somatomedins, *Mech. Ageing Dev.* **15:**165.

Forman, L. J., Sonntag, W. E., Miki, N., Van Vugt, D. A., and Meites, J., 1981, Increase in immunoreactive β-endorphin in the plasma of old male rats; Presence of a higher molecular weight form, *Proc. 11th Annual Meeting, Soc. for Neuroscience*, Los Angeles, California.

Forman, L. J., Sonntag, W. E., Gottschall, P. E., Trapp, J. M., and Meites, J., 1982, Pulsatile and CNS drug stimulated GH secretion in young and old female rats (submitted for publication).

Frantz, A. G., and Rabkin, M. T., 1964, Human growth hormone: Clinical measurement response to hypoglycemia and suppression by corticosteroids, *N. Engl. J. Med.* **271:**1375.

Frantz, A. G., and Rabkin, M. T., 1965, Effects of estrogen and sex difference on secretion of human growth hormone, *J. Clin. Endocrinol. Metabol.* **25:**1470.

Frohman, L. A., and Bernardis, L. L., 1968, Growth hormones and insulin levels in weanlings, *Endocrinology* **82:**1125.

Frohman, L. A., Bernardis, L. L., and Kant, K., 1968, Hypothalamic stimulation of growth hormone secretion. *Science* **162:**580.

Furuhjelm, M., 1966, Urinary excretion of hormones during the climacteric, *Acta Obstet. Gynecol. (Scand.)* **45:**352–365.

Goodman, H. M., a963, Effects of chronic growth hormone treatment on lipogenesis by rat adipose tissue, *Endocrinology* **72:**95–99.

Goodman, H. M., 1969, The effects of epinephrine on glycerol production in segments of adipose tissue preincubated with dexamethasone and growth hormone, *Proc. Soc. Exp. Biol. Med.* **130:**909–912.

Govoni, S., Spano, P. F., and Trabucchi, M., 1978, [³H]haloperidol and [³H]spiroperidol binding in rat striatum during aging, *J. Pharmacol.* **30**:448.

Greenberg, L. H., and Weiss, B., 1978, β-adrenergic receptors in aged rat brain: Reduced number and capacity of pineal gland to develop supersensitivity, *Science* **201**:61.

Greenspan, F. S., Li, C. H., Simpson, M. E., and Evans, H. M., 1950, Growth hormone, in: *Hormone Assay* (C. W. Emmens, eds.), Academic Press, New York, p. 274.

Grinna, L. W., and Barber, A. A., 1972, Age-related changes in membrane lipid content and enzyme activities, *Biochim. Biophys, Acta* **288**:347–353.

Grossman, A., Stubbs, W. A., Gaillard, R. C., De Litala, G., Rees, L. H., and Besser, G. M., 1981, Studies of the opiate control of prolactin, GH and TSH, *Clin. Endocrinol.* **14**:381–386.

Hallgren, H. M., Buckley, E. C., III, Gilbertsen, C. A., and Yunis, E. J., 1973, Lymphocyte phytohemagglutinin responsiveness, immunoglobulins and auto-antibodies in aging human, *J. Immunol.* **111**:1101–1107.

Hammond, J., and Marshall, F., 1952, The life cycle, in: *Marshall's Physiology of Reproduction*, II (A. Parkes, ed.), Longmans, Green, New York, pp. 793–846.

Hardin, J. A., Chuseo, T. M., and Steinberg, A. D., 1973, Suppressor cells in the graft-vs.-host reaction, *J. Immunol.* **111**:650–651.

Hartog, J., Graafer, M. A., and Fraser, R., 1964, Effect of corticosteroids on serum growth hormone, *Lancet* **7356**:376.

Heidrick, M. L., and Makinodan, T., 1973, Presence of impairment of humoral immunity in nonadherent spleen cells of old mice, *J. Immunol.* **111**:1502–1506.

Henneman, P. H., and Wallach, S., 1957, The use of androgens and estrogens and their metabolic effects. A review of the prolonged use of estrogen and androgen in post-menopausal and senile osteoporosis, *Arch. Int. Med.* **100**:715–723.

Hervas, F., Morreale de Escobar, G., and Escobar del Rey, F., 1975, Rapid effects of single small doses of L-thyroxine and triiodo-L-thyronine on growth hormone, as studied in the rat by radioimmunoassay, *Endocrinology* **97**:91.

Himsworth, H. P., and Kerr, R. B., 1939, Age and insulin sensitivity, *Clin. Sci.* **4**:153–157.

Hintz, R. L., Clemmons, D. R., and Van Wyk, J. J., 1972, Growth hormone induced somatomedin-like activity from liver, *Pediat. Res.* **6**:353.

Hjalmarson, A., 1968, Sensitivity of the rat diaphragm to growth hormones. III. Biphasic action of growth hormone *in vitro* on amino acid uptake and pentose uptake. *Acta Endocrinol.* (Suppl.) **126**:1–17.

Hori, Y., Perkins, E. H., and Halstall, M. K., 1973, Decline in phytohemagglutinin responsiveness of spleen cells from aging mice, *Proc. Soc. Exp. Biol. Med.* **144**:48–53.

Huang, H. H., and Meites, J., 1975, Reproductive capacity of aging female rats, *Neuroendocrinology* **17**:289–295.

Huang, H. H., Simpkins, J. W., and Meites, J., 1979, Hypothalamic norepinephrine and dopamine turnover in ovariectomized old rats treated with gonadal steroids, *APS Specialty Meeting*, Michigan State University, Fed. Proc.

Huang, H. H., Steger, R. W., and Meites, J., 1980, Capacity of old versus young male rats to release thyrotropin (TSH), thyroxine (T_4) and triiodothyronine (T_3) in response to differential stimuli, *Exp. Aging Res.* **6**:3–12.

Imura, H., Nakai, Y., Yoshimi, T., 1973, Effect of 5-hydroxytryptophan (5-HTP) on growth hormone and ACTH release in man, *J. Clin. Endocrinol. Metabol.* **36**:204–266.

Iwatsubo, H., Omori, K., Okada, Y., Fuckuchi, M., Miyai, K., Abe, H., and Kumahara, Y., 1967, Human growth hormone secretion in primary hypothyroidism before and after treatment, *J. Clin. Endocrinol. Metabol.* **27**:1751.

Jacobs, P. A., Brunton, M., and Court-Brown, W. M., 1964, Cytogenetic studies in leu-kocytes on the general population: Subjects of ages 65 years or more, Ann. Hum. Genet. 27:353–365.

Jefferson, L. S., and Korner, A., 1967, A direct effect of growth hormone on the incor-poration of precursors into proteins and nucleic acids of perfused rat liver, Biochem. J. 104:826–832.

Jelinkova, M., and Hrůza, Z., 1964, Decreased effect of norepinephrine and growth hor-mone on the release of free fatty acids in old rats, Physiol. Bohemoslov. 13:327.

Johanson, A. J., and Blizzard, R. M., 1981, Low somatomedin-C levels in older men rise in response to growth hormone administration, Johns Hopkins Med. J. 149:115.

Kalk, W., Vinick, A., Pimstone, B., and Jackson, W., 1973, Growth hormone response to insulin hypoglycemia in the elderly, J. Gerontol. 28:431.

Kasting, N. W., Martin, J. B., and Arnold, M. A., 1981, Pulsatile somatostatin release from the median eminence of the unanesthetized rat and its relationship to plasma growth hormone levels, Endocrinology 109:1739.

Kato, R., and Takanaka, A., 1968a, Metabolism of drugs in old rats (II) Metabolism in vivo and effect of drugs in old rats, Jap. J. Pharmacol. 18:389.

Kato, R., and Takanaka, A., 1968b, Effect of phenobarbital on electron transport system, oxidation and reduction of drugs in liver microsomes of rats of different ages, J. Biochem. 63:406–408.

Kato, H. P., Youlton, R., Kaplan, S. L., and Grumbach, M. M., 1969, Growth and growth hormone. III. Growth hormone release in children with primary hypothyroidism and thyrotoxicosis, J. Clin. Endocrinol. Metabol. 29:346.

Kato, Y., Dupre, J., and Beck, J. C., 1973, Plasma growth hormone in the anesthetized rat: Effects of dibutyral cyclic AMP, prostaglandin E, adrenergic agents, vasopressin, chlorpromazine, amphetamine and L-dopa, Endocrinology 93:135–146.

Kipnis, D. M., and Reiss, E., 1960, The effect of cell structure and growth hormone on protein synthesis in striated muscle, J. Clin. Invest. 39:1002.

Klug, T. C., and Adelman, R. C., 1977, Evidence for a large thyrotropin and its accu-mulation during aging in rats, Biochem. Biophys. Res. Commun. 77:1431.

Knobil, E., and Hotchkiss, J., 1964, Growth hormone, Annu. Rev. Physiol. 26:47–74.

Kostyo, J. L., 1968, Rapid effects of growth hormone on amino acid transport and protein synthesis, Ann. N.Y. Acad. Sci. 148:389–407.

Kostyo, J. L., and Nutting, D. F., 1974, Growth hormone and protein metabolism in: Handbook of Physiology, Section 7: Endocrinology, Vol. 4, American Physiological Soc., Washington, D.C., pp. 187–210.

Kostyo, J. L., and Reagan, C. R., 1976, The biology of growth hormone, Pharmacol. Ther. Part B 2:591–604.

Kostyo, J. L., and Rillema, J. A., 1971, In vitro effect of growth hormone on the number and activity of ribosomes engaged in protein synthesis in the isolated rat diaphragm, Endocrinology 88:1054–1062.

Kostyo, J. L., Hotchkiss, J., and Knobil, E., 1959, Stimulation of amino acid transport in isolated diaphragm by growth hormone added in vitro, Science 130:1653–1654.

Krieger, D. T., and Glick, S. M., 1972, Growth hormone and cortisone responsiveness in Chusing's syndrome: Relation to a possible central nervous system etiology, Am. J. Med. 52:25.

Kritchevsky, D., 1978, How aging affects cholesterol metabolism, Postgrad. Med. 63:133.

Lal, S., Dela Vega, C. E., and Sourkes, T. L., 1972, Effect of apomorphine on human growth hormone secretion, Lancet 7778:661.

Lal, S., Martin, J. B., and Dela Vega, C. E., 1975, Comparison of the effect of apomorphine and L-dopa on serum growth hormone levels in normal men, *Clin. Endocrinol.* **4:**277.

Lal, S., Nari, N. P. V., Cervantes, P., Pulman, J., and Guyda, H., 1979. Effects of naloxone and levallorphan on serum prolactin concentrations and apomorphine-induced growth hormone secretion, *Acta Psychiat. (Scand.)* **59:**173.

Lansing, A. I., 1948, Evidence for aging as a consequence of growth cessation, *Proc. Natl. Acad. Sci. (Wash.)* **34:**304.

Laron, A., Doron, M., and Arnikan, B., 1970, Plasma growth hormone in men and women over 70 years of age, in: *Medicine and Sports, Physical Activity and Aging*, Vol. 4, Karger, New York, p. 126.

Levine, R., 1980, Metabolic and lipid metabolism in the aged, in: *Aging—Its Chemistry* (A. A. Dietz, ed.), Am. Assoc. for Clin. Chem., Washington, D. C., pp. 107–113.

Lindeman, R. D., Van Buren, H. C., and Raisz, L. G., 1960, Osmolar renal concentrating ability in healthy young men and hospitalized patients without renal disease, *N. Engl. J. Med.* **262:**1306–1309.

Lindeman, R. D., Lee, T. D., Jr., Yiengst, M. J., and Shock, N. W., 1966, Influence of age, renal disease, hypertension, diuretics, and calcium on the antidiuretic response to suboptimal infusions of vasopressin, *J. Lab. Clin. Med.* **68:**206–223.

Ljungquist, A., and Lagergren, C., 1962, Normal intrarenal arterial pattern in adult and aging human kidney. A microangiographical and histological study, *J. Anat. (Lond.)* **96:**285–298.

Longscope, C., 1973, Effect of HCG on plasma steroid levels in young and old men, *Steroids* **21:**583–592.

Lucke, C., and Glick, S. M., 1971, Effect of medroxyprogesterone acetate on the sleep-induced peak of growth hormone secretion, *J. Clin. Endocrinol. Metabol.* **33:**851.

MacGillivray, M. H., Aceto, T., Jr., and Frohman, L. A., 1968, Plasma growth hormone responses and growth retardation in hypothyroidism, *Am. J. Dis. Child.* **115:**273.

Maggi, A., Schmidt, M. J., Ghetti, B., and Enna, S. J., 1979, Effects of aging on neurotransmitter receptor binding in rat and human brain, *Life Sci.* **24:**367.

Makinodan, T., and Peterson, W. J., 1964, Growth and senescence of the primary antibody-forming potential of the spleen, *J. Immunol.* **93:**886–896.

Marelli, G., 1968, Influenza dell'ormone somatotropo sul filtrato glomerulare E Sul Tm glucosio nel vecchio. *Acta. Gerontol.* **18:**71.

Martin, J. B., 1974, The role of hypothalamic and extrahypothalamic structures in the control of growth hormone secretion, in: *Advances in Human Growth Hormone Research* (S. Raiti, ed.), NIH, Washington, D.C., p. 223.

Martin, J. B., 1976, Brain regulation of growth hormone secretion in: *Frontiers of Neuroendocrinology* (L. Martini and W. Ganong, eds.), Raven Press, New York, p. 129.

Martin, J. B., 1979, Brain mechanisms for integration of growth hormone secretion *The Physiologist* **22:**23.

Martin, J. B., Tolis, G., Woods, I., and Guyda, H., 1979, Failure of naloxone to influence physiological growth hormone and prolactin secretion, *Brain Res.* **168:**210.

McCay, C. M., Crowell, M. F., and Maynard, L. A., 1935, The effect of retarded growth upon the length of the lifespan and upon ultimate body size, *J. Nutrition* **10:**63.

McConaghey, P., and Sledge, C. B., 1970. Production of sulphation factor by perfused liver, *Nature* **225:**1249.

Meites, J., and Sonntag, W. E., 1981, Hypothalamic hypophysiotrophic hormones and neurotransmitter regulation. Current Views, *Annu. Rev. Pharmacol. Toxicol.* **21:**295.

Meites, J., Huang, H. H., and Simpkins, J. W., 1978, Recent studies on neuroendocrine control of reproductive senescence in rats, in: *The Aging Reproductive System, Aging,* Vol. 4 (E. L. Schneider, ed.), Raven Press, New York, p. 213.

Merimee, T. J., Finesberg, S. E., and Tyson, J. E., 1969, Fluctuation of human growth hormone secretion during menstrual cycle: Response to arginine, *Metabolism* **18:**606.

Miller, D., and Payne, P., 1968, Longevity and protein intake, *Exp. Gerontol.* **3:**231.

Miller, J. H., McDonald, R. K., and Shock, N. W., 1952, Age changes in the maximal rate of renal tubular reabsorption of glucose, *J. Gerontol.* **7:**196 200.

Mims, R. B., Stein, R. B., and Bethune, J. E., 1973, The effect of a single dose of L-dopa on pituitary hormones in acromegaly, obesity and in normal subjects, *J. Clin. Endocrinol. Metabol.* **37:**34.

Morely, J. E., Baranetsky, N. G., Wingert, T. O., Carlson, H. E., Hershmann, J. M., Melmed, S., Levin, S. R., Jamison, K. R., Weitzman, R., Chang, R. J., and Varrner, A. A., 1980, Endocrine effects of naloxone-induced opiate receptor blockade, *J. Clin. Endocrinol. Metabol.* **50:**251–257.

Moses, A. C., Nissley, S. P., Passamani, J., and White, R. M., 1979, Further characterization of growth hormone-dependent somatomedin binding proteins in rat serum and demonstration of somatomedin binding proteins produced by rat liver cells in culture, *Endocrinology* **104:**536.

Mueller, G. P., Simpkins, J. W., Meites, J., and Moore, K. E., 1976, Differential effects of dopamine agonists and haloperidol on release of prolactin, thyroid stimulating hormone, growth hormone and luteinizing hormone in rats, *Neuroendocrinology* **20:**121.

Müller, E. E., Brambilla, F., Cavagnini, F., Peracchi, M., and Panerai, A., 1974, Slight effect of L-tryptophan on growth hormone release in normal human subjects, *J. Clin. Endocrinol. Metabol.* **39:**1–5.

Nakai, Y., Imura, H., Sakurai, H., Kurahachi, H., and Yoshimi, T., 1974, Effect of cyproheptadine on human growth hormone secretion, *J. Clin. Endocrinol. Metabol.* **38:**446.

Nicholson, J., Garside, P. S., Siegel, M., Spencer, W., Steiner, P. M., and Glueck, C. J., 1979, Lipid and lipoprotein distribution in octo- and nonagenarians, *Metabolism* **28:**51.

Noall, M. W., Riggs, T. R., Walker, L. M., and Christensen, H. N., 1957, Endocrine control of amino acid transfer. Distribution of an unmetabolizable amino acid, *Science* **126:**1002–1005.

Northrop, J. H., 1917, The effect of prolongation of the period of growth on the total duration of life, *J. Biol. Chem.* **32:**123.

O'Sullivan, J. B., 1974, Age gradient in blood glucose levels, *Diabetes* **23:** 713–715.

O'Sullivan, J. B., Mahan, C. M., Freedlender, A. E., and Smith, G., 1971, Effect of age on carbohydrate metabolism, *J. Clin. Endocrinol. Metabol.* **33:**619–623.

Pandian, M. R., and Talwar, G. P., 1971, Effect of growth hormone on the metabolism of thymus and on the immune response against sheep erythrocytes, *J. Exp. Med.* **134:**1095–1113.

Peake, G. T., Birge, C. A., and Daughaday, W. H., 1973, Alterations of radioimmunoassayable growth hormone and prolactin during hypothyroidism, *Endocrinology* **92:**487.

Pecile, A., Müller, E., Falconi, G., and Martini, L., 1965, Growth hormone releasing activity of hypothalamic extracts at different ages, *Endocrinology* **77:**241–246.

Peter, C. P., 1973, Possible immune origin of age-related pathological changes in long-lived mice, *J. Gerontol.* **28:**265–275.

Phillips, L. S., Herington, A. C., Karl, I. E., and Daughaday, W. H., 1976, Comparison of somatomedin activity in perfusates of normal and hypophysectomized rat livers with and without added growth hormone, *Endocrinology* **98:**606.

Pierpaoli, W., and Sorkin, E., 1968, Hormones and immunologic capacity. I. Effect of heterologous antigrowth hormone (ASTH) antiserum on thymus and peripheral lymphatic tissue in mice. Induction of a wasting syndrome, *J. Immunol.* **101**:1036.

Pierpaoli, W., Baroni, C., Fabris, N., and Sorkin, E., 1969, Reconsistution of antibody production in hormonally deficient mice by somatotropic hormone, thyrotropic hormone and thyroxine, *Immunology* **16**:217.

Pincus, G., Romonoff, L. P., and Carol, J., 1954, The excretion of urinary steroids by men and women of various ages, *J. Gerontol.* **9**:113–132.

Pirke, K. M., and Doerr, P., 1973, Age-related changes and interrelations between plasma testosterone, oestradiol and testosterone binding globulin in normal adult males, *Acta Endocrinol.* **74**:792–800.

Price, G. B., and Makinodan, T., 1972, Immunologic deficiencies in senescence. I. Characterization of intrinsic deficiencies, *J. Immunol.* **108**:403–412.

Prinz, P., Halter, K., Raskind, M., Cunningham, G., and Karacna, I., 1981, Aging, sleep and diurnally varying hormones in man, in: *Biochemical Mechanisms in Aging, Conf. Proc., 1980* (R. T. Schimke, ed.), U.S. Dept. of Health and Human Services, PHS, Washington, D.C., NIH Publication No. 81-2194, pp. 618–628.

Rabinowitz, D., Merimee, T. J., Maffezzolo, R., and Burgess, J. A., 1966, Patterns of hormonal release after glucose, protein and glucose plus protein, *Lancet* **7461**:454.

Rabinowitz, D., Merimee, T. J., Nelson, J. K., Schultz, R. B., and Burgess, J. A., 1968, The influence of proteins and amino acids on growth hormone release in man, in: *Growth Hormone* (A. Pecile and E. E. Müller, eds.), North-Holland: Excerpta Medica Found., Amsterdam, p. 105.

Rasmussen, H., 1974, Parathyroid hormone, calcitonin, and the calciferols, in: *Textbook of Endocrinology*, (R. H. Williams, Ed.), W. B. Saunders, Philadelphia, pp. 660–773.

Reichlin, S., 1966, Regulation of somatotrophic hormone secretion, in: *The Pituitary Gland* (G. W. Harris and B. T. Donovan, eds.), Butterworths, London, p. 270.

Rice, R. W., and Critchlow, V., 1976, Extrahypothalamic control of stress induced inhibition of growth hormone secretion in the rat, *Endocrinology* **99**:970.

Richardson, A., 1981, A comprehensive review of the scientific literature on the effect of aging on protein synthesis, in: *Biological Mechanisms of Aging, Conf. Proc., 1980* (R. T. Schimke, ed.), U. S. Dept. of Health and Human Services, PHS, Washington, D.C., NIH Publication No. 81-2194, pp. 339–358.

Richman, R. A., Weiss, J. P., Hochberg, Z., and Florini, J. R., 1981, Regulation of growth hormone release: Evidence against negative feedback in rat pituitary cells, *Endocrinology* **108**:2287–2292.

Riegle, G. D., and Miller, A. E., 1978, Aging effects on the hypothalamic-hypophyseal-gonadal control system in the rat, in: *The Aging Reproductive System* (E. L. Schneider, ed.), Raven Press, New York, pp. 159–192.

Riggs, T. R., and Walker, L. M., 1960, Growth hormone stimulation of amino acid transport into rat tissues *in vivo*, *J. Biol. Chem.* **235**:3603–3607.

Rinderknecht, E., and Humbel, R. E., 1978a, The amino acid sequence of human insulin-like growth factor I, and its structural homology with proinsulin, *J. Biol. Chem.* **253**:2769.

Rinderknecht, E., and Humbel, R. E., 1978b, Primary structure of human insulin-like growth factor II, *FEBS. Lett.* **89**:283.

Ribier, C., Vale, W., Ling, N., Brown, M., and Guillemin, R., 1977, Stimulation *in vivo* of the secretion of prolactin and growth hormone by β-endorphin, *Endocrinology* **100**:238–241.

Roberts-Thomson, I. C., Whittingham, S., Youngchaiyud, U., and Mackay, I. R., 1974, Aging immune response, and mortality, *Lancet* **7877**:368–370.

Robinson, D. S., Nies, A., Davis, J., Bunney, W. E., Davis J. M., Colburn, R. W., Bourne, H. R., Shaw, D. M., and Coppen, A. J., 1972, Aging, monoamines and monoamine oxidase levels, *Lancet* **7745:**290–291.

Rockstein, M., Chesky, J. A., and Sussman, M. L., 1977, Comparative biology and evolution of aging, in: *Handbook of the Biology of Aging* (C. E. Finch and L. Hayflick, eds.), Van Nostrand, New York, p. 3.

Root, A. W., 1972, Chemical and biological properties of growth hormone, in: *Human Pituitary Growth Hormone*, Charles C. Thomas, Springfield, Illinois, p. 3.

Root, A. W., and Oski, F. A., 1969, Effects of human growth hormone in elderly males, *J. Gerontol.* **24:**94.

Rouser, G., and Yamamoto, Y., 1968, Curvilinear regression course of human brain lipid changes with age, *Lipids* **3:**284–287.

Rowe, J. W., Andres, R., Tobin, J. D., Norris, A. H., and Shock, N. W., 1976, The effect of age on creatinine clearance in men: A cross-sectional and longitudinal study, *J. Gerontol.* **31:**155–163.

Salmon, W. D., and Daughaday, W. H., 1957, A hormonally controlled serum factor which stimulated sulphate incorporation by cartilage *in vitro*, *J. Lab. Clin. Med.* **49:**825.

Sandberg, H., Hashimine, N., Maeda, S., Symons, D., and Zarodnick, J., 1973, Effect of an oral glucose load on serum immunoreactive insulin free fatty acid, growth hormone and blood sugar level in young and elderly subjects, *J. Am. Geriat. Soc.* **21:**433.

Sassin, J. F., Parker, D. C., Mace, J. W., Gotlin, R. W., Johnson, L. C., and Rossman, L. G., 1969, Human growth hormone release: Relation to slow-wave sleep and sleep-waking cycles, *Science* **165:**513.

Saunders, A., Terry, L. C., Audet, J., Brazeau, P., and Martin, J. B., 1976, Dynamic studies of growth hormone and prolactin secretion in the female rat, *Neuroendocrinology* **21:**193–203.

Saxton, J. A., 1945, Nutrition and growth and their influence on longevity in rats, *Biol. Symp.* **11:**177.

Schalch, D. S., Heinrich, U. E., Draznin, B., Johnson, C. J., and Miller, L. L., 1979, Role of the liver in regulating somatomedin activity-hormonal effects on the synthesis and release of insulin-like growth factor and its carrier protein by the isolated perfused rat liver, *Endocrinology* **104:**1143.

Sedlin, E. D., Villanueva, A. R., and Frost, H. M., 1963, Age variations in the specific surface of Howship's lacunae as an index of human bone resorption, *Anat. Record.* **146:**201–207.

Sharr, C. J., Frederickson, R. C. A., Dininger, N. B., and Jackson, L., 1977, Enkephalin analogues and naloxone modulate the release of growth hormone and prolactin-evidence for regulation by an endogenous opioid peptide in brain, *Life Sci.* **21:**853–860.

Silverstone, F. A., Brandfonbrener, M., Shock, N. W., and Yiengst, M. J., 1957, Age differences in the intravenous glucose tolerance tests and the response to insulin, *J. Clin. Invest.* **36:**504–514.

Simon, S. M., Schiffer, M., Glick, S. M., and Schwartz, E., 1967, Effect of medroxypro-gesterone acetate upon stimulated release of growth hormone in men, *J. Clin. Endocrinol. Metabol.* **27:**1633.

Simpkins, J. W., Mueller, G. P., Huang, H. H., and Metes, J., 1977, Evidence for depressed catecholamine and enhanced serotonin metabolism in aging male rats: Possible relation to gonadotropin secretion, *Endocrinology* **100:**1672.

Sladek, J., and Hoffman, G., 1980, Immunocytochemical localization of LHRH and so-matostatin in the hypothalamus of old female rats, *Neurobiol. Aging* **1:**34.

Smythe, G. A., and Lazarus, L., 1974, Supression of human growth hormone secretion by melatonin and cyproheptadine, *J. Clin. Invest.* **54:**116–121.

Smythe, G. A., Brandstater, J. F., and Lazarus, L., 1975, Serotonergic control of rat growth hormone secretion, *Neuroendocrinology* **17:**245–257.

Sonntag, W. E., Steger, R. W., Forman, L. J., and Meites, J., 1980, Decreased pulsatile release of growth hormone in old male rats, *Endocrinology* **107:**1875.

Sonntag, W. E., Forman, L. J., Miki, N., Steger, R. W., Ramos, T., Arimura, A., and Meites, J., 1981, Effects of CNS active drugs and somatostatin antiserum on growth hormone release in young and old male rats, *Neuroendocrinology* **33:**73.

Sonntag, W. E., Forman, L. J., Miki, N., Trapp, J. M., Gottschall, P. E., and Meites, J., 1982a, L-dopa restores amplitude of growth hormone pulses in old male rats to that observed in young male rats, *Neuroendocrinology* **34:**163.

Sonntag, W. E., Forman, L. J., Trapp, J. M., and Hylka, V., 1982b, Regulation of LHRH receptors in old male rats: Relation to the release of LH, *34th Annual Meeting of The Endocrine Soc.* (Abst.), San Francisco, California.

Spiler, I. J., and Molitch, M. E., 1980, Lack of modulation of pituitary hormone stress response by neural pathways involving opiate receptors, *J. Clin. Endocrinol. Metabol.* **50:**516.

Streeten, D. H. P., Gerstein, M. M., Mamor, B. M., and Doisy, R. J., 1965, Reduced glucose tolerance in elderly human subjects, *Diabetes* **14:**579–583.

Stubbs, W. A., Jones, A., Edwards, C. R. W., Delitala, G., Jeffcoat, W. J., Rattner, S. J., and Besser, G. M., 1978, Hormonal and metabolic responses to an enkephalin analogue in normal man, *Lancet* **8102:**1225.

Stuchlikova, E., Hruskova, J., Hruza, Z., Jelinkova, M., Novak, P., and Soukupova, K., 1966, Effect of adrenalin on lipolysis in glycogenolysis in relation to age and stress, *Exp. Gerontol.* **2:**15–21.

Takahashi, K., Kipnis, D. M., and Daughaday, W. H., 1968, Growth hormone secretion during sleep, *J. Clin Invest.* **47:**2079.

Takazakura, E., Wasabu, N., Handa, A., Takada, A., Shinoda, A., and Takeuchi, J., 1972, Intrarenal vascular changes with age and disease, *Kidney Int.* **2:**224–230.

Takuchi, A., Suzuki, M., and Tsuchiya, S., 1978, Effects of thyroidectomy on the secretory profiles of growth hormone, thyrotropin and corticosterone in the rat, *Endocrinology (Jpn.)* **25:**381.

Tannenbaum, G. S., 1980, Evidence for auto-regulation of growth hormone secretion via the central nervous system, *Endocrinology* **107:**2117–2120.

Tannenbaum, G. S., and Martin, J. B., 1976, Evidence for an endogenous ultradian rhythm governing growth hormone secretion in the rat, *Endocrinology* **98:**562.

Tannenbaum, G. S., Panerai, A. E., and Frisen, H. G., 1979, Failure of β-endorphin antiserum, naloxone, and naltrexone to alter physiological growth hormone and insulin secretion, *Life Sci.* **25:**1983–1990.

Tannenbaum, G. S., Ling, N., and Brazeau, P., 1981, Dynamic time course studies of the effects of somatostatin-28 and somatostatin-25 on pituitary and pancreatic hormone release, *63rd Annual Meeting of The Endocrine Soc.* (Abst.) Cincinnati, Ohio.

Thompson, E. N., and Williams, R., 1965, Effect of age on liver function with particular reference to bromsulphalein excretion, *Gut* **6:**266–269.

Thompson, R. G., Rodriquez, A., Kowarski, A., Migeon, C. L., and Blizzard, R. M., 1972, Integrated concentrations of growth hormone correlated with plasma testosterone and bone age in preadolescent and adolescent males, *J. Clin. Endocrinol. Metabol.* **35:**334.

Tonna, E. A., 1977, Aging of skeletal-dental systems and supporting tissues, in: *Handbook of the Biology of Aging* (C. E. Finch and L. Hayflick, eds.), Van Nostrand Reinhold, New York, pp. 470–495.

Tonna, E. A., and Cronkite, E. P., 1961, Autoradiographic studies of cell proliferation in the periosteum of intact and fractured femora of mice utilizing DNA labeling with [H^3]-thymidine, *Proc. Soc. Exp. Biol. Med.* **107:**719–721.

Tonna, E. A., and Pillsbury, N., 1959, Mitochondrial changes associated with aging of periosteal osteoblasts, *Anat. Record.* **134:**739–760.

Van Wyk, J. J., and Underwood, L. E., 1975, Relation between growth hormone and somatomedin, *Annu. Rev. Med.* **26:**427–441.

Van Wyk, J. J., Underwood, L. E., Hintz, R. L., Clemmons, D. R., Voina, S. J., and Weaver, R. P., 1974, The somatomedins: A family of insulin-like hormones under growth hormone control, *Rec. Prog. Horm. Res.* **30:**259.

Vermeulen, A., Rubens, R., and Verdonck, L., 1972, Testosterone secretion and metabolism in male senescence, *J. Clin. Endocrinal. Metabol.* **34:**730–735.

Vidalon, C., Khurana, R., Chae, S., Gregick, C., Stephans, T., Nolan, S., and Danowski, T., 1973, Age-related changes in growth hormone in non-diabetic women, *J. Am. Geriat. Soc.* **21:**253.

Vijayan, E., Krulich, L., and McCann, S. M., 1978, Catecholaminergic regulation of TSH and growth hormone release in ovariectomized and ovariectomized steroid-primed rats, *Neuroendocrinology* **26:**174.

Wakabayashi, I., Demura, R., Miki, N., Ohmura, E., Miyoshi, H., and Shizume, K., 1980, Failure of naloxone to influence plasma growth hormone, prolactin, and cortisol secretions induced by insulin hypoglycemia, *J. Clin. Endocrinol. Metabol.* **50:**597.

Weil, R., 1965, Pituitary growth hormone and intermediary metabolism I. The hormonal effect on the metabolism of fat and carbohydrate, *Acta Endocrinol.* (Suppl.) **98:**1–92.

Winkler, B., Steele, R., and Altszuler, N., 1969, Effects of growth hormone administration on free fatty acid and glycerol turnover in the normal dog, *Endocrinology* **85:**25–30.

Winterer, J. C., Steffee, W. P., Davy, W., Perera, A., Uauy, R., Scrimshaw, N. S., and Young, V. R., 1976, Whole body protein turnover in aging man, *Exp. Gerontol.* **11:**79–87.

Young, V. R., Stefee, W. P., Pencharz, P. G., Winterer, J. C., and Scrimshaw, N. S., 1975, Total human body protein synthesis in relation to protein requirements at various ages, *Nature* **253:**192.

CHAPTER 15

Changes in Hypothalamic Control of ACTH and Adrenal Cortical Functions during Aging

GAIL D. RIEGLE

1. Introduction

Early identification of endocrine regulation of body function, including growth, metabolism, and reproduction, has historically generated several hypotheses suggesting that changes in endocrine function were closely related to biological aging. Many early gerontologists hypothesized that reductions of metabolic and reproductive endocrine secretion were directly involved in the decline in function which occurs in most organ systems during aging. Except for the menopausal loss of ovarian steroids, the current understanding of the effects of aging on endocrine function indicates that clear hormonal deficiencies rarely occur. However, it became evident that subtle alterations in endocrine function can contribute to deterioration of physiological functions with aging, keeping the hypothesis of endocrine involvement viable.

Involvement of adrenocortical glucocorticoid hormones in metabolic homeostasis and the relationship of this hormone system to the body's defense against stress continue to make age-related studies of the pituitary-adrenocortical system attractive. Stress-induced stimulation of the pituitary-adrenal control system has been shown to be connected with the ability of people and animals to survive stress. A higher rate of mortality is associated with surgical and other forms of stress in the elderly (Blichert-Toft, 1978), supporting the hypothesis of age effects on the function of this system.

GAIL D. RIEGLE • Department of Physiology, Michigan State University, East Lansing, Michigan 48824.

The objective of this chapter is to review the effects of biological aging on neuroendocrine factors believed to regulate hypothalamic secretion of substances which control pituitary ACTH synthesis and secretion. However, since we recognize that these brain functions are in turn influenced by adrenocortical and pituitary inputs, this chapter will also consider aspects of age alterations in all components of the control system.

2. Adrenal Gland Anatomy

In most species, changes in adrenal gland morphology with age are not dramatic. Adrenal glands from several species show increased connective tissue content with age (Cooper, 1925; Jayne, 1953; Blichert-Toft, 1978). There is also an increased amount of adrenocortical age pigment or lipochrome granules with increased age (Reichel, 1968; Szabo *et al.*, 1970). Changes in adrenal gland size with aging varies considerably among species. In birds, the size of the adrenals are decreased with age (Bourne, 1967). Although aged male beagle dogs had smaller adrenals, female beagle adrenal weights were increased with age (Das and Magilton, 1971). Adrenal weights and cortical widths were similar in young and aged humans (Galloway *et al.*, 1965; Haugen, 1973).

The effect of age on adrenal morphology in the rat appears more variable than in other species. Female rate adrenals are larger than those of the male, with the increase in size occurring as a function of estrogen availability. Dunihue (1965) found atrophied zona glomerulosa tissue in aged rats. With increasing age female rat adrenals show pathological changes in capillary walls which leads to a clinical condition termed peliosis, associated with extreme capillary dilatation and substantial increases in gland size (Dhom *et al.*, 1981). These changes in adrenal capillaries were not associated with changes in resting blood corticosterone or the acute increase in blood corticosterone following ACTH or stress treatment. Schriefers *et al.* (1972) reported estrogen induction of adrenal hyperemia and increased capillary permeability in aged female rats, suggesting that the adrenal peliosis of the aged female rat could be due to the increased estrogenicity of the constant estrus aging female rat. In humans, the formation of functional adrenocortical nodules, which apparently develop secondarily to systemic hypertension, is characteristic of increasing age (Dobbie, 1969). In summary, these data indicate that although there are substantial structural alterations in adrenal tissue of some species with increasing age, these changes have not been consistently associated with changes in basal adrenal glucocorticoid secretion.

3. Anterior Pituitary Anatomy

The limited data available from human subjects suggest that relatively minor changes in anterior pituitary structure occur in aged individuals (Monroe, 1951; Verzár, 1966). The number, appearance, and distribution of secretory granules in anterior pituitary cells were not different in 32-month-old as compared to young rats (Balagh *et al.*, 1970). The most common anatomical alteration occurring in the pituitary of aging rats is the appearance of tumors (Saxton and Graham, 1944; Griesbach, 1967). Meites *et al.* (1978) associated the relatively high incidence of pituitary tumors in aging rats to increased prolactin and decreased gonadotropin secretion.

Although Verzár (1966) indicated uncertainties about the effect of age on pituitary ACTH content, it is becoming clear that anterior pituitary hormone content is not a precise measure of gland function. The effect of age on pituitary responsiveness to stimulation and inhibition is of importance in considering age effects on the function of this control system and will be considered in detail in subsequent sections of this review.

4. Hypothalamic Structure and Hormone Content

Comparatively less information is known concerning direct aging effects on hypothalamic anatomy. Although it is accepted that neuronal loss occurs with age in many brain areas (Andrew, 1956), hypothalamic neuronal numbers seem to be less affected by aging. Buttlar-Brentans (1954) and Andrew (1956) reported no age modifications in cell numbers in human hypothalamic supraoptic and paraventricular nuclei. In contrast, Frolkis (1976) found larger, more dense secretory granules in supraoptic and paraventricular nuclei of aged rats. His 24-month-old rats also had smaller cellular nuclei in their hypothalamic regions which he interpreted as evidence for decreased neurosecretory activity in these hypothalamic neurons.

In a more recent study, Hsu and Peng (1978) considered age effects on several rat hypothalamic nuclei. They found significant decreases in neuronal densities in the medial preoptic area, the anterior hypothalamic area, and the arcuate nucleus. On the other hand, no change in neuronal density was found in the supraoptic, paraventricular, ventromedial, or dorsomedial nuclei.

Although there have been several recent reports of age-related alterations in hypothalamic releasing-hormone content, age changes in hypothalamic content of ACTH-controlling substances have not been reported. In summary, there is no conclusive evidence at present that changes in hypothalamic structure are involved in age-related changes in hypothalamic-pituitary-adrenal control systems.

5. Adrenal Steroid Secretion and Basal Blood Concentrations

One of the most significant alterations in hormone function occurring in aging humans is the decrease in adrenal androgen secretion and blood concentration. Adrenal secretion of dehydroepiandrosterone increases sharply (Fig. 1) during puberty and falls off dramatically in aging men and women (Vihko, 1966, Smith *et al.*, 1975). This steroid practically disappears from the circulation in some older people (Migeon *et al.*, 1957; Smith *et al.*, 1975). Although its biological significance is unknown,

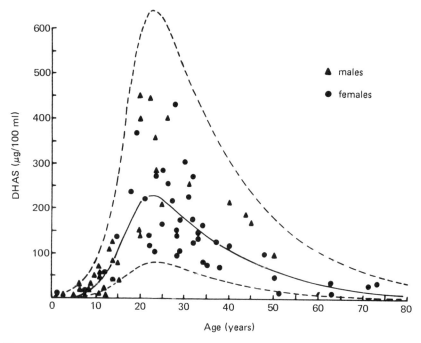

Fig. 1. Normal serum concentration of dehydroepiandrosterone sulfate from 18 months to 73 years. Solid line represents exponential mean; dashed lines ± 1.96 standard deviations. (From Smith *et al.*, 1975.)

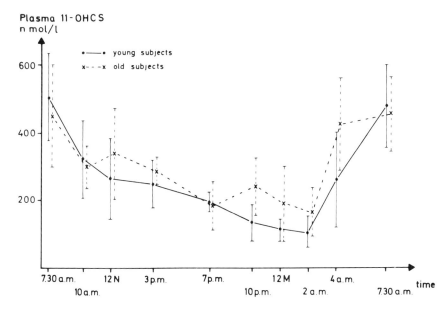

Fig. 2. Nycothermal rhythm of 11-OHCS concentrations in plasma in 11 young and five elderly healthy subjects. The average values are given. The vertical bar represents 1 SD. (From Blichert-Toft, 1978.)

this decline in adrenal androgen secretion is more consistent and far exceeds age alteration in other adrenal steroids.

The effect of age on glucocorticoid function has received widespread attention. Most studies show similar plasma cortisol concentrations and similar diurnal rhythms (Fig. 2) of blood cortisol concentrations in young and aged human subjects (Blichert-Toft *et al.,* 1970; Blichert-Toft, 1975; Jensen and Blichert-Toft, 1971). Although basal blood cortisol concentrations remain remarkably stable in aging subjects, Romanoff *et al.* (1961) found that aged men had about a 25% decrease in 24-h secretory rate of cortisol when compared to young men. The reduced secretory rate for cortisol with aging is accompanied by an almost identical decline in cortisol metabolism and excretion (Romanoff *et al.,* 1958; West *et al.,* 1961; Moncloa *et al.,* 1963). In addition, these studies showed that the excretion of glucocorticoid metabolites and cortisol secretory rates were not different in young and aged subjects if these variables were expressed per unit of creatinine excretion. Although considerable significance was initially attached to the creatinine relationship, its biological significance is questionable since creatinine excretion reflects muscle mass, and the liver rather than the muscles, is the primary site of cortisol metabolism. Collectively, these data suggest that the resting, nonstimulated adrenocortical control system is normally responsive to control input, reacting to the reduced rate of cortisol metabolism by reducing cortisol secretion.

In a series of experiments we showed similar resting blood glucocorticoid concentrations in young and aged cattle (Riegle and Nellor, 1967), goals (Riegle et al., 1968), and rats (Hess and Riegle, 1970). Although Landfield (1978) has proposed an increase in resting corticosterone with biological aging in the rat, our studies (Hess and Riegle, 1970; Hess and Riegle, 1972; Riegle and Hess, 1972; Riegle, 1973) and others (Tang and Phillips, 1978; Wilson et al., 1981) have shown no consistent change in basal corticosterone concentrations in aging rats of either sex. In contrast to Landfield's hypothesis, Wilson et al., (1981) found reduced basal corticosterone in the afternoon in 25-month-old as compared to 2-month-old male rats. In summary, there is only minimal evidence that steady-state, resting concentrations of adrenal glucocorticoids are altered by increasing age in mammalian species. These data suggest normalcy of basal adrenocortical control system function in nonstressed aging subjects, and suggest that if significant age-related alterations in this control system occur, they are evident only at times when the system is stimulated or inhibited.

6. Adrenocortical Response to ACTH

Age alterations in adrenocortical control system responsiveness to regulatory input have most often been measured as changes in blood glucocorticoid concentrations in response to the stimulation or inhibition of the system. A consistent problem with the interpretation of these data is that differences in blood hormone concentrations could reflect alterations in adrenal response to ACTH or changes in hypothalamic-pituitary response to their control inputs. Although it is generally accepted that ACTH is the primary regulator of adrenal cortex function, Engeland et al. (1975) suggested another factor which could potentially influence this endocrine function. They reported that the adrenal hypertrophy following unilateral adrenalectomy occurred without measurable changes in peripheral corticosterone or ACTH concentration, and the ability to increase gland size still was operative in hypophysectomized rats. This group proposed a neurally mediated hypothalamic regulation of adrenal function which could interact with more classically adreno-cortical responses to ACTH.

Although Moncloa *et al.* (1963) reported age-related decreases in both 17β-hydroxycorticosterone excretion and adrenocortical respon-siveness to multiple levels of ACTH stimulation in men ranging from 20–85 years of age, Blichert-Toft *et al.* (1970) and West *et al.* (1961) found similar increases in blood cortisol after ACTH stimulation of the adrenals of aged subjects. Adrenocortical secretion of dehydroepian-drosterone is also stimulated by ACTH. Although blood levels of this hormone are increased following ACTH stimulation, the response is delayed as compared to subjects, and the increase in dehydroepian-drosterone remains low in the aged, never approaching blood concen-trations of the hormone found in young subjects (Blichert-Toft *et al.*, 1970).

Adrenocortical response to ACTH is more variable in other species. In our first studies of aging effects on adrenocortical function, we found sharply reduced increases in blood glucocorticoids following ACTH in-fusion in aged cattle and goats compared to young subjects of these species (Riegle and Nellor, 1967; Riegle *et al.*, 1968). This decrease in adrenocortical reserve capacity in aged animals was accompanied by greatly increased connective tissue infiltration of the adrenal cortices of these animals, with only restricted nodules of normally appearing ad-renocortical tissue remaining (Riegle and Nellor, 1965). These studies suggested that these species encountered a primary adrenocortical fail-ure with increased biological age.

In our rat studies we found small but statistically significant de-creases in the increase in plasma corticosterone following acute ACTH injection into aged, as compared to young rats of both sexes (Hess and Riegle, 1970). In a separate study we treated young and aged male and female rats with 20 U ACTH/kg/day for six weeks. These ACTH treat-ments resulted in sharply increased serum corticosterone concentrations which were sustained throughout the treatment regime in both age groups. In a more recent study, Pritchett *et al.* (1979) studied *in vitro* respon-siveness of adrenal tissue from 60- and 340-day-old rats. They found significantly less corticosterone secretion from the adrenal tissue of the older group in response to both ACTH and cyclic AMP, and reduced adrenal tissue accumulation of cyclic AMP following ACTH treatment.

In summary, these data indicate that although some indices of ad-renal responsiveness to ACTH may be altered with aging in the rat and in humans, these species retain a high degree of responsiveness into old age and it is unlikely that changes in adrenal cortical response, as measured by blood hormone concentration, significantly contributes to age changes in endocrine function.

7. Responsiveness of the Hypothalamic-Pituitary Unit

Current understanding of the regulation of ACTH secretion suggests that the activity of the hypothalamic-pituitary unit controlling ACTH secretion is controlled by the combined effects of glucocorticoid negative feedback and a central neural stimulating system which responds to an internal circadian rhythm and is activated by physical and psychogenic stressors. The similarity of the circadian pattern of plasma cortisol and serum ACTH concentrations in young and elderly subjects has been interpreted to indicate no age-related changes in diurnal ACTH secretion in humans (Blichert-Toft, 1975). On the other hand, Wilson *et al.* (1981) found a smaller increase in evening as compared to morning plasma corticosterone in aged, as compared to young male rats, suggesting an alteration in the diurnal pattern of ACTH secretion in the older group. Interestingly, Dallman *et al.* (1978) found a 2.5-fold increase in rat adrenocortical responsiveness to ACTH with lights off, as compared to lights on, that was not associated with changes in plasma ACTH. These data support their previous hypothesis that factors other than ACTH secretion are involved in regulation of the adrenal cortex (Engeland *et al.*, 1975).

Several stimulators of hypothalamic-pituitary adrenocortical secretion have been used to study the effects of age on the ability of this system to respond to stimuli. Although aging human subjects have not had adrenocortical assessments made after direct stress under control conditions, the effects of several indirect stressors have been studied. Asnis *et al.* (1981b) reported that 50% of patients with endogenous depression have increased blood cortisol concentrations. These depressed patients were also more resistant to insulin induced hypoglycemia (Swami *et al.*, 1981). Age effects on these changes in serum cortisol have recently been reported. Mean 24-hr serum cortisol levels in depressed patients rose from 5 μg/dl in a young group (38 years, mean age) to 9 μg/dl in the older groups (60 years, mean age; Asnis *et al.*, 1981a). These changes were ascribed to increased ACTH secretion in the older group rather than to alterations in cortisol clearance, since psychotherapy restored cortisol values to normal in all age groups.

Insulin-induced hypoglycemia is a recognized stimulator of hypothalamic-pituitary-adrenal secretion. Several groups have used insulin responsiveness as an indicator of hypothalamic-pituitary ACTH reserve in aged human subjects (Friedman *et al.*, 1969; Cartlidge *et al.*, 1970; Muggo *et al.*, 1975; Blichert-Toft, 1978). These studies uniformly indicate identical insulin-induced hypoglycemia and similar increases in blood cortisol following hypoglycemia in young, middle-aged, and old individuals.

Hypothalamic-pituitary responsiveness to metyrapone-induced decreases in cortisol secretion has also been measured as a function of age in human subjects. Metyrapone acts to decrease cortisol concentration by enzymatic inhibition of 11-hydroxylase and as a stimulator of cortisol metabolism. Blichert-Toft (1975) has shown nearly identical adrenocortical response to metyrapone (Fig. 3), again indicating normal hypothalamic-pituitary responsiveness to reduced glucocorticoid feedback in human subjects.

Hypothalamic-pituitary-adrenal response to surgery is another measure of function that can be assessed during aging. An extensive study of this response in aging human subjects was reported by Blichert-Toft (1975). They measured the effect of elective surgical stress acutely during surgery and for six postoperative days. Serial blood samples taken during the operations showed similar increases in plasma cortisol in young and aged groups. On the other hand, the total increment of plasma cortisol on the day of surgery was higher in the aged group, and the evening plasma cortisol concentration remained higher in the aged than in the young group for 4 additional postoperative days (Fig. 4; Blichert-Toft, 1975). The aged group also had a larger increase in 11-desoxycortisol

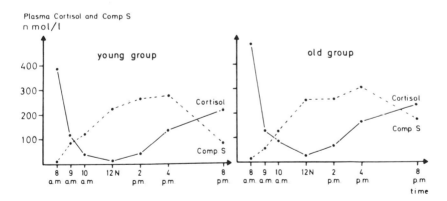

Fig. 3. Changes in cortisol and compound S concentrations in plasma in 16 young and 11 elderly volunteers during and after intravenous infusion and metyrapone 17.5 mg/Kg bw/hr, from 8:00 a.m. to 12:00 noon. Average values are recorded. (From Blichert-Toft, 1978.)

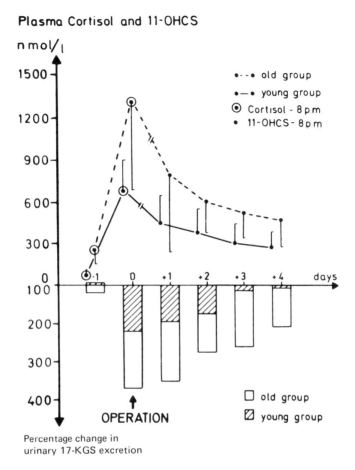

Fig. 4. The average evening values of plasma cortisol prior to surgery and on the day of surgery are seen uppermost in the figure followed by the average evening values of 11-OHCS determined during the ensuing four postoperative days in 15 elderly and 20 young elective patients. Vertical bars denote 1 SD. At the bottom of the figure, the percentage change in urinary 17-KGS excretion is seen. Patients and conditions as above. (From Blichert-Toft, 1978.)

than the young subjects following an intravenous metyrapone test on day 5 after surgery. The results of this study suggest no impairment in the ability of the hypothalamic-pituitary-adrenal control system of elderly subjects to sustain surgical stress, as indicated by the increase in hormone secretion. The ability of this control system to show higher plasma cortisol during the surgery and postoperative recovery period, and the larger response to metyrapone postoperatively, suggests that the aged hypothalamic-pituitary unit either secretes more ACTH in response to this stress, or that the control system is less sensitive to glucocorticoid negative feedback in the aged.

Several studies have suggested age alterations in hypothalmic-pituitary responsiveness in the laboratory rat. Our initial experiments showed only modest decreases in the increase in plasma corticosterone following ether stress in aged rats (Hess and Riegle, 1970). On the other hand, Wilson *et al.* (1981) showed smaller increases in both serum ACTH and plasma corticosterone in aged, as compared to young male rats, following controlled ether stress. This study also showed similar *in vitro* responsiveness of young and aged rat pituitaries to vasopressin stimulation of ACTH secretion, suggesting that the age difference in stress responsiveness of the rat was primarily due to reduced ability of the hypothalamus to secrete ACTH-stimulating factors. In a similar study, Tang and Phillips (1978) reported that although aged male rats had higher pre-stress serum ACTH concentrations than young rats, the older rats showed smaller increases in serum ACTH concentrations 2.5 and 15 min after initiation of a stress stimulation.

In another of our early experiments we tested the effect of long-term stimulation of the hypothalamic-pituitary-adrenal system in the rat (Hess and Riegle, 1972). Young and aged male and female groups received daily subcutaneous depot injections of 20 u of ACTH/kg for 6 weeks. At 2-week intervals the adrenocortical control mechanism response to ether vapor stress was tested (Figs. 5 and 6). Although chronic ACTH activation of the adrenocortical control system resulted in smaller ether stress-induced increases in plasma corticosterone in young ACTH injected rats than in their non-ACTH-treated controls, the adrenocortical responsiveness of the aged groups was not different from their control group. The decreased responsiveness of the young rats to ether stress suggested that the hypothalamic-pituitary corticotropin control mechanism of the young rats was responding differently to the chronically increased blood corticosterone concentrations following prolonged adrenocortical activation than the control system of the old rats.

The apparent decrease in sensitivity of the aged rat hypothalamic-pituitary control unit to corticosterone negative feedback was tested by measuring its responsiveness to stress following acute and chronic treatment with the synthetic glucocorticoid, dexamethasone (Riegle and Hess, 1972). Both acute and chronic dexamethasone injections produced greater inhibition of ether stress-induced increases in plasma corticosterone in young than in aged rat groups, supporting the hypothesis of the previous study (Fig. 7).

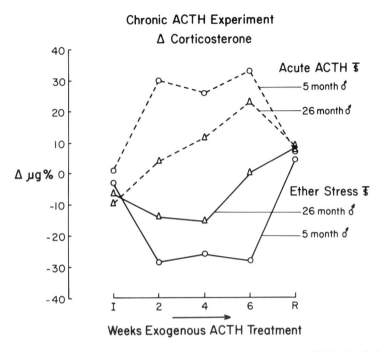

Fig. 5. Adrenocortical responsiveness to ether stress and acute ACTH stimulation in young and aged male rats receiving 10 units of depot ACTH/day for 6 weeks. The stress treatment consisted of anesthesia level of ether vapor exposure at 40 min, 10 min, and at the time of blood sample collection. Acute ACTH response was measured in terms of plasma corticosterone concentration 1 hr after subcutaneous injection of 10 U/Kg bw of ACTH. Adrenal responsiveness to stress and ACTH was measured before chronic adrenal stimulation, after 2, 4, and 6 weeks of treatment and after 2 weeks of posttreatment recovery. (From Hess and Riegle, 1972.)

In another experiment we tested the effects of chronic stress-induced increases in corticosterone secretion on the adrenocortical control system of young and aged male and female rats (Riegle, 1973). Rats received twice daily 2-hr restraint stress treatments for 20 days. Restraint stress is intense, resulting in a maximal stimulation of adrenocortical secretion in all groups throughout the experiment. Adrenocortical response, in terms of the magnitude of the increase in plasma corticosterone secreted in response to the stress, was decreased during the experiment in all stressed groups. The decrease in responsiveness was greater in the young than in the aged groups. This study suggested that corticosteroid feedback from chronic stress activation of the adrenal cortex results in incomplete inhibition of the adrenocortical control

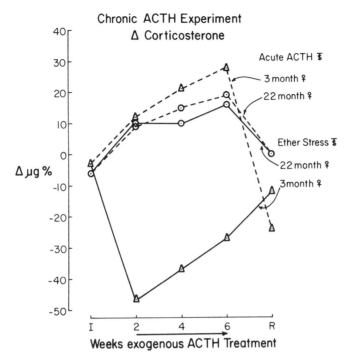

Fig. 6. Adrenocortical responsiveness to ether stress and acute ACTH stimulation in young and aged female rats receiving 6 units of depot ACTH/day for 6 weeks. Experimental conditions as described in Fig. 5. (From Hess and Riegle, 1972.)

mechanism. The increased inhibition of the adrenals of the young rats supports the concept of decreased adrenocortical control system sensitivity during aging.

In summary, these data indicate that there are age-related changes in adrenocortical control systems. Most studies in a variety of species suggest little change in basal or resting glucocorticoid concentrations with increasing age. Although there are some reports of reduced adrenocortical responsiveness to ACTH stimulation, most studies indicate a high degree of adrenocortical responsiveness in old age. The most consistent change in adrenocortical function with age appears to involve a change in negative feedback responsiveness to increased blood corticosteroids following adrenocortical activation. These changes may result in aged individuals being exposed to higher glucocorticoid activity under stress conditions. Precise neuroendocrine mechanisms involved in this change during aging remain to be elucidated.

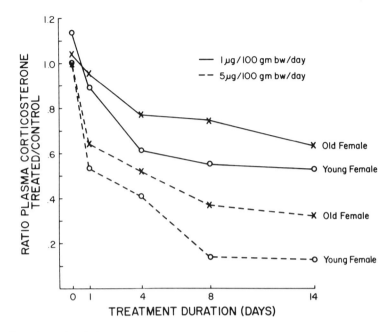

Fig. 7. The ratio of plasma corticosterone in young and old rats subjected to ether stress before and after 1, 4, 8, and 14 days of 1.0 and 5.0 μg of dexamethosone/100 gm bw.

8. Neuroendocrine Control of Corticotropin-Releasing Hormone

Considerable new information has recently been added to our understanding of the biochemistry and physiology of ACTH and the neuroendocrine control of ACTH secretion. It has been demonstrated that ACTH and lipotropin are contained within a common precursor glycosylated molecule referred to as 31K ACTH/endorphin, or proopiocortin (Mains *et al.*, 1977; Rubinstein et al., 1978). This precursor molecule is believed to be the source of a variety of pituitary and neuroendocrine secretions including ACTH which in turn is a source of α-melanocyte-stimulating hormone (MSH) and β-lipotropin, portions of which can be converted to γ-lipotropin, β-endorphin and β-MSH. Krieger (1980) has shown that immunoassayable quantities of ACTH, α-MSH and β-endorphin are present in the hypothalamus and can be synthesized by pituitary and brain neurons of several mammalian species including the rat and human. Although there is some preliminary evidence that ACTH and the MSH molecules may function in certain behavioral systems such as avoidance behavior or learning, concepts of ACTH functioning as a peptidergic neurotransmitter remain speculative.

Another area of neuroendocrinology where there has been recent significant advances, concerns the identification of corticotropin-releasing hormone. The secretion of ACTH appears to be regulated by excitatory hypothalamic stimulation (Weiner and Ganong, 1978). The posterior pituitary hormone, vasopressin, has been associated with increased pituitary-adrenal secretions. Aizawa *et al.* (1982) have recently shown that vasopressin and related peptides have direct pituitary activity in cultured pituitary cells, suggesting that this peptide can directly simulate ACTH secretion separate from its function as a vasopressor or a neurotransmitter.

In addition to the ACTH-stimulating activity of vasopressor, a 41 amino acid polypeptide with ACTH-regulating activity has recently been isolated from hypothalamic tissue (Vale *et al.*, 1981; Rivier *et al.*, 1982). Rivier *et al.* (1982) recently reported a dose-response relationship for this peptide as a stimulator of corticosterone secretion in rats. In addition, they found that this molecule was without effect on corticosterone secretion in hypophysectomized rats and that dexamethasone pretreatment decreased the ACTH release stimulated by the peptide.

Another factor which complicates our understanding of the neuroendocrine control of ACTH in some species is the recognition that ACTH is secreted from both the anterior and intermediate lobes of the pituitary. There is a dopaminergic innervation of the intermediate pituitary lobe, and dopamine has been reported to inhibit the release of ACTH from the intermediate pituitary *in vitro* (Fischer and Moriarty, 1977). This neurotransmitter function could be an important regulatory factor in species with functional intermediate pituitary function.

In a recent review, Ganong (1980) hypothesizes four possible sites of action for neurotransmitters affecting corticotropin-releasing hormone: (1) the neurotransmitters may act directly on the pituitary after transport via the hypothalamic-hypophysial portal vascular system, (2) they may act by axoaxonic synaptic action on corticotropin-releasing hormone neurons in the median eminence, (3) they may act by axodendritic termination on cell bodies in more distal portions of the hypothalamus, and (4) they may function by a paracrine rather than a synaptic fashion on corticotropin-releasing hormone neurons. Ganong (1980) points out that there is no evidence for a direct neurotransmitter effect on pituitary ACTH secretion, and since most drug studies of neurotransmitter regulation of corticotropin-releasing hormone secretion suggests their activity occurs within the blood-brain barrier, Ganong concluded there is little evidence for axoaxonic effect. On the other hand, Tilders *et al.* (1982) have recently concluded that circulating epinephrine from sympathoadrenal secretion can stimulate pituitary-adrenal activity. Since epinephrine does not easily pass the blood-brain barrier and the pituitary-adrenal system is sensitive to low levels of circulating epinephrine, they concluded the β-adrenergic receptors affecting this system are located outside the blood-brain barrier, presumably in the median eminence. Tilders *et al.* (1982) also point out that since adrenal medullary secretions are not required for stimulation of pituitary-adrenal secretions, there must be corollary neuroendocrine mechanisms involved in ACTH regulation. It is obvious from the above data that even the anatomical relationship of where neurotransmitter regulation of ACTH secretion occurs is controversial.

Although hypothalamic-pituitary-adrenal regulation was one of the first of the neuroendocrine systems studied, there remains a great deal of conflict and controversy concerning mechanisms of neural regulation of this system. In their review, Martin *et al.* (1977) summarized their perspective by suggesting that understanding of neurotransmitter regulation of the corticotropin-releasing hormone and ACTH secretion was probably the most difficult of all anterior pituitary hormones. It is still uncertain which neurotransmitters and which regulatory pathways are involved. However, pharmacological data suggests a variety of different transmitters participate in the regulation of this system.

It is agreed that ACTH and adrenal glucocorticoid secretion involves both a circadian rhythm and a series of eight to nine episodial cycles (Weitzman *et al.*, 1971). The episodic bursts appear to be independent of stress and circulating cortisol concentration persisting in Addison's disease at a much higher level of ACTH secretion. Although it has been shown that the diurnal rhythm of ACTH can be blocked by lesions in the anterior hypothalamus (Martin *et al.*, 1977), the neural control of the episodic release and circadian rhythms involve brain centers higher than the hypothalamus.

Although the control of ACTH secretion clearly involves centers outside the hypothalamus, much of the basal hypothalamus also influences regulation of corticotropin-releasing hormone secretion. The physiological effects of hypothalamic isolation have been variable (Martin *et al.*, 1977). Total disconnection of the hypothalamus from the brain, blocks the pituitary-adrenal response to a variety of stressors including cold, surgical trauma, and acoustic stimuli. On the other hand, ether stress is apparently sensed locally, requiring only the hypothalamus to activate the adrenal control system, and certain stressors such as hemorrhage, endotoxin, and laparotomy have been suggested to affect ACTH secretion independently of the hypothalamus (Kendall, 1971).

A large number of studies have considered the effects of alteration of catecholamine function on hypothalamic-pituitary-adrenal function. Corticotropin-releasing factor is not affected by incubation of rat hypothalamic tissue with dopamine or norepinephrine (Jones et al., 1976). Alpha-methyl-tyrosine-induced decreases in hypothalamic dopamine and norepinephrine have been shown to increase corticosterone secretion in the rat (VanLoon, 1973). L-Dopa treatment reversed the effect of alpha-methyl tyrosine and selective depletion of dopamine did not affect adrenal function (VanLoon, 1973). In addition, amphetamine lowers resting ACTH secretion and inhibits ACTH increases in response to stress (Bhattacharya and Marks, 1969) and 6-hydroxydopamine injection into the third ventricle of the rat depletes hypothalamic norepinephrine and increases corticosterone secretion (Cuello et al., 1974). There is also considerable data suggesting an α-adrenergic inhibition of ACTH secretion in the dog (Weiner and Ganong, 1978; Ganong, 1980). Collectively, these experiments suggest an inhibitory role for norepinephrine on ACTH secretion. However, Martin et al. (1977) found increased ACTH release following epinephrine and norepinephrine infusion into the basal hypothalamus, norepinephrine implants into the median eminence and selected extrahypothalamic regions of the cat brain (Kreiger and Kreiger, 1970), and norepinephrine injection into the hypothalamus of the guinea pig (Naumenko, 1968) stimulates ACTH release. In addition, treatment with the α-adrenergic agonist clonidine had no effect on cortisol secretion in humans (Lal et al., 1975). Apomorphine, L-dopa, or clonidine had no effect on non-human primate cortisol secretion (Chambers and Brown, 1976), but L-dopa alone was reported to potentiate the ACTH response to metyrapone (Hsu et al., 1976). The above reports indicate a clear conflict concerning the role of catecholamines in the regulation of ACTH secretion which may in part be species specific.

There has also been considerable debate about the effects of serotonin on ACTH secretion. Treatment with the serotonin precursor 5-hydroxytryptophan has been reported to stimulate increases in plasma ACTH in humans (Imura et al., 1973). Inhibition of serotonin with centrally acting drugs reduced metyrapone-induced increase in ACTH secretion (Cavagnini et al., 1975) and insulin-induced hypoglycemic stimulation of cortisol secretion in humans (Plonk et al., 1974). On the other hand, serotoninergic inhibitors did not block the increase in ACTH secretion stimulated by vasopressin in humans (Cavagnini et al., 1976), suggesting either multiple hypothalamic mechanisms for ACTH stimulation or direct vasopressin effects on pituitary ACTH secretion.

Serotonin has also been associated with activation of the pituitary-adrenal system in other species. Administration of 5-hydroxytryptophan was found to increase hypothalamic serotonin concentration and serum corticosterone in deafferentated rats (Popova *et al.*, 1972). Jones *et al.* (1976) reported increased corticotropin-releasing activity from hypothalamic tissue incubated with serotonin. In addition, direct implantation of serotonin into regions of guinea pig (Naumenko, 1968) and cat brains (Kreiger and Kreiger, 1970) increased plasma concentrations of glucocorticoids. On the other hand, Jones *et al.* (1976) found that treatment with cholinergic antagonists blocked the *in vitro* stimulatory effect of serotonin, which was interpreted to suggest a cholinergic mediation of the serotonin effect.

There is also considerable evidence for an inhibitory effect of serotonin in pituitary-adrenal function. In contrast to the studies of Jones *et al.* (1976), Vermes *et al.* (1972) reported decreased ACTH secretion after serotonin treatment of rat hypothalamic-pituitary incubates. This group also reported reduced stress-induced increases in corticosterone following serotonin implantation into the medial hypothalamus (Vermes and Telegdy, 1972). In another study, this group reported a serotoninergic role in stress regulation of adrenal function, proposing a decrease in brain serotonin with stress and a corticosteroid-induced increase in serotonin synthesis (Vermes *et al.*, 1973). In a series of studies in the dog, Ganong (1980) reported an inhibitory role for 5-hydroxytryptophan on control of ACTH secretion. On the other hand, he concluded that the inhibition was not due to a direct effect of serotonin since treatment with the serotonin-blocking drug, metergoline, did not effect the 5-hydroxytryptophan response. Ganong summarized his data by concluding there was no evidence that increased central release of serotonin stimulates or inhibits corticotropin-releasing hormone secretion in dogs.

Intraventricular injection of histamine in dogs increased plasma ACTH and corticosteroid concentrations (Rudolph *et al.* 1979). Treatment of the dogs with mepyramine, a histamine receptor blocker, prevented histamine-induced stimulation of pituitary-adrenal function (Rudolph *et al.*, 1979). On the other hand, mepyramine treatment did not block stress-induced increases in ACTH secretion, leading Ganong (1980) to conclude that these experiments did not show that histamine is an obligatory mediator in stress stimulation of the hypothalamic-pituitary-adrenal system.

Acetylcholine and angiotensin II are other neurotransmitters for which there is some evidence for stimulatory effects on the pituitary-adrenal system. Acetylcholine has been reported to stimulate corticotropin-releasing factor secretion from rat hypothalamic incubates (Jones *et al.*, 1976). In addition, blocking acetylcholine metabolism with neostigmine (Naumenko, 1967) or carbachol stimulation of cholinergic receptors following intraventricular injection (Abe and Hiroshige, 1974), elevated plasma corticosteroid concentrations. Although systemic administration of angiotensin II has been reported to increase ACTH (Ramsay *et al.*, 1978), other studies showed an inhibition of ACTH by systemic angiotensin II treatment (Semple *et al.*, 1979). Direct intraventricular injection of angiotensin II stimulated increased ACTH secretion (Reid, 1977; Maran and Yates, 1977). However, Ganong (1980) found no effect on corticosteroid secretion in surgically stressed dogs following intraventricular injection of the angiotensin receptor blocking drug, saralasin.

Most of the above studies have attempted to identify stimulatory effects of neurotransmitters on corticotropin-releasing hormone secretion. γ-aminobutyric acid is one hypothalamic transmitter that consistently appears to inhibit the hypothalamic-pituitary-adrenal system. γ-aminobutyric acid has an inhibitory effect on corticotropin-releasing hormone secretion from incubated rat hypothalamic tissue (Jones *et al.*, 1976). Two antagonists of this transmitter, picrotoxin, and bicuculline, prevented corticosterone release inhibition following intraventricular γ-aminobutyric acid infusion (Makara and Stark, 1974). In addition, the ability of dexamethasone to inhibit ACTH secretion was blocked by treatment with mercaptopropionic acid, a specific inhibitor of glutamic acid decarboxylase.

9. Summary

The neurotransmitter relationship to control of hypothalamic corticotropin-releasing factor and ACTH secretion is complex. Most known hypothalamic neurotransmitters have been shown to have effects on at least some aspects of this system. Although most data suggest excitatory effects of neurotransmitters on ACTH release, the activities and interactions of all of these transmitters remain controversial and suggest multiple pathways of neurological activation of the hypothalamic-pituitary system. Lack of understanding of basic neuroendocrine control of pituitary ACTH secretion has made it impossible to relate changes in neuroendocrine function to age alterations in hypothalamic-pituitary-adrenal function. A substantial amount of information suggests significant age-related differences in hypothalamic-response to a variety of control inputs. However, a precise description of aging effects on neuroendocrine regulation of ACTH secretion requires a better understanding of both age effects on neurotransmitters and neurotransmitter effect on ACTH secretion.

10. References

Abe, K., and Hiroshige, T., 1974, Changes in plasma corticosterone and hypothalamic CRF levels following intraventricular injection or drug-induced changes of brain biogenic amines in the rat, *Neuroendocrinology* **14**:195.

Aizawa, T., Tasuda, N., Greer, M. A., and Sawyer, W. H., 1982, *In vivo* adrenocorticotropin-releasing activity of neurohypophyseal hormones and their analogs, *Endocrinology* **110**:98.

Andrew, W., 1956, Structural alterations with aging in the nervous system, *J. Chronic Dis.* **3**:575.

Asnis, G. M., Sachar, E. J., Halbreich, U., Nathan, R. S., Novacenko, H., and Ostrow, L. C., 1981a, Cortisol secretion in relation to age in major depression, *Psychosomat. Med.* **43**:235.

Asnis, G. M., Sachar, E. J., Halbreich, U., Nathan, R. S., Ostrow, L., and Halpern, E. J., 1981b, Cortisol secretion and dexamethasone response in depression, *Am. J. Psychiat.* **138**:1218.

Balagh, A., Takacs, I., Ladanyi, D., and Arvay, A., 1970, Electron microscopic studies of the adenohypophysis of aged rats, *Gerontol. Clinica* **16**:313.

Bhattacharya, A. N., and Marks, B. H., 1969, Effects of paragyline and amphetamine upon acute stress response in rats, *Proc. Soc. Exp. Biol. Med.* **130**:1194.

Blichert-Toft, M., 1975, Secretion of corticotrophin and somatotrophin by the senescent adenohypophysis in man, Thesis, *Acta Endocrinol. (Kbh.)* (Suppl.) **195**:1.

Blichert-Toft, M., 1978, The adrenal glands in old age, in: *Geriatric Endocrinology* (R. B. Greenblatt, ed.), Raven Press, New York, p. 81.

Blichert-Toft, M., Blichert-Toft, B., and Jensen, H. K., 1970, Pituitary-adrenocortical stimulation in the aged as reflected in levels of plasma cortisol and compound S, *Acta Chir. Scand.* **136**:665.

Bourne, G. H., 1967, Aging changes in the endocrines, in: *Endocrines and Aging* (L. Gitman, ed.), Charles C. Thomas, Springfield, Illinois.

Buttlar-Brentans, K., 1954, Zar Lebensgeschichte des Nuclear basilis, tubermammalaris, supraopticus und paraventriculus unter normalen und pathogener Bedingungen, *J. Hirnforschi.* **1**:337.

Cartlidge, N. E. F., Black, M. M., Hall, M. R. P., and Hall, P., 1970, Pituitary function in the elderly, *Gerontol. Clin.* **12**:65.

Cavagnini, F., Panerai, A. E., Valentini, F., Bulgheroni, P., Peracchi, M., and Pinto, M., 1975, Inhibition of ACTH response to oral and intravenous metyrapone by antiserotoninergic treatment in man, *J. Clin. Endocrinol. Metabol.* **41**:143.

Cavagnini, F., Raggi, U., Micossi, P., DiLandro, A., and Invitti, C., 1976, Effect of the antiserotoninergic drug, metergoline, on the ACTH and cortisol response to insulin hypoglycemia and lucine-vasopressin in man, *J. Clin. Endocrinol. Metabol.* **43**:306.

Chambers, J. W., and Brown, G. M., 1976, Neurotransmitter regulation of growth hormone and ACTH in the rhesus monkey: Effects of biogenic amines, *Endocrinology* **98**:420.

Cooper, E. R. A., 1925, *The Histology of the More Important Human Endocrine Organs at Various Age,* Oxford University Press, London.

Cuello, A. C., Shoemaker, W. J., and Ganong, W. F., 1974, Effect of 6-hydroxydopamine on hypothalamic norepinephrine and dopamine content, ultrastructure of the median eminence, and plasma corticosterone, *Brain Res.* **78:**57.

Dallman, M. F., Engeland, W. C., Rose, J. C., Wilkenson, C. W., Shinako, J., and Siedenberg, F., 1978, Nycthemeral rhythms in adrenal responsiveness to ACTH, *Am. J. Physiol.* **235:**R210.

Das, L. N., and Magilton, J. H., 1971, Age changes in the relationship among endocrine glands of the beagle, *Exp. Gerontol.* **6:**297.

Dhom, G., Hahback, C., Mausle, E., Scheir, O., and Ueberberg, H., 1981, Peliosis of the female adrenal cortex of the aging rat, *Virchows Arch.* **36:**195.

Dobbie, J. W., 1969, Adrenocortical nodular hyperplasia: The aging adrenal, *J. Pathol.* **99:**1.

Dunihue, F. W., 1965, Reduced juxtaglomeular cell granularity, pituitary neurosecretory material, and width of the zona glomerulosa in aging rats, *Endocrinology* **77:**948.

Engeland, W. C., Shinsako, J., and Dallman, M. F., 1975, Corticosteroids and ACTH are not required for compensatory adrenal growth, *Am. J. Physiol.* **229:**1461.

Fischer, J. L., and Moriarty, C. M., 1977, Control of bioactive corticotropin release from the neuro-intermediate lobe of the rat pituitary *in vitro*, *Endocrinology* **100:**1047.

Friedman, M., Green, M. F., and Sharland, D. E., 1969, Assessment of hypothalamic-pituitary-adrenal function in the geriatric age group, *J. Gerontol.* **24:**292.

Frolkis, V. V., 1976, The hypothalamic mechanisms of aging, in: *Hypothalamus, Pituitary and Aging* (A. V. Everitt and J. H. Burgess, eds.), C. C. Thomas, Springfield, p. 614.

Galloway, N. O., Foley, C. F., and Lagerbloom, P., 1965, Uncertainties in geriatric data: II. Organ size, *J. Am. Geriat. Soc.* **13:**20.

Ganong, W. F., 1980, Neurotransmitters and pituitary function: Regulation of ACTH secretion, *Fed. Proc.* **39:**2923.

Griesbach, W. E., 1967, Basophil adenomata in the pituitary glands of 2-year-old male Long–Evans rats, *Cancer Res.* **27:**1813.

Haugen, O. A., 1973, The adrenal glands of elderly men in relation to abnormal prostatic growth, *Acta Pathol. Microbiol. Scand.* **81:**831.

Hess, G. D., and Riegle, G. D., 1970, Adrenocortical responsiveness to stress and ACTH in aging rats, *J. Gerontol.* **25:**354.

Hess, G. D., and Riegle, G. D., 1972, Effects of chronic ACTH stimulation on adrenocortical function in young and aged rats, *Am. J. Physiol.* **222:**1458.

Hsu, K. K., and Peng, M. T., 1978, Hypothalamic neuron number of old female rats, *Gerontology* **24:**434.

Hsu, T-H., Hsu, C-K., and Gann, D. S., 1976, Potentiation of ACTH response to metyrapone by L-Dopa in the monkey, *Endocrinology* **99:**1115.

Imura, H., Nakai, Y., and Yoshimi, T., 1973, Effect of 5-hydroxytryptophan (5-HTP) on growth hormone and ACTH release in man, *J. Clin. Endocrinol. Metabol.* **36:**204.

Jayne, E. P., 1953, Cytology of the adrenal gland of the rat at different ages, *Anat. Rec.* **115:**459.

Jensen, H. K., and Blichert-Toft, M., 1971, Serum corticotrophin, plasma cortisol, and urinary excretion of 17-ketogenic steroids in the elderly (age group: 66–94 years), *Acta Endocrinol.* **66:**25.

Jones, M., Hillhouse, E., and Burden, J., 1976, The secretion of corticotropin-releasing hormone *in vitro*, in: *Frontiers in Neuroendocrinology* (L. Martini and W. F. Ganong, eds.), Raven Press, New York, p. 195.

Kendall, J. W., 1971, Feedback control of adrenocorticotropin hormone secretion, in: *Frontiers in Neuroendocrinology* (L. Martini and W. F. Ganong, eds.), Oxford University Press, New York, p. 177.

Krieger, D. T., 1980, Pituitary hormones in the brain: What is their function, *Fed. Proc.* **39**:2937.

Krieger, H. P., and Krieger, D. T., 1970, Chemical stimulation of the brain: Effect on adrenal corticoid release, *Am. J. Physiol.* **218**:1632.

Lal, S., Tolis, G., Martin, J. B., Brown, G. M., and Guyda, H., 1975, Effect of clonidine on growth hormone, prolactin, luteinizing hormone, follicle stimulating hormone and thyroid stimulating hormone in the serum of normal men, *J. Clin. Endocrinol. Metabol.* **41**:827.

Landfield, P. W., 1978, An endocrine hypothesis of brain aging and studies of brain-endocrine correlations and monosynaptic neurophysiology during aging, in: *Parkinson's Disease II: Aging and Neuroendocrine Relationships*, C. Finch, D. Potter, and A. Kenny, eds., Plenum Press, New York, p. 179.

Mains, R. E., Eipper, B. A., and Ling, M., 1977, Common precursor to corticotropins and endorphins, *Proc. Natl. Acad. Sci. USA* **74**:3014.

Makara, G. B., and Stark, E., 1974, Effect of gamma-aminobutyric acid (GABA) and GABA antagonist drugs on ACTH release, *Neuroendocrinology* **16**:178.

Maran, J. W., and Yates, F. E., 1977, Cortisol secretion during intrapituitary infusion of angiotensin II in conscious dogs, *Am. J. Physiol.* **233**:F273.

Martin, J. B., Reichlin, S., and Brown, G. M., 1977, Regulation of ACTH secretion and its disorders, in: *Clinical Neuroendocrinology*, F. A. Davis, Philadelphia, p. 179.

Meites, J., Huang, H. H., and Simpkins, J. W., 1978, Recent studies on neuroendocrine control of reproductive senescence in rats, in: *The Aging Reproductive System* (E. L. Schneider, ed.), Raven Press, New York, p. 213.

Migeon, C. J., Keiler, A. R., Lawrence, B., and Shepard, T. H., 1957, Dehydroepiandrosterone and androsterone levels in human plasma, *J. Clin. Endocrinol.* **17**:1051.

Moncloa, F., Gomez, R., and Pretell, E., 1963, Response to corticotropin and correlation between secretion of creatinine and urinary steroids and between the clearance of creatinine and urinary steroids in aging, *Steroids* **1**:437.

Monroe, R. T., 1951, *Diseases of Old Age*, Harvard University Press, Cambridge.

Muggo, M., Fedele, P., Tiergo, A., Molinari, M., and Crepaldi, G., 1975, Human growth hormone and cortisol response to insulin stimulation in aging, *J. Gerontol.* **30**:546.

Naumenko, E. V., 1967, Role of adrenergic and cholinergic structures on the control of the pituitary-adrenal system, *Endocrinology* **80**:69.

Naumenko, E. V., 1968, Hypothalamic chemoreactive structures and the regulation of pituitary-adrenal function: Effects of local injections of norepinephrine carbachol and serotonin into the brain of guinea pigs with intact brains and after mesencephalic transection, *Brain Res.* **11**:1.

Plonk, J. W., Bivens, C. H., and Feldman, J. M., 1974, Inhibition of hypoglycemia-induced cortisol secretion by the serotonin antagonist cyproheptadine, *J. Clin. Endocrinol. Metabol.* **38**:836.

Popova, N. K., Moslova, L. N., and Naumenko, E. V., 1972, Serotonin and the regulation of the pituitary-adrenal system for deafferentation of the hypothalamus, *Brain Res.* **47**:61.

Pritchett, J. F., Sartin, J. L., Marple, D. N., Harper, W. L., and Till, M. L., 1979, Interaction of aging with *in vitro* adrenocortical responsiveness to ACTH and cyclic AMP, *Horm. Res.* **10**:96.

Ramsay, D. J., Keil, L., Sharpe, M. C., and Shinsako, J., 1978, Angiotensin. II. infusion increases vasopressin, ACTH, and 11-hydroxycorticosteroid secretion, *Am. J. Physiol.* **234**:R66.

Reichel, W., 1968, Lipofuscin pigment accumulation and distribution in five rat organs as a function of age, *J. Gerontol.* **23**:145.

Reid, I. A., 1977, Is there a brain renin-angiotension system?, *Circ. Res.* **41**:147.

Riegle, G. D., 1973, Chronic stress effects on adrenocortical responsiveness in young and aged rats, *Neuroendocrinology* **11**:1.

Riegle, G. D., and Hess, G. D., 1972, Chronic and acute dexamethasone suppression of stress activation of the adrenal cortex in young and aged rats, *Neuroendocrinology* **9**:175.

Riegle, G. D., and Nellor, J. E., 1967, Changes in pituitary-adrenal function during aging in cattle, *J. Gerontol.* **22**:83.

Riegle, G. D., and Nellor, J. E., 1965, Adrenal-pituitary axis and aging in cattle, *Physiologist* **8**:366.

Riegle, G. D., Prezekop, F., and Nellor, J. E., 1968, Changes in adrenocortical responsiveness to ACTH infusion in aging goats, *J. Gerontol.* **23**:187.

Rivier, C., Brownstein, M., Spiess, J., Rivier, J., and Vale, W., 1982, *In vivo* corticotropin-releasing factor-induced secretion of adrenocorticotropin, β-endorphin, and corticosterone, *Endocrinology* **110**:272.

Romanoff, L. P., Rodriquez, R. M., Seelye, J. M., Parent, C., and Pincus, G., 1958, The urinary excretion of tetrahydrocortisol, 3-allotetrahydrocortisol, and tetrahydrocortisone in young and elderly men and women, *J. Clin. Endocrinol.* **18**:1285.

Romanoff, L. P., Morris, C. W., Welch, P., Rodriques, R. M., and Pincus, G., 1961, The metabolism of corticol-4-C[14] in young and elderly men, *J. Clin. Endocrinol.* **21**:1413.

Rubinstein, M., Stein, S., and Udenfriend, S., 1978, Characterization of proopiocortin, a precursor to opioid peptides and corticotropin, *Proc. Natl. Acad. Sci. USA* **75**:669.

Rudolph, C., Richards, G. E., Kaplan, S., and Ganong, W. F., 1979, Effect of intraventricular histamine on hormone secretion in dogs, *Neuroendocrinology* **29**:169.

Saxton, J. A., and Graham, J. B., 1944, Chromophobe adenoma-like lesions in the rat hypophysis, *Cancer Res.* **4**:168.

Schriefers, H., Hoff, H. G., Ghrof, R., and Ockenfels, H., 1972, Geschlechts und altersabhangige Entwicklung des Aktivitats-musters von Enzymen des Steroidhormon-Stoffwechsels in der Ratten leber nach neonatalan Eingriff in die sexuelle Differenzierung, *Acta Endocrinol.* **69**:789.

Semple, P. L., Buckingham, J. C., Mason, P. A., and Frazier, R., 1979, Suppression of plasma ACTH concentrations by angiotensin II infusion in normal humans and in a subject with a steroid 17 α-hydroxylase defect, *Clin. Endocrinol.* **10**:137.

Smith, M. R., Rudd, B. T., Shirley, A., Rayner, P. H. W., Williams, J. W., Duignan, N. W., and Bertrand, P. V., 1975, A radioimmunoassay for the estimation of serum dehydroepiandrosterone sulfate in normal and pathological sera, *Clin. Chim. Acta* **65**:5.

Swami, N. R., Sachar, E. J., Asnis, G. M., Halbreich, U., and Halpern, F. S., 1981, Insulin insensitivity and cortisol secretion in depressed patients, *Psychiat. Res.* **4**:2911.

Szabo, R., Dzsinich, D., Okros, I., and Stark, E., 1970, The ultrastructure of the aged rat zona fasciculata under various stressing procedures, *Exp. Gerontol.* **5**:335.

Tang, F., and Phillips, J. G., 1978, Some age-related changes in pituitary-adrenal function in the male laboratory rat, *J. Gerontol.* **33**:377.

Tilders, F. J. H., Berkenbosch, F., and Smelik, P. G., 1982, Adrenergic mechanisms involved in the control of pituitary-adrenal activity in the rat: A β-adrenergic stimulating mechanism, *Endocrinology* **110**:114.

Vale, W., Spiess, J., Rivier, C., and Rivier, J., 1981, Characterization of a 41 residue ovine hypothalamic peptide that stimulates the secretion of corticotropin and β-endorphin, *Science* **213**:1394.

VanLoon, G. R., 1973, Brain catecholamines and ACTH secretion, in: *Frontiers in Neuroendocrinology* (W. F. Ganong and L. Martini, eds.), Oxford University Press, New York, p. 209.

Vermes, I., and Telegdy, G., 1972, Effect of intraventricular injection and intrahypothalamic implantation of serotonin on the hypothalamic-hypophyseal adrenal system in the rat, *Acta Physiol. Acad. Sci. Hung.* **42**:49.

Vermes, I., Telegdy, G., and Lissak, K., 1972, Inhibitory action of serotonin on the hypothalamus-induced ACTH release, *Acta Physiol. Acad. Sci. Hung.* **41**:95.

Vermes, I., Telegdy, G., and Lissak, K., 1973, Correlation between hypothalamic serotonin content and adrenal function during acute stress: Effect of adrenal corticosteroids on hypothalamic serotonin content, *Acta Physiol. Acad. Sci. Hung.* **43**:33.

Verzár, F., 1966, Anterior pituitary function in age, in: *The Pituitary Gland*, Vol. 2 (B. T. Donovan and G. W. Harris, eds.), University of California Press, Berkeley, p. 444.

Vihko, R., 1966, Gas chromatographic-mass spectrometric studies on solvolyzable steroids in human peripheral plasma, *Acta Endocrinol. (Kbh.)* **52**(Suppl. 109):1.

Weiner, R. I., and Ganong, W. F., 1978, Role of brain monoamines and histamine in regulation of anterior pituitary secretion, *Physiol. Rev.* **58**:905.

Weitzman, E. D., Fukushima, D., Nogeire, C., Roffwang, H., Gallagher, T. F., and Hellman, L., 1971, Twenty-four hour pattern of the episodic secretion of cortisol in normal subjects, *J. Clin. Endocrinol Metabol.* **33**:14.

West, C. D., Brown, H., Simons, E. L., Carter, D. B., Kumagai, L. I., and Englert, E., Jr., 1961, Adrenocortical function and cortisol metabolism in old age, *J. Clin. Endocrinol.* **21**:1197.

Wilson, M. M., Keith, L. D., Levitt, G. R., and Greer, S., 1981, Altered regulation of the pituitary-adrenal system of female rats during aging, *Gerontologist* (Abst.) **21**.

CHAPTER 16

Relation of the Neuroendocrine System to the Development of Mammary Tumors in Rats during Aging

CLIFFORD W. WELSCH and CHARLES F. AYLSWORTH

1. Hormones and the Genesis and Growth of Carcinogen-Induced Rat Mammary Carcinomas

Among the vast array of rodent models of human breast cancer, the carcinogen-induced, i.e., MCA, DMBA, MNU, rat mammary tumor model has received the greatest attention, particularly from those who are interested in the hormonal control of this disease. The popularity of this experimental tumor system stems from the realization that this model closely parallels the human disease, as judged by significant morphological and physiological criteria. For example, carcinogen-induced rat mammary carcinomas appear to arise from the ductal elements of the mammary gland (Russo *et al.*, 1977), and most human breast carcinomas also appear to be of ductal origin (Wellings *et al.*, 1975). A crucial viral component has not been clearly demonstrated in this model (Chopra and Taylor, 1970), nor has such a factor been unequivocally demonstrated in the human disease (McGrath and Soule, 1977). Most of the rat mammary carcinomas induced by chemical carcinogens are hormone (pituitary and ovarian) responsive (Welsch, 1982) as are a significant fraction of human breast carcinomas (Segaloff, 1975) Furthermore, carcinogens such as DMBA and MNU are relatively specific for the mam-

CLIFFORD W. WELSCH and CHARLES F. AYLSWORTH • Department of Anatomy, Michigan State University, East Lansing, Michigan 48824.

mary gland (other organs are not often involved) and a single injection of either one of these carcinogens is tumorigenic in the rat, allowing one to examine separately the initiation and promotional phases of this neoplastic process (Welsch *et al.*, 1980, 1981).

The hormones which appear to be most crucial for the genesis, progression, and growth of the carcinogen-induced rat mammary carcinoma are prolactin, estrogen, and progesterone. The ensuing discussion will focus on these hormones. Other hormones, e.g., the androgens (Young *et al.*, 1965), growth hormone (Li and Yang, 1974), thyroid hormones (Newman and Moon, 1968), glucocorticoids (Aylsworth *et al.*, 1980), and insulin (Heuson *et al.*, 1972a), have also been reported to influence this tumorigenic process as have certain hormones of the central nervous system, e.g., dopamine (Quadri *et al.*, 1973), norepinephrine (Hodson *et al.*, 1978a), serotonin (Hodson *et al.*, 1978b), melatonin (Tamarkin *et al.*, 1981), the opiates (Aylsworth *et al.*, 1979b), GnRH (DeSombre *et al.*, 1976) and TRH (Chen *et al.*, 1977). These hormones will not be discussed in this communication as they appear to influence this tumorigenic process by an indirect and/or permissive action.

1.1. Role of Prolactin, Estrogen, and Progesterone in the Initiation of Carcinogen-Induced Rat Mammary Carcinomas

Ovariectomy of female rats several weeks prior to DMBA administration completely prevents the induction of mammary carcinomas (Dao, 1962; Welsch *et al.*, 1968). Mammary carcinomas fail to develop in these animals despite grafting of ovaries at varying periods of time following carcinogen treatment. If ovariectomy is performed only 1 or 2 weeks prior to DMBA treatment and ovaries are transplanted after carcinogen treatment, mammary carcinoma incidence is sharply reduced but not completely prevented (Dao, 1962). Thus, a diminished but enduring effect of the ovaries for a period of 1 or 2 weeks postcastration is observed. These are important observations, for they clearly demonstrate the necessity of ovarian hormones for initiation of chemical carcinogenesis of the mammary gland.

Results of treatment of ovariectomized rats with estrogen or progesterone prior to carcinogen administration, in an effort to delineate the relative contributions of these hormones in this tumorigenic event, are sparse and difficult to interpret. The daily administration of estradiol to ovariectomized rats for 7 days before and after DMBA treatment increased mammary tumor incidence when compared to ovariectomized controls (Talwalker *et al.*, 1964). Administration of progesterone to ovariectomized or ovariectomized-adrenalectomized rats beginning 2 days before carcinogen treatment and for the duration of the study only slightly increased mammary carcinoma incidence (Jabara and Harcourt, 1971) when compared with ovariectomized or ovariectomized-adrenalectomized controls. In each study, mammary tumor incidence in the hormonally treated ovariectomized rats was considerably less than that observed in intact control animals. In ovariectomized rats, multiple and concurrent treatment with MCA and estrogen or progesterone sharply increased mammary carcinoma incidence when compared with ovariectomized control rats treated only with the carcinogen (Huggins et al., 1959a). Evaluation of these studies is difficult, for the endocrine system of the ovariectomized rats after carcinogen treatment is abnormal; therefore, the promoting phase of this tumorigenic process is also altered. Nevertheless, the observations that estrogen replacement therapy of ovariectomized rats prior to carcinogen treatment at least partially restores mammary tumorigenesis and that the administration of estrogen antagonists, e.g., tamoxifen (Terenius, 1971; Welsch et al., 1982), nafoxidine (Heuson et al., 1972b), and MER-25 (Kledzik et al., 1974) prior to carcinogen treatment sharply reduces mammary tumor incidence, provide substantial evidence that estrogen is an important ovarian hormone for the initiation of chemical carcinogenesis of the rat mammary gland. Furthermore, neonatally androgenized rats, a syndrome characterized by a lack of ovulation associated with an absence of ovarian corpora lutea and constant keratinized vaginal mucosa, are relatively refractory to the carcinogenic action of DMBA (Kovacs, 1965). The endocrine imbalance in these animals is characterized by normal or moderately elevated blood levels of estrogen and prolactin and negligible levels of progesterone (Christakos et al., 1976; Yoshida et al., 1980). However, when these rats are given progesterone after carcinogen treatment, mammary carcinoma incidence returns to normal (Yoshida et al., 1980), thus providing evidence that progesterone is not essential for the initiating phase of chemical carcinogenesis of the rat mammary gland. Enhancement by progesterone of mammary carcinogenesis in ovariectomized rats can be explained, at least in part, by the metabolic conversion of this steroid to estrogen. Protection from chemical carcinogenesis of the rat mammary gland by early ovariectomy cannot be attributed to a deficiency in prolactin secretion, as ovariectomized rats bearing multiple prolactin-secreting pituitary homografts and treated with DMBA do not develop mammary carcinomas (Welsch et al., 1968).

Hypophysectomy of female rats prior to or during carcinogen treatment completely prevents the subsequent development of mammary carcinomas (Moon et al., 1952; Noble and Walters, 1954; Huggins et al., 1959b). To our knowledge, only one laboratory has attempted hormonal replacement therapy of carcinogen-treated hypophysectomized rats. Young (1961) reported enhancement of MCA-induced mammary tumorigenesis in hypophysectomized rats by concurrent treatment with estradiol, progesterone, and bovine growth hormone. Mammary carcinomas developed in five of the nine treated rats. The purity of the growth hormone preparation, however, was not stated. Due to the conspicuous dearth of experimentation of this type, the pituitary hormones prerequisite to or essential for the initiation of chemical carcinogenesis of the rat mammary gland remain to be determined.

In 50- to 65-day-old *intact* female Sprague–Dawley rats treated with maximally tolerated doses of chemical carcinogens, e.g., DMBA, mammary carcinoma incidence is 90–100%. Treatment of these rats with relatively high doses of estrogen, progesterone, and/or prolactin, prior to carcinogen treatment, has a profound inhibitory effect on the genesis of these neoplasms (Welsch *et al.*, 1968; Clemens *et al.*, 1968; Welsch and Meites, 1970; Kledzik *et al.*, 1974), as does pretreatment with certain steroid-containing oral contraceptives (Welsch and Meites, 1969). Furthermore, mammary glands of a pregnant or lactating rat are relatively resistant to chemical carcinogenesis (Dao *et al.*, 1960). Conversely, administration of drugs which inhibit the secretion of prolactin or which act as estrogen antagonists to intact rats prior to carcinogen treatment sharply reduces the subsequent development of mammary tumors (Clemens and Shaar, 1972; Kledzik *et al.*, 1974; Welsch *et al.*, 1979, 1981, 1982; Terenius, 1971; Heuson *et al.*, 1972b). Thus, it is clear that a moderate level of pituitary and ovarian hormone secretion is prerequisite for fulfillment of the initiating events of mammary gland carcinogenesis. Excess or deficient secretions of these hormones appear to render the mammary gland refractory to the action of the carcinogen. Mechanistically it is conceivable that the altered hormonal milieu may quantitatively reduce the morphological structures of the mammary gland most sensitive to chemical carcinogenesis (Russo and Russo, 1980). Alternatively, the altered hormonal environment may effect carcinogen metabolism (Fysh and Okey, 1979).

1.2. Role of Prolactin, Estrogen, and Progesterone in Growth Promotion of Carcinogen-Induced Rat Mammary Carcinomas

Hypophysectomy, ovariectomy, or antiestrogen treatment of rats bearing carcinogen-induced, e.g., DMBA, MCA, mammary carcinomas results in a rapid and pronounced regression of these neoplasms (Huggins *et al.*, 1959a; Sterental *et al.*, 1963; Welsch *et al.*, 1973; Jordan *et al.*, 1980). In accord, the administration of moderate amounts of estrogen

(Sterental *et al.*, 1963) or progesterone (Jabara, 1967; McCormick and Moon, 1967; Jabara and Harcourt, 1970) to rats bearing these carcinomas results in a significant increase in tumor growth. Large doses of estrogen, on the other hand, inhibit the growth of these neoplasms, an effect which appears to be augmented by progesterone supplementation (Huggins *et al.*, 1962). Oral contraceptives, such as Enovid (norethynodrel and mestranol), also stimulate growth of these neoplasms (Welsch and Meites, 1969). Estrogen-induced growth of rat mammary carcinoma, however, requires the presence of a functional pituitary gland as these tumors will not grow in estrogen treated hypophysectomized rats (Sterental *et al.*, 1963). Thus, estrogen-activated growth of DMBA induced rat mammary carcinomas is pituitary hormone dependent.

The pituitary hormone which appears to be most important for growth of carcinogen-induced rat mammary carcinoma is prolactin (Welsch and Nagasawa, 1977). The importance of this pituitary peptide for growth of these neoplasms is demonstrated by studies showing that the suppression of the secretion of this hormone by ergot alkaloids inhibits the growth of these tumors (Welsch *et al.*, 1973). The administration of this hormone stimulates tumor growth not only in intact female rats (Welsch *et al.*, 1969), but in ovariectomized (Welsch *et al.*, 1969), ovariectomized-adrenalectomized (Nagasawa and Yanai, 1970), and ovariectomized-adrenalectomized-hypophysectomized (Pearson *et al.*, 1960) rats as well. Thus, it appears that prolactin can stimulate growth of these tumors even in animals deficient in ovarian steroids, at least for an initial period of time. Ovarian steroids may be essential, however, for prolonged growth of these neoplasms, even in animals with increased secretory rates of prolactin (Sinha *et al.*, 1973). An exception to this concept is the observation by Kim and Furth (1960) showing that secretions from a prolactin and growth hormone secreting transplantable pituitary tumor (MtTF4) can enhance development and growth of rat mammary carcinoma in hypophysectomized or ovariectomized animals, even when the pituitary tumor is transplanted to these animals as late as 30–50 days after endocrine ablation. Thus, the secretions from this pituitary tumor appear to be capable of stimulating mammary carcinoma growth even in animals deficient in ovarian steroids. Furthermore, carcinogen-induced rat mammary carcinoma cells may remain dormant for periods of 7 months or more and still respond to the growth-promoting influence of the secretory products of transplantable pituitary tumors (Yokoro *et al.*, 1977).

Although it is certain that progesterone is a growth stimulant of carcinogen-induced rat mammary carcinoma, the precise role of this hormone in this tumorigenic process remains uncertain because a portion of this hormone can be metabolically converted to estrogen. Nevertheless, an important role for progesterone *per se* in the growth of carcinogen-induced rat mammary carcinomas is suggested by the study of Yoshida *et al.* (1980). It was demonstrated that the chronic administration of progesterone, for varying time periods after carcinogen treatment, to neonatally androgenized rats resulted in a marked increase in mammary carcinoma development and growth. Neonatally androgenized rats have moderately elevated secretory rates of estrogen and prolactin and minimal progesterone secretion. It is doubtful that the estrogenic metabolic by products of progesterone metabolism could quantitatively contribute to the existing hyperestrogenemia in the androgenized animals. Pregnancy, an endocrine state in the rat characterized by increased secretion of progesterone, estrogen, and prolactin, including placental hormones (Sakamoto *et al.*, 1979), promotes exuberant growth of carcinogen-induced rat mammary carcinomas (Dao and Sunderland, 1959). Unlike pregnancy, lactation results in reduced growth and often regression of rat mammary carcinomas induced by chemical carcinogens (Dao and Sunderland, 1959). This phenomenon, perhaps, can best be explained by a deficiency in ovarian hormone secretion, in particular progesterone (McCormick and Moon, 1967), and/or by enhanced adrenal corticoid secretion (Aylsworth *et al.*, 1979a). The administration of progesterone to ovariectomized lactating rats bearing carcinogen-induced mammary carcinomas restores growth of these neoplasms (McCormick and Moon, 1967), whereas, the administration of adrenal corticoids to rats bearing these tumors causes tumor regression (Aylsworth *et al.*, 1980). Thus, for optimal growth of carcinogen-induced rat mammary carcinomas, enhanced secretion of prolactin, estrogen, *and* progesterone appears to be necessary. Under certain conditions, however, hyperprolactinemia (or enhanced pituitary secretions), even in animals lacking ovarian secretion, may be all that is necessary for enhanced growth of these tumors.

1.3. Neuroendocrine Relationships to the Initiation and Promotion of Carcinogen-Induced Rat Mammary Carcinomas

Physiological and pharmacological states that alter the activity of most hypothalamic neurotransmitters and neurohormones can influence the initiation and growth-promotion of carcinogen-induced mammary tumors in the rat. Most of these effects are mediated indirectly through an alteration of anterior pituitary secretion of prolactin and/or gonadotropins which in turn control gonadal steroid secretion.

Both enhancement and inhibition of hypothalamic dopaminergic activity before and during carcinogen administration inhibits mammary tumorigenesis. Treatment with L-Dopa, to increase hypothalamic dopaminergic activity, for 20 days prior to and through 20 days following DMBA administration, inhibits mammary tumor development (Kledzik *et al.*, 1974). Similar treatment with haloperidol, a specific dopamine receptor blocker, to reduce hypothalamic dopaminergic activity, also inhibits DMBA-induced mammary tumorigenesis (Kledzik *et al.*, 1974). Also, placement of hypothalamic lesions to reduce dopaminergic activity, prior to carcinogen administration inhibits subsequent mammary tumorigenesis (Welsch *et al.*, 1969).

Administration of drugs such as pimozide and perphenazine, which decrease hypothalamic dopaminergic activity, after carcinogen administration, i.e., during the promotional phase of mammary tumorigenesis, enhances the development and growth of mammary tumors (Hodson *et al.*, 1978a; Pearson *et al.*, 1969). Conversely, increasing hypothalamic dopaminergic activity by administration of dopamine agonists, such as L-Dopa, piribedil, or various ergot alkaloids, inhibits the growth of developing carcinogen-induced mammary tumors (Quadri *et al.*, 1973; Hodson *et al.*, 1978a; Heuson *et al.*, 1972b; Welsch *et al.*, 1979). Since treatments that increase hypothalamic dopaminergic activity decrease serum prolactin and treatments that decrease hypothalamic dopaminergic activity increase serum prolactin levels, it has been concluded that the effects of dopamine agonists and antagonists on the initiation and growth-promotion of carcinogen-induced mammary tumors are mediated by concurrent changes in circulating prolactin levels (Welsch and Nagasawa, 1977).

Other hypothalamic neurotransmitters and neurohormones have also been shown to influence the growth promotion of carcinogen-induced mammary tumors in rats via their effect on pituitary prolactin secretion. Increasing hypothalamic norepinephrine activity by administration of clonidine, an α-adrenergic agonist, inhibits the growth of DMBA-induced mammary tumors and decreases serum prolactin levels (Hodson *et al.*, 1978a). Decreasing hypothalamic serotonin activity by administration of parachlorophenylalanine (PCPA) also inhibits DMBA-induced mammary tumor growth and decreases serum prolactin levels (Hodson *et al.*, 1978b). Administration of opiate antagonists, such as naloxone and naltrexone to decrease endogenous opiate peptide activity, inhibits DMBA-induced mammary tumor growth and decreases serum prolactin levels (Aylsworth *et al.*, 1979b). Thyrotropin-releasing hormone (TRH) enhances DMBA-induced mammary tumor growth and increases serum prolactin levels (Chen *et al.*, 1977). Melatonin inhibits DMBA-induced mammary tumorigenesis and is stated to decrease serum prolactin levels (Tamarkin *et al.*, 1981), but there is evidence to the contrary on prolactin secretion. Administration of high doses of gonad-otropin-releasing hormone (GnRH) analogs inhibit mammary tumor growth and cause regression of established mammary tumors, apparently by decreasing the secretion of gonadal steroids and prolactin (DeSombre *et al.*, 1976).

In summary, alterations in hypothalamic function resulting in either an increase or decrease in circulating prolactin levels prior to or during carcinogen administration to rats inhibits subsequent mammary tumor development. Alterations in hypothalamic function after carcinogen administration resulting in elevated serum prolactin and/or estrogen levels stimulates mammary tumorigenesis, whereas changes in hypothalamic function resulting in a decrease in circulating levels of these hormones inhibits mammary tumor development and growth.

2. Age-Associated Changes in Pituitary-Ovarian Activity of Rats

2.1. Changes in Estrous Activity in Aging Female Rats

The aging female rat shows a gradual decline in reproductive function associated with a decline in the number of ovulations, a decrease in the litter size and a disruption in the estrous cycling pattern. Changes in the estrous cycling of senescent rats, as described by vaginal cytology, have been reported (Ingram, 1959; Mandl, 1961; Aschheim, 1961, 1976; Block, 1961; Huang and Meites, 1975; Meites and Huang, 1976). In general, between 8–15 months of age, the regular 4–5-day cyclic pattern of the normal estrous cycle becomes increasingly irregular and lengthened, usually due to an increase in the duration of the estrous or diestrous stages. Between 12–24 months of age, the predominant estrous smear pattern is characterized by constant vaginal cornification. This state of constant estrus (CE) is an anovulatory reproductive period in which the ovaries contain many well-developed and some cystic follicles and no corpora lutea. In most aging rats, the CE reproductive state is followed by repetitive, spontaneous pseudopregnancies (RPP) of varying length (12–30 days) in which the vaginal smear pattern is characterized predominantly by leukocytes (diestrus). The ovaries of the RPP rat, in contrast to the CE rat, have many functional corpora lutea which secrete large amounts of progesterone. These prolonged pseudopregnancies are interspersed by ovulations and 1- to 2-day estrous vaginal smears. Senile RPP rats are often observed to revert to the CE state or to irregular cycling. However, not all animals will show both the RPP and the CE reproductive states during their lifespans but may show only one or the other. Furthermore, a few rats may continue to cycle, although irregularly, for their entire lifespan and not exhibit these estrous cycle changes.

Most rats 2–3 years of age are characterized by a permanent senescent (anestrous) reproductive state. Unlike the old RPP rats, a permanent leukocytic (diestrus) vaginal smear which is not interspersed by ovulations or estrous smears, is observed in the anestrous rat. The ovaries of the anestrous rat are largely atrophic, secreting very little estrogen or progesterone. Prolactin-secreting adenomas are quite common in the anestrous rat. In summary, with advancing age, most female rats progress from regular to irregular estrous cycles to a state of constant estrus (CE), to a state of repetitive pseudopregnancy (RPP), and finally to an anestrous state (Huang and Meites, 1975; Meites and Huang, 1976; Lu et al., 1979).

In the following section the endocrine profiles of the senile laboratory rat are summarized. Changes in the secretory patterns of prolactin, estrogen, and progesterone are discussed as these hormones are of primary importance in murine mammary tumorigenesis. Details of the changes in the hormonal status of the aging female rat and the neuroendocrine mechanisms by which these changes are manifested are presented elsewhere in this volume and will not be addressed here. With advancing age and loss of the estrous cycling activity of the female rat, there is generally a concurrent loss in the cyclic pituitary-ovarian profiles observed in normal mature rats. Prolactin, gonadotropins, and gonadal steroids, which are secreted in definite cyclic patterns in the young, regular-cycling animal are generally secreted in a more static or constant fashion in the old rat. With advancing age, there is an additional increase in the incidence of pituitary pathology which is most often manifested as a prolactin-secreting pituitary adenoma.

2.2. Changes in Serum Estrogens in Aging Female Rats

The secretory pattern of estradiol in young, normal estrous cycling rats has been described (Butcher et al., 1974; Steger et al., 1979; Huang et al., 1978). Estradiol levels are lowest (17 pg/ml) during the estrous stage of the cycle and progressively increase during metestrus and diestrus to reach peak levels (88 pg/ml) at noon of proestrus (Butcher et al., 1974). Estrone levels in young, cycling rats are elevated during diestrus at day 2, but do not show the dramatic cyclic pattern as observed with estradiol (Lu et al., 1979).

Estradiol levels in old CE rats appear to be moderately elevated with respect to basal levels observed in young cycling rats during estrus and metestrus. Steger *et al.* (1979) and Huang *et al.* (1978) reported estradiol levels in old (20–24 months) CE rats comparable to diestrus at day 2 estradiol levels in normal cycling 4- to 5-month-old rats. Lu *et al.* (1979) observed an elevation of estradiol levels in old (16–30 months) CE rats above the basal levels of estrus or diestrus at day 1 in young cycling rats. According to Wilkes *et al.* (1978), estradiol levels in 24-month-old CE rats are equivalent to the levels of estradiol observed in young cycling rats during the morning of proestrus. This elevation of estradiol in CE rats, however, appears to be dependent upon the age of the rat since middle-aged (10–13 months) CE rats have estradiol levels which are reduced when compared to old CE rats and are more comparable to basal levels observed in young cyclic animals during the estrous stage of the cycle (Wilkes *et al.*, 1978; Lu *et al.*, 1979). Changes in circulating estrone levels in CE rats are similar to those observed with estradiol. That is, in middle-aged (11–16 months) CE rats, circulating estrone is reduced to near basal levels observed in young cycling rats during estrus and diestrus at day 1, whereas in old (25–30 months) CE rats estrone levels are moderately elevated (Lu *et al.*, 1979).

Changes in circulating estrogen levels during RPP are not as clear as during CE. Huang *et al.* (1978) and Steger *et al.* (1979) report moderately elevated estradiol levels in 20- to 24-month-old RPP rats which are similar to those observed in old (20–24 months) CE rats and young cycling rats during the diestrous at day 2 stage of the cycle. However, Lu *et al.* (1979) found that estradiol levels in old (27–30 months) RPP rats were similar to the basal levels in young rats during estrus and diestrus at day 1 and were significantly lower than CE rats of similar age. Wilkes *et al.* (1978) has also reported that estradiol levels were significantly lower in 30-month-old RPP rats when compared to regular cycling 6- and 12-month-old rats on the morning of proestrus. It appears, therefore, that circulating estradiol levels in RPP rats are either similar or slightly reduced when compared to the moderately elevated estradiol levels in CE rats.

Serum estradiol levels in anestrous rats are significantly reduced when compared to levels in CE or RPP rats and are similar to basal levels observed in young cyclic rats during the estrous stage of the cycle (Huang *et al.*, 1978; Steger *et al.*, 1979). Lu *et al.* (1979) similarly reported a decrease in circulating estradiol levels in old (30–33 months) anestrous rats when compared to CE rats. However, in this study, serum estradiol levels in the anestrous rats were equivalent to those observed in RPP rats.

2.3. Changes in Serum Progesterone in Aging Female Rats

The progesterone profile of young normal estrous cycling rats is characterized by a large surge of the hormone which peaks during the afternoon of proestrus, a smaller, more prolonged surge of the hormone from late metestrus to early diestrus, and a return to basal hormone levels during late diestrus, early proestrus, and estrus (Butcher *et al.*, 1974). Circulating progesterone levels are generally thought to be reduced in CE rats primarily due to the absence of corpora lutea in their ovaries. Huang *et al.* (1978) showed serum progesterone levels in old (20–24 months) CE rats to be significantly lower than basal progesterone levels in young (4–5 months) cycling rats. Chan and Leatham (1977) have also reported a reduction in serum progesterone in 18-month-old CE rats when compared to 4-month-old cycling rats in estrus. Wilkes *et al.* (1978) have also shown circulating progesterone levels in 12- and 24-month-old CE rats to be decreased when compared to young cycling rats on the morning of proestrus. Other investigators, however, have not shown this reduction in circulating progesterone in old CE rats, but report progesterone levels to be similar to the basal levels observed in young cycling rats during estrus (Steger *et al.*, 1979; Lu *et al.*, 1979). A more dramatic change observed in the CE rat is the sharply reduced level of 20α-OH-progesterone. Minimal levels of 20α-OH-progesterone are reported by Lu *et al.*, (1979) in old (11–30 months) CE rats which are greatly reduced when compared to all stages of the estrous cycle. In addition, Wilkes *et al.* (1978) observed a 95% reduction in circulating 20α-OH-progesterone in both middle-aged (12 months) and old (24 months) CE rats compared to young cycling rats on the morning of proestrus.

The progesterone profile in RPP rats is clearly elevated, presumably due to the presence of many functional corpora lutea in the ovaries of these animals. Progesterone levels in RPP rats are significantly elevated above basal levels observed in young cycling rats during estrus, diestrus, or the morning of estrus, and in many cases may approach or exceed the peak levels of progesterone observed during the afternoon of proestrus (Steger *et al.*, 1979; Huang *et al.*, 1978; Wilkes *et al.*, 1978; Lu *et al.*, 1979). Additionally, Fayein and Aschheim (1980) have shown that progesterone levels observed during spontaneous pseudopregnancy in 24-month-old rats are similar to the elevated levels of progesterone occurring as a result of induced pseudopregnancy in young (10 months) rats. Consequently, circulating progesterone levels in old RPP are also markedly elevated when compared to progesterone levels in CE rats of a comparable age (Riegle and Miller, 1978; Huang *et al.*, 1978; Wilkes *et al.*, 1978; Steger *et al.*, 1979; Lu *et al.*, 1979).

Progesterone levels are markedly reduced in the anestrous rat, presumably due to the pronounced atrophy of the ovaries in these animals. Huang *et al.* (1978) and Steger *et al.* (1979) show progesterone levels in the anestrous rat to be significantly lower than basal levels of progesterone in cycling young rats, and also lower than old RPP and CE rats. Lu *et al.* (1979), however, report circulating progesterone levels in the anestrous rat to be similar to basal levels observed in old CE and young cycling rats in estrus. 20α-OH-progesterone levels are markedly reduced in the anestrous rat (Lu *et al.*, 1979).

2.4. Changes in Serum Prolactin in Aging Female Rats

The secretory pattern of prolactin in young normal estrous cycling female rats is characteristically at basal levels throughout the metestrous and diestrous stages of the estrous cycle, followed by a surge of the hormone during the afternoon of proestrus and often a second surge during the afternoon of estrus (Butcher *et al.*, 1974). Elevated pituitary and serum prolactin levels in old as compared to young rats have been reported by many investigators (Clemens and Meites, 1971; Shaar *et al.*, 1975). More specifically, circulating levels of prolactin have been reported to be elevated in old CE rats when compared to morning estrous and proestrous levels in young rats (Huang *et al.*, 1978; Wilkes *et al.*, 1978). Lu *et al.* (1979) report three- to fourfold increases in serum prolactin levels in 25- to 30-month-old CE rats with normal pituitaries when compared to basal levels of 4- to 5-month-old normal cycling rats. Serum prolactin levels are further elevated in similarly aged CE rats with hemorrhagic pituitaries (Lu *et al.*, 1979). However, the elevation of serum prolactin in CE rats appears to be related to the age of the animal rather than solely to the state of reproductive senescence since younger (11–16 months) CE rats have normal basal prolactin levels (Lu *et al.*, 1979; Wilkes *et al.*, 1978). A report by Damassa *et al.* (1980) suggests that serum prolactin levels in old CE rats without pituitary pathology, are not statistically elevated, but rather, consist of a major diurnal surge at 1400–1700 hr and a smaller nocturnal surge at 0200–0500 hr. CE rats that have pituitary tumors and/or lesions exhibit static serum prolactin levels which are greatly elevated.

Most evidence suggests that serum prolactin levels in aging RPP rats are elevated but not to the degree as observed in the CE or anestrous rat. Lu *et al.* (1979) and Wilkes *et al.* (1978) report circulating prolactin levels in RPP rats, devoid of pituitary pathology, are significantly higher than basal serum prolactin levels in young cycling rats, but lower than serum prolactin levels in CE rats with similar pituitary histology and age. In contrast, Huang *et al.* (1976) show serum prolactin levels in old (22–24 months) RPP rats to be approximately the same as young (4–5 months) cycling rats on the morning of estrus. Serum prolactin levels in the RPP rat, devoid of pituitary pathology, do not appear to be statistically elevated, but rather, show a major nocturnal surge from 0200–0500 and a smaller diurnal surge from 1400–1700 (Damassa *et al.*, 1980). As in the CE rat, RPP rats with pituitary tumors and/or lesions have greatly elevated serum prolactin levels without surges (Damassa *et al.*, 1980).

The anestrous rat characteristically has the highest serum prolactin levels associated with a very high incidence of pituitary tumors (Huang and Meites, 1975). Huang *et al.* (1976) report serum prolactin levels in old (26–30 months) anestrous rats to be two times higher than old (22–24 months) CE rats and four to eight times higher than in RPP and young cycling rats. In this study, all anestrous rats had large, tumorous pituitaries. Similarly Lu *et al.* (1979) show greatly elevated serum prolactin levels in 30- to 33-month-old anestrous rats, all of which have hemorrhagic pituitaries. In summary, the degree to which circulating prolactin levels are elevated in the aging female rat depends on the age, presence, or absence of pituitary pathology, as well as the state of reproductive senescence.

3. Incidence of Mammary Tumors in Aging Female Rats: Hormonal Implications

While some differences exist, significant numbers of mammary tumors arise spontaneously in most strains of aging female rats (Noble and Cutts, 1959). These tumors begin appearing at approximately 300 days of age. Thereafter, a gradual but steady increase in the incidence of these neoplasms, as a function of age, is observed. Mammary tumor incidence in Sprague–Dawley rats allowed to live a maximum life span is approximately 70%, and mean age of mammary tumor appearance in these animals is approximately 2 years (Durbin *et al.*, 1966). Histologically, both benign and carcinomatous mammary tumors occur spontaneously. However, the majority of these neoplasms are benign fibroadenomas (Welsch *et al.*, 1970a,b).

As previously discussed, moderate (normal) secretions of prolactin, estrogen, and progesterone appear to be prerequisite for maximal sensitivity of the rat mammary gland to polycyclic hydrocarbon carcinogenesis. A marked increase or decrease in levels of these hormones appears to impede the initiating events of this neoplastic process. Thus, young estrous cycling female rats appear to be more sensitive to chemical carcinogenesis of the mammary gland than are aged rats (Huggins *et al.*, 1961), rats in constant estrus (Kovacs, 1965), pseudopregnant rats (Dao *et al.*, 1960), ovariectomized rats (Welsch *et al.*, 1968), or hypophysectomized rats (Moon *et al.*, 1952). It is tempting to conclude, therefore, that the initiating events of spontaneous mammary gland tumorigenesis in the rat may have occurred early in the lifetime of that animal, i.e., during the period of normal estrous cycles. Such a conclusion must be considered tenuous at best for it has been reported recently that young and old rats are equally sensitive to the mammary carcinogenic effects of whole body X-irradiation (Shellabarger, 1981) and topically (in contrast to i.v. or i.g. applications) applied polycyclic hydrocarbons such as DMBA (Sinha and Dao, 1980).

In contrast to the hormonal factors involved in initiation, the most efficacious promoting hormonal milieu in rat mammary gland carcinogenesis appears to be increased secretion of prolactin, estrogen, and progesterone. Markedly enhanced blood levels of prolactin (Welsch *et al.*, 1969), estrogen (Sterental *et al.*, 1963), or progesterone (Jabara, 1967), within a physiological range, invariably promote increased growth of polycyclic hydrocarbon-induced mammary gland tumors. Perhaps the most exuberant growth of these neoplasms occurs during enhanced secretion of all three hormones as in late pseudopregnancy or pregnancy (Dao and Sunderland, 1959). It is doubtful that an increased secretory rate of the ovaries, in the absence of pituitary gland secretion, will promote growth of these neoplasms (Sterental *et al.*, 1963). Conversely, the secretory products from pituitary gland tumors, even in the absence of ovarian secretion, appears to be a potent growth-promoting hormonal milieu for the polycyclic hydrocarbon mammary tumor model (Kim and Furth, 1960).

The hormonal milieu of the constant estrus (CE), repetitive pseudopregnant (RPP), and anestrous rat would, therefore, appear to be conducive to increased growth of carcinogen-induced mammary tumors. The RPP rat, i.e., basal or slightly increased secretory rates of estrogen and prolactin and large increases in progesterone (Huang *et al.*, 1978; Steger *et al.*, 1979; Lu *et al.*, 1979, and the anestrous rat, i.e., large increased secretory rates of prolactin particularly in animals with adenomatous pituitaries and very little estrogen and progesterone (Huang *et al.*, 1978; Lu *et al.*, 1979, would appear to have the more effective endocrinic mammary tumor growth-promoting environment when compared with the CE rat, i.e., moderately increased secretory rates of estrogen and prolactin and little progesterone (Huang *et al.*, 1978; Lu *et al.,* 1979). In the older rat, most often, the endocrine state of CE precedes RPP, the latter followed by the anestrous state. Thus, the most effective tumor growth-promoting physiological state, i.e., RPP and anestrous, occurs very late in the lifespan of the aging female rat, a time period in which the occurrence of mammary tumors is most frequent (Durbin *et al.,* 1966). It appears, therefore, that the endocrinic state of the old rat is quite conducive to mammary tumor growth promotion. An intense and prolonged hyperprolactinemia may be all that is required for increased growth of previously initiated or transformed mammary epithelial cells. It is well-known that a prolonged hyperprolactinemia in rats (Welsch *et al.,* 1970a,b) and mice (Muhlbock and Boot, 1959) sharply increases the incidence of spontaneous mammary tumors, whereas, a prolonged drug-induced hypoprolactinemia, virtually completely blocks this neoplastic process (Welsch and Gribler, 1973). Whether or not the potential mammary growth-promoting effects of the endocrinic states of CE, RPP, or anestrus influence or alter the susceptibility of the mammary gland to initiating events (chemical, physical, and/or viral) remains to be determined. It has been proposed that the mitotic state of the mammae is a critical determinant for the initiation of this neoplastic process (Nagasawa and Yanai, 1974; Russo and Russo, 1978). Although it is uncertain as to whether or not the altered hormonal milieu of the old rat imparts increased sensitivity of the mammary gland to oncogenic initiating agents, it certainly appears that this altered hormonal state is an effective and potent growth promoter of the initiated (transformed) mammary epithelial cell.

4. References

Aschheim, P., 1961, La pseudogestation a repetition chez les rats seniles, *C. R. Acad. Sci.* **253:**1988–1990.

Aschheim, P., 1976, Aging in the hypothalamic-hypophyseal ovarian axis in the rat, in: *Hypothalamus, Pituitary and Aging* (A. V. Everitt and J. A. Burgess, eds.), Charles C. Thomas, Springfield, Illinois, pp. 376–418.

Aylsworth, C. F., Hodson, C. A., Berg, C., Kledzik, G., and Meites, J., 1979a, Role of adrenals and estrogen in regression of mammary tumors during postpartum lactation in the rat, *Cancer Res.* **39:**2436–2439.

Aylsworth, C. F., Hodson, C. A., and Meites, J., 1979b, Opiate antagonists can inhibit mammary tumor growth in rats, *Proc. Soc. Exp. Biol. Med.* **161:**18–20.

Aylsworth, C. F., Sylvester, P. W., Leung, F. C., and Meites, J., 1980, Inhibition of mammary tumor growth by dexamethasone in rats in the presence of high serum prolactin levels, *Cancer Res.* **40:**1863–1866.

Block, V. S., 1961, Untersuchungen uber das genitale altern des rattenweibshens, *Gerontologia* **5:**55–62.

Butcher, R. L., Collings, W. E., and Fugo, N. W., 1974, Plasma concentration of LH, FSH, prolactin, progesterone, and estradiol-17β throughout the 4-day estrous cycle of the rat, *Endocrinology* **94:**1704–1708.

Chan, S. W. C., and Leathem, J. H., 1977, Aging and ovarian steroidogenesis in the rat, *J. Gerontol.* **32:**395–401.

Chen, H. J., Bradley, C. J., and Meites, J., 1977, Stimulation of growth of carcinogen-induced mammary cancers in rats by thyrotropin-releasing hormone, *Cancer Res.* **37:**64–66.

Chopra, H., and Taylor, D. J., 1970, Virus particles in rat mammary tumors of varying origin, *J. Natl. Cancer Inst.* **44:**1141–1147.

Christakos, S., Sinha, D., and Dao, T. L., 1976, Neonatal modification of endocrine functions and mammary carcinogenesis in the rat, *Brit. J. Cancer* **34:**58–63.

Clemens, J. A., and Meites, J., 1971, Neuroendocrine status of old constant estrous rats, *Neuroendocrinology* **7:**249–256.

Clemens, J. A., and Shaar, C. J., 1972, Inhibition by ergocornine of initiation and growth of 7,12-dimethylbenzanthracene-induced mammary tumors in rats: Effect of tumor size, *Proc. Soc. Exp. Biol. Med.* **139:**659–662.

Clemens, J. A., Welsch, C. W., and Meites, J., 1968, Effects of hypothalamic lesions on incidence and growth of mammary tumors in carcinogen treated rats, *Proc. Soc. Exp. Biol. Med.* **127:**969–972.

Damassa, D. A., Gilman, D. P., Lu, K. H., Judd, H. L., and Sawyer, C. H., 1980, The twenty-four hour pattern of prolactin secretion in aging female rats, *Biol. Reprod.* **22:**571–575.

Dao, T. L., 1962, The role of ovarian hormones in initiating the induction of mammary cancer in rats by polynuclear hydrocarbons, *Cancer Res.* **22:**973–981.

Dao, T. L., and Sunderland, H., 1959, Mammary carcinogenesis by 3-methylcholanthrene. I. Hormonal aspects in tumor induction and growth, *J. Natl. Cancer Inst.* **23:**567–585.

Dao, T. L., Bock, F. G., and Greiner, M. J., 1960, Mammary carcinogenesis by 3-methylcholanthrene. II. Inhibitory effect of pregnancy and lactation on tumor induction, *J. Natl. Cancer Inst.* **25:**991–1003.

DeSombre, E. R., Johnson, E. S., and White, W. F., 1976, Regression of rat mammary tumors effected by a gonadoliberin analog, *Cancer Res.* **36:**3830–3833.

Durbin, P. W., Williams, M. H., Jeung, N., and Arnold, J. S., 1966, Development of spontaneous mammary tumors over the life-span of the female Charles River (Sprague–Dawley) rat: The influence of ovariectomy, thyroidectomy, and adrenalectomy-ovariectomy, *Cancer Res.* **26:**400–411.

Fayein, N. A., and Aschheim, P., 1980, Age-related temporal changes of levels of circulating progesterone in repeatedly pseudopregnant rats, *Biol. Reprod.* **23:**616–620.

Fysh, J. M., and Okey, A. B., 1979, Aryl hydrocarbon (benzopyrene) hydroxylase in rat mammary tissue during pregnancy and lactation, *Can. J. Physiol. Pharmacol.* **57:**112–117.

Heuson, J. C., Legros, N., and Heimann, R., 1972a, Influence of insulin administration on growth of the 7,12-dimethylbenzanthracene-induced mammary carcinoma in intact, oophorectomized and hypophysectomized rats, *Cancer Res.* **32:**233–238.

Heuson, J. C., Waelbroeck, C., Legros, N., Gallez, G., Robyn, C., and L'Hermite, M., 1972b, Inhibition of DMBA-induced mammary carcinogenesis in the rat by 2-Br-α-ergocryptine (CB-154), an inhibitor of prolactin secretion, and by nafoxidine (U-11, 100A), an estrogen antagonist, *Gynecol. Invest.* **2:**130–137.

Hodson, C. A., Mioduszewski, R., and Meites, J., 1978a, Effects of catecholaminergic drugs on growth of carcinogen-induced mammary tumors in rats, *IRCS Med. Sci.* **6:**399.

Hodson, C. A., Simpkins, J. W., and Meites, J., 1978b, Effect of brain serotonin reduction on growth of carcinogen-induced mammary tumors in rats, *IRCS Med. Sci.* **6:**398.

Huang, II. H., and Meites, J., 1975, Reproductive capacity of aging female rats, *Neuroendocrinology* **17**:289–295.

Huang, H. H., Marshall, S., and Meites, J., 1976, Capacity of old versus young female rats to secrete LH, FSH, and Prolactin, *Biol. Reprod.* **14**:538–543.

Huang, H. H., Stegar, R. W., Bruni, J. F., and Meites, J., 1978, Patterns of sex steroid and gonadotropin secretion in aging female rats, *Endocrinology* **103**:1855–1859.

Huggins, O., Briziarelli, G., and Sutton, H., 1959a, Rapid induction of mammary carcinoma in the rat and the influence of hormones on the tumors, *J. Exp. Med.* **109**:25–42.

Huggins, C., Grand, L. C., and Brillantes, F. P., 1959b, Critical significance of breast structure in the induction of mammary cancer in the rat, *Proc. Natl. Acad. Sci. USA* **45**:1294–1300.

Huggins, C., Grand, L. C., and Brillantes, F. P., 1961, Mammary cancer induced by a single feeding of polynuclear hydrocarbons, and its suppression, *Nature* **189**:204–207.

Huggins, C., Moon, R. C., and Morii, S., 1962, Extinction of experimental mammary cancer. I. Estradiol-17β and Progesterone, *Proc. Natl. Acad. Sci. USA* **48**:379–386.

Ingram, D. L., 1959, The vaginal smear of senile laboratory rats, *J. Endocrinol.* **19**:182–188.

Jabara, A. G., 1967, Effects of progesterone on 9,10-dimethylbenzanthracene-induced mammary tumours in Sprague–Dawley rats, *Brit. J. Cancer* **21**:418–429.

Jabara, A. G., and Harcourt, A. G., 1970, The effects of progesterone and ovariectomy on mammary tumours induced by 7,12-dimethylbenzanthracene in Sprague–Dawley rats, *Pathology* **2**:115–123.

Jabara, A. G., and Harcourt, A. G., 1971, Effects of progesterone, ovariectomy and adrenalectomy on mammary tumours induced by 7,12-dimethylbenzanthracene in Sprague–Dawley rats, *Pathology* **3**:209–214.

Jordan, V. C., Allen, K. E., and Dix, C. J., 1980, Pharmacology of tamoxifen in laboratory animals, *Cancer Treat. Rep.* **64**:745–759.

Kim, U., and Furth, J., 1960, Relation of mammary tumors to mammotropes. II. Hormone responsiveness of 3-methylcholanthrene induced mammary carcinomas, *Proc. Soc. Exp. Biol. Med.* **103**:643–645.

Kledzik, G. S., Bradley, C. J., and Meites, J., 1974, Reduction of carcinogen-induced mammary cancer incidence in rats by early treatment with hormones or drugs, *Cancer Res.* **34**:2953–2956.

Kovacs, K., 1965, Effect of androgenisation on the development of mammary tumours in rats induced by the oral administration of 9,10-dimethyl-1,2-benzanthracene, *Brit. J. Cancer* **19**:531–537.

Li, C. H., and Yang, W., 1974, The effect of bovine growth hormone on growth of mammary tumors in hypophysectomized rats, *Life Sci.* **15**:761–764.

Lu, K. H., Hopper, B. R., Vargo, T. M., and Yen, S. S. C., 1979, Chronological changes in sex steroid, gonadotropin, and prolactin secretion in aging female rats displaying different reproductive states, *Biol. Reprod.* **21**:193–203.

Mandl, A. M., 1961, Cyclical changes in the vaginal smears of senile nulliparous and multiparous rats, *J. Endocrinol.* **22**:257–268.

McCormick, G. M., and Moon, R. C., 1967, Hormones influencing postpartum growth of 7,12-dimethylbenzanthracene rat mammary tumors, *Cancer Res.* **27**:626–631.

McGrath, C. M., and Soule, H. D., 1977, An inquiry into the involvement of nonhuman breast cancer viruses in the human disease: Virus expression in malignant breast ductal stem cells, in: *Origins of Human Cancer*, Cold Spring Harbor Laboratory, Cold Spring Harbor, New York, pp. 1287–1303.

Meites, J., and Huang, H. H., 1976, Relation of the neuroendocrine system to loss of reproductive function in aging rats, in: *Neuroendocrine Regulation of Fertility* (T. C. Anand Kumar, ed.), Karger, Basel Press, New York, pp. 246–258.

Moon, H. D., Simpson, M. E., and Evans, H. M., 1952, Inhibition of methylcholanthrene carcinogenesis by hypophysectomy, *Science* **116**:331.

Muhlbock, O., and Boot, L. M., 1959, Induction of mammary cancer in mice without the mammary tumor agent by isografts of hypophysis, *Cancer Res.* **19**:402–412.

Nagasawa, H., and Yanai, R., 1970, Effects of prolactin or growth hormone on growth of carcinogen-induced mammary tumors of adreno-ovariectomized rats, *Int. J. Cancer* **6**:488–495.

Nagasawa, H., and Yanai, R., 1974, Frequency of mammary cell division in relation to age: Its significance in the induction of mammary tumors by carcinogen in rats, *J. Natl. Cancer Inst.* **52**:609–610.

Newman, W. C., and Moon, R. C., 1968, Chemically induced mammary cancer in rats with altered thyroid function, *Cancer Res.* **28**:864–868.

Noble, R. L., and Cutts, J. H., 1959, Mammary tumors of the rat: A review, *Cancer Res.* **19**:1125–1139.

Noble, R. L., and Walters, J. H., 1954, The effect of hypophysectomy on 9,10-dimethyl-1,2-benzanthracene induced carcinogenesis, *Proc. Amer. Assoc. Cancer Res.* **1**:35.

Pearson, O. H., Llerena, O., Llerena, L., Molina, A., and Butler, T., 1969, Prolactin-dependent rat mammary cancer: A model for man? *Trans. Assoc. Am. Physicians* **82**:225–238.

Quadri, S. K., Kledzik, G. S., and Meites, J., 1973, Effects of L-dopa and methyl-dopa on growth of mammary cancers in rats, *Proc. Soc. Exp. Biol. Med.* **142**:759–761.

Riegle, G. D., and Miller, A. E., 1978, Age effects on the hypothalamic-pituitary-gonadal control system in the rat, *Adv. Exp. Med. Biol.* **113**:159–178.

Russo, J., and Russo, I. H., 1978, DNA labelling index and structure of the rat mammary gland as determinants of its susceptibility to carcinogenesis, *J. Natl. Cancer Inst.* **61**:1451–1459.

Russo, J., and Russo, I. H., 1980, Influence of differentiation and cell kinetics on the susceptibility of the rat mammary gland to carcinogenesis, *Cancer Res.* **40**:2677–2687.

Russo, J., Saby, J., Isenberg, W., and Russo, I. H., 1977, Pathogenesis of mammary carcinomas induced in rats by 7,12-dimethylbenzanthracene, *J. Natl. Cancer Inst.* **59**:435–445.

Sakamoto, S., Imamura, Y., Sassa, S., and Okamoto, R., 1979, DMBA induced mammary tumor and hormone environment in the rat during pregnancy, postpartum, and long term lactation, *Toxicol. Lett.* **4**:237–240.

Segaloff, A., 1975, Hormonal therapy of breast cancer, *Cancer Treat. Rev.* **2**:129–135.

Shaar, C. J., Euker, J. S., Riegle, G. D., and Meites, J., 1975, Effects of castration and gonadal steroids on serum luteinizing hormone and prolactin in old and young rats, *J. Endocrinol.* **66**:45–51.

Shellabarger, C. L., 1981, Pituitary and steroid hormones in radiation-induced mammary tumors, in: *Hormones and Breast Cancer*, Banbury Report #8 (M. C. Pike, P. K. Siiteri, and C. W. Welsch, eds.), Cold Spring Harbor Laboratory, Cold Spring Harbor, New York, pp. 339–351.

Sinha, D. K., and Dao, T. L., 1980, Induction of mammary tumors in aging rats by 7,12-dimethylbenzanthracene: Role of DNA synthesis during carcinogenesis, *J. Natl. Cancer Inst.* **64**:519–521.

Sinha, D., Cooper, D., and Dao, T. L., 1973, The nature of estrogen and prolactin effect on mammary tumorigenesis, *Cancer Res.* **33**:411–414.

Steger, R. W., Huang, H. H., and Meites, J., 1979, Relation of aging to hypothalamic LHRH content and serum gonadal steroids in female rats, *Proc. Soc. Exp. Biol. Med.* **161**:251–254.

Sterental, A., Dominguez, J. M., Weissman, C., and Pearson, O. H., 1963, Pituitary role in the estrogen dependency of experimental mammary cancer, *Cancer Res.* **23**:481–484.

Talwalker, P. K, Meites, J., and Mizuno, H., 1964, Mammary tumor induction by estrogen or anterior pituitary hormones in ovariectomized rats given 7,12-dimethylbenzan-thracene, *Proc. Soc. Exp. Biol. Med.* **116**:531–534.

Tamarkin, L., Cohen, M., Roselle, D., Rerchert, C., Lippman, M., and Chabner, B., 1981, Melatonin inhibition and pinealectomy enhancement of 7,12-dimethylbenzanthra-cene-induced mammary tumors in the rat, *Cancer Res.* **41**:4432–4436.

Terenius, L., 1971, Effect of anti-oestrogens on initiation of mammary cancer in the female rat, *Eur. J. Cancer* **7**:65–70.

Wellings, S. R., Jensen, H. M., and Marcum, R. G., 1975, An atlas of subgross pathology of the human breast with special reference to possible precancerous lesions, *J. Natl. Cancer Inst.* **55**:231–273.

Welsch, C. W., 1982, Hormones and murine mammary tumorigenesis: An historical per-spective, in: *Hormonal Regulation of Experimental Mammary Tumors* (B. S. Leung, ed.), Eden Press, Philadelphia, pp. 1–30.

Welsch, C. W., and Gribler, C., 1973, Prophylaxis of spontaneously developing mammary carcinoma in C3H/HeJ female mice by suppression of prolactin, *Cancer Res.* **33**:2939–2946.

Welsch, C. W., and Meites, J., 1969, Effects of a norethynodrel-mestranol combination (Enovid) on development and growth of carcinogen-induced mammary tumors in female rats, *Cancer* **23**:601–607.

Welsch, C. W., and Meites, J., 1970, Effects of reserpine on development of 7,12-dime-thylbenzanthracene induced mammary tumors in female rats, *Experientia* **26**:1133–1134.

Welsch, C. W., and Nagasawa, H., 1977, Prolactin and murine mammary tumorigenesis: A review, *Cancer Res.* **37**:951–963.

Welsch, C. W., Clemens, J. A., and Meites, J., 1968, Effects of multiple pituitary homografts or progesterone on 7,12-dimethylbenzanthracene-induced mammary tumors in rats, *J. Natl. Cancer Inst.* **41**:465–471.

Welsch, C. W., Clemens, J. A., and Meites, J., 1969, Effects of hypothalamic and amygdaloid lesions on development and growth of carcinogen-induced mammary tumors in the female rat, *Cancer Res.* **29**:1541–1549.

Welsch, C. W., Jenkins, T. W., and Meites, J., 1970a, Increased incidence of mammary tumors in the female rat grafted with multiple pituitaries, *Cancer Res.* **30**:1024–1029.

Welsch, C. W., Nagasawa, H., and Meites, J., 1970b, Increased incidence of spontaneous mammary tumors in female rats with induced hypothalamic lesions, *Cancer Res.* **30**:2310–2313.

Welsch, C. W., Iturri, G., and Meites, J., 1973, Comparative effects of hypophysectomy, ergocornine and ergocornine-reserpine treatments on rat mammary carcinoma, *Int. J. Cancer* **12**:206–212.

Welsch, C. W., Brown, C. K., Goodrich-Smith, M., Van, J., Denenberg, B., Anderson, T. M., and Brooks, C. L., 1979, Inhibition of mammary tumorigenesis in carcinogen-treated Lewis rats by suppression of prolactin secretion, *J. Natl. Cancer Inst.* **63**:1211–1214.

Welsch, C. W., Brown, C. K., Goodrich-Smith, M., Chiusano, J., and Moon, R. C., 1980, Synergistic effect of chronic prolactin suppression and retinoid treatment in the prophylaxis of N-methyl-N-nitrosourea-induced mammary tumorigenesis in female Sprague–Dawley rats, *Cancer Res.* **40**:3095–3098.

Welsch, C. W., Goodrich-Smith, M., and Brown, C. K., 1981, The prophylaxis of rat and mouse mammary gland tumorigenesis by suppression of prolactin secretion: A reap-praisal, *Breast Cancer Res. Treat.* **1**:225–232.

Welsch, C. W., Goodrich-Smith, M., Brown, C. K., Mackie, D., and Johnson, D., 1982, 2-Bromo-α-ergocryptine (CB-154) and tamoxifen (ICI 46,474) induced suppression of the genesis of mammary carcinomas in female rats treated with 7,12-dimethylbenzanthracene (DMBA): A comparison, *Oncology* **39:**88–92.

Wilkes, M. M., Lu, K. H., Fulton, S. L., and Yen, S. S. C., 1978, Hypothalamic-pituitary-ovarian interactions during reproductive senescence in the rat, *Adv. Exp. Med. Biol.* **113:**127–147.

Yokoro, K., Nakano, M., Ito, A., Nagao, K., Kodama, Y., and Hamada, K., 1977, Role of prolactin in rat mammary carcinogenesis: Detection of carcinogenicity of low dose carcinogens and of persisting dormant cancer cells, *J. Natl. Cancer Inst.* **58:**1777–1783.

Yoshida, H., Fukunishi, R., Kato, Y., and Matsumoto, K., 1980, Progesterone-stimulated growth of mammary carcinomas induced by 7,12-dimethylbenzanthracene in neonatally androgenized rats, *J. Natl. Cancer Inst.* **65:**823–828.

Young, S., 1961, Induction of mammary carcinoma in hypophysectomized rats treated with 3-methylcholanthrene, estradiol-17β, progesterone and growth hormone, *Nature* **190:**356–357.

Young, S., Baker, R. A., and Helfenstein, J. E., 1965, The effects of androgens on induced mammary tumours in rats, *Brit. J. Cancer* **19:**155–159.

CHAPTER 17

Relation of the Neuroendocrine System to Development of Prolactin-Secreting Pituitary Tumors

DIPAK K. SARKAR, PAUL E. GOTTSCHALL, and
JOSEPH MEITES

1. Introduction

Prolactin (PRL)-secreting tumors are the most common pituitary tumor type seen in rats, mice, and man (Ito *et al.*, 1972; Post *et al.*, 1980; Schechter *et al.*, 1981; Meites, 1981). Pituitary tumors that secrete growth hormone (GH), adrenocorticotropic hormones (ACTH), and thyroid-stimulating hormone (TSH) also occur in animals and man, and some pituitary tumors secrete several of these hormones simultaneously. In rodents, the incidence of the tumors increases with advancing age, but in human subjects, PRL-secreting pituitary microadenomas occur in young, as well as older individuals, and may increase with aging (Post *et al.*, 1980). Whereas macroscopic pituitary tumors appear most frequently in aging rats and mice, such tumors are much less common in human subjects.

Women with prolactinomas may show symptoms of ammenorrhea and galactorrhea, and men may exhibit impotence and decreased libido, due to the antigonadotropic effects of high PRL secretion. Many individuals with PRL-secreting microadenomas show no obvious symptoms. Old rats bearing PRL-secreting pituitary tumors invariably exhibit derangements of reproductive function including loss of cycles, enlarge-

DIPAK K. SARKAR ● Department of Reproductive Medicine, University of California, San Diego, California 92093. PAUL E. GOTTSCHALL and JOSEPH MEITES ● Department of Physiology, Neuroendocrine Research Laboratory, Michigan State University, East Lansing, Michigan 48824.

ment or tumorous development of the mammary glands, and in males, a decrease of spermatogenesis and testosterone secretion.

Tumors of the pituitary may occur spontaneously, or they can be induced experimentally in animals by treatment with carcinogenic agents (radiation, chemicals, and viruses), or estrogen (E_2). It has been suggested that development of spontaneous tumors may be due to a sustained imbalance of the mechanisms regulating pituitary secretion (Furth *et al.*, 1973). Evidence will be presented here showing that spontaneous prolactinomas in old rats, occur in part at least, as a result of a defect in the neuroendocrine mechanism that inhibits PRL secretion, leading to chronic stimulation of PRL-secreting cells.

2. Regulation of Prolactin Secretion

Since the mechanisms controlling PRL secretion are believed to be involved in development of prolactinomas, it is important to briefly review the control of PRL secretion. This subject has been reviewed extensively in animals and man (Meites, 1977; Lancranjan and Friesen, 1978; Neill, 1980; Besser *et al.*, 1980; Clemens and Shaar, 1980). Secretion of PRL is mainly controlled by hypothalamic neurotransmitters and hypophysiotrophic hormones. The most important hypothalamic inhibitory neurotransmitter for PRL secretion is dopamine (DA), whose major mode of action is directly on the lactotrophs of the pituitary to inhibit PRL secretion. Dopamine has been detected in the pituitary portal circulation in amounts sufficient to directly depress anterior pituitary (AP) PRL secretion (Eskay *et al.*, 1975; Neill, 1980). There is also some evidence for the existence of one or more PRL-release inhibiting factors (PIFs) that are different from DA, although DA can account for most of the inhibitory influence from the hypothalamus. There is also evidence for the presence of a PRL-releasing factor (PRF) in the hypothalamus that is different from TRH, both of which can increase PRL secretion. However, a physiological role for TRH in PRL release has not been definitely established, and under most conditions when PRL is released, there is no change in TSH secretion or TSH secretion is actually reduced. Hypothalamic neurotransmitters that can promote PRL secretion include serotonin and the endogenous opiates, both of which have been shown to be involved in physiological states when PRL secretion is increased. Substances, such as vasoactive intestinal peptide (VIP), neurotensin, substance P, and histamine have been reported to promote PRL secretion. However, none of these latter substances have yet been shown to be involved in the physiological release of PRL.

There is convincing evidence that E_2 is an important promoter of PRL secretion in animals and in man. Estrogen can directly stimulate the AP to increase synthesis and release of PRL under both *in vitro* and *in vivo* conditions. This was first demonstrated in our laboratory by culture or incubation of rat AP tissue, together with small amounts of E_2, and also after injection of E_2 in hypophysectomized-ovariectomized rats with a pituitary graft underneath the kidney capsule (Nicoll and Meites, 1962; Lu *et al.*, 1971). The finding that E_2 can act directly at the AP to stimulate synthesis and release of PRL in rats has been confirmed by other investigators (Raymond *et al.*, 1978).

Estrogen has also been shown to act via the hypothalamus to promote PRL release. Short-term E_2 administration was reported to deplete PRL-inhibiting activity of the hypothalamus (Ratner and Meites, 1964), which in the light of present knowledge is probably mainly dopamine. Acute treatment with E_2 decreases the release of DA in pituitary portal blood (Cramer *et al.*, 1979a). Estrogen can antagonize the inhibitory action of DA on PRL release at the AP level (Raymond *et al.*, 1978; Gudelsky *et al.*, 1981). Ergocornine, a dopaminergic agent that can directly inhibit PRL release by the incubated pituitary, was shown to prevent E_2-induced release of PRL in an *in vitro* incubation system (Lu *et al.*, 1971). In addition to its antidopaminergic activity and its direct action on the pituitary, E_2 also may promote PRL secretion by increasing hypothalamic PRF activity (Nagasawa *et al.*, 1969). The mechanism of action of long-term exposure to E_2 on PRL secretion is unclear, but is discussed in detail in the latter part of this chapter. Progesterone and testosterone are much less effective than E_2 for stimulating PRL secretion *in vivo*, but do not act on PRL secretion *in vitro* (Meites, 1975).

Prolactin can inhibit its own secretion when present in the circulation in relatively large amounts through a "short-loop-feedback" mechanism, involving DA. Thus, injection of exogenous PRL increased release of DA into the portal blood and decreased rat serum PRL concentration (Gudelsky and Porter, 1980; Sarkar *et al.*, 1982a). Also, PRL can increase PIF activity and DA turnover in the median eminence of rats (Welsch *et al.*, 1968; Fuxe *et al.*, 1969; Gudelsky *et al.*, 1976).

It has been shown that PRL secretion increases progressively in aging female and male rats (Meites 1982). In general, the increase in blood PRL level is greater in aging female than in aging male rats. The increase of PRL in the aging female is usually greatest in anestrous rats, and is often associated with the presence of PRL-secreting pituitary tumors. The rise in blood PRL levels in aging females occurs during a period of declining E_2 secretion by the ovaries, and in aging male rats showing reduced testosterone secretion by the testes. There is evidence that the increase in PRL secretion in old rats is associated with a decrease in hypothalamic PIF activity and an increase in brain opiates and serotonin (Simpkins *et al.*, 1977; Steger *et al.*, 1980; Forman *et al.*, 1981).

3. Spontaneous Pituitary Tumors in Animals and Man

Spontaneous pituitary tumors are common in aging female and male rats. The incidence of these tumors in female rats is 10–86%, depending on the strain of rat, and increases with advancing age. Development of spontaneous pituitary tumors in mice is more infrequent (0.25–10%), except in some inbred strains such as the NZY (25%) and C57BL/6J (80%). Pituitary tumors are rare in rodents before 1 year of age, and usually appear between 2–3 years of age. Most of these tumors are lactotrophic (Russfield, 1966; Ito *et al.*, 1972; Furth *et al.*, 1973; Schechter *et al.*, 1981).

Recently, there has been an increased interest in human pituitary tumors because of autopsy findings of frequent microadenomas in individuals with a normal sized sella turcica (Hardy, 1980). The incidence of these microadenomas in human subjects at autopsy is stated to be 3–25% (Post *et al.*, 1980; Hardy, 1980). Most of these microadenomas are chromophobic, but may secrete relatively large amounts of PRL, GH, ACTH, or other hormones. Their incidence increases with age, although they are common in younger individuals. Large pituitary tumors in human patients are relatively rare (Post *et al.*, 1980).

Morphologically, the endocrine status of a pituitary adenoma may be identified by using a combination of techniques. Electron microscopic and immunocytochemical techniques can differentiate between the various adenohypophysial hormone-secreting adenomas, including prolactinomas. The common hematoxylin and eosin stains differentiate between acidophils (GH and PRL) and nonacidophilic cells which include the chromophobes and basophils (ACTH, LH, FSH, and TSH). When cells are highly stimulated as in the tumorous state, the release of hormone may deplete the cytoplasm of secretory granules and therefore the cells appear to be chromophobic. This is the reason that, until radioimmunoassays (RIAs) and sophisticated morphological techniques became available, human microadenomas were considered to be "nonfunctional" tumors. Since neoplastic cells are highly active, and quickly release most of the hormones produced, immunohistochemical procedures normally produce pale staining in neoplastic areas. Discrete neoplastic sites in the pituitary may be more easily identified in the future by development of monoclonal antibodies against different hormone-secreting tumor cells with specific surface antigens. These techniques should help to establish more accurately the true incidence of prolactinomas and other pituitary hormone-secreting tumors in human subjects.

4. Experimental Induction of Pituitary Tumors

A variety of experimental procedures have been used to study pituitary adenomas in animals, principally rats and mice, including the use of E_2, radiation, transplantation of pituitary (mice), and treatment with chemical carcinogens. Chemical carcinogens have been used infrequently for induction of such tumors.

4.1. Estrogen-Induced Pituitary Tumors

Experimentally induced pituitary tumors were first reported after chronic E_2 administration to female mice (Cramer and Horning, 1936) and rats (McEuen et al., 1936). The stimulatory effects of E_2 on pituitary tumor formation can be exerted, directly on the pituitary, since tumors were induced in pituitary grafts placed underneath the kidney capsule of intact rats after long-term E_2 treatment (Welsch et al., 1971; Fig. 1). Involvement of the hypothalamus in pituitary tumorigenesis and growth is also indicated by experiments showing that, size and incidence of tumors were greater in the in situ pituitary than when the pituitary is grafted underneath the kidney capsule (Welsch et al., 1971). The kidney may exert some protective action against E_2 on the grafted pituitary, since E_2 can be metabolized in the kidney (Bulfield and Nahum, 1978) and therefore may be less effective in this site. Also, the hypothalamic influence would be lacking. Prolactin-releasing activity in the hypothalamus was reported to increase in rats with E_2-induced in situ pituitary tumors (Nakagawa et al., 1980), which may contribute to the greater size and number of these tumors.

4.2. Irradiation-Induced Pituitary Tumors

Thyrotropic hormone-secreting tumors can be induced by administering a large dose of ^{131}I to mice (Gorbman, 1949), by surgical removal of the thyroid gland, by administering a goitrogenic food (Furth and Clifton, 1966), or by maintaining rats on an iodine deficient diet (Axelrod and LeBlond, 1955). Ionizing radiation increases the incidence of pituitary tumors in rats and mice and most of these tumors are PRL and GH secretors (Upton and Furth, 1953). Radiation may be the only pro-

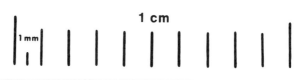

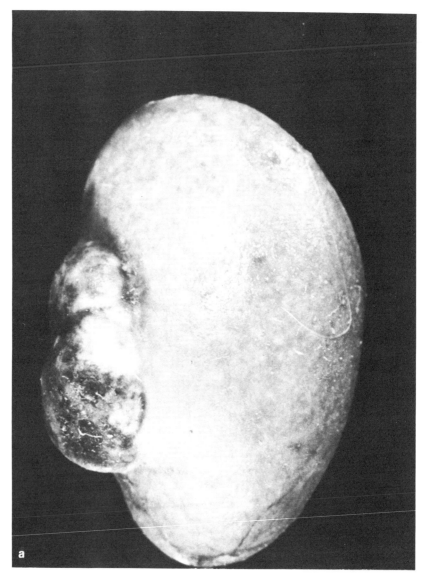

Fig. 1. (a) A representative kidney subcapsular tumorous pituitary homograft, and (b) a stimulated pituitary homograft, from female Sprague–Dawley rats treated for 16 months with diethylstilbesterol. (Reproduced from Welsch *et al.*, 1971.)

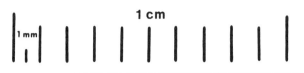

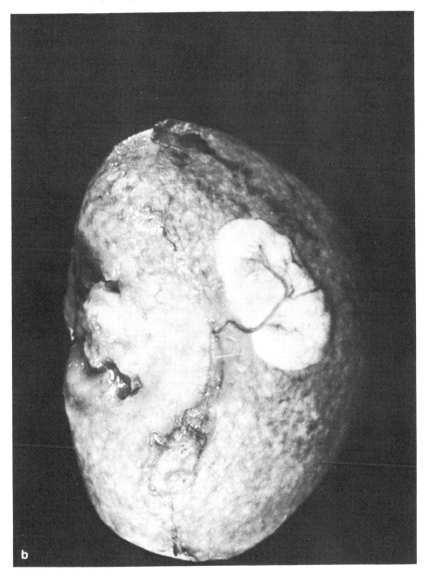

Fig. 1. *(Continued)*

cedure by which adrenocorticotropic pituitary tumors can be induced (Furth and Clifton, 1966).

4.3. Transplantation of Pituitary

Transplantation of a normal pituitary under the kidney capsule in mice results in the development of prolactinomas (Mühlbock and Boot, 1959). Ovariectomy of female mice decreased the incidence of tumorigenesis in the grafted pituitary (Clifton, 1963), indicating a role for E_2. In the rat, there is little evidence for tumor formation in the grafted pituitary. In the Sprague-Dawley strain of rats, pituitary size is reduced long after it is transplanted beneath the kidney capsule (Everett, 1954; Welsch *et al.*, 1971). In Fischer strain rats, pituitaries grafted beneath the kidney capsule for a shorter time showed no hyperplasia unless exogenous E_2 was administered (Clifton and Furth, 1961). On the other hand, when pituitaries from Fischer rats were isografted intramuscularly for 10 months, an occasional pituitary tumor was seen (Furth *et al.*, 1973). Further studies of pituitary grafts in genetically inbred rats need to be performed in order to determine whether PRL-secreting microadenomas might be formed without E_2 administration. Increased number and size of PRL-secreting cells were recently reported in grafted pituitaries in hypophysectomized rats by Rossi *et al.* (1977).

5. Hypothalamic Relationships in Development of Prolactin-Secreting Pituitary Tumors

Tumorigenesis in nonendocrine tissues is usually initiated by extrinsic carcinogenic agents. In endocrine glands, including the pituitary, initiation of tumorigenesis may occur not only by intrusion of a carcinogen, but also can be the consequence of an abnormality in its internal control mechanisms. Since pituitary gland function is controlled by interactions among the hypothalamo-pituitary-target gland system, any sustained alterations in this system may result in a neoplasm of the pituitary, perhaps by replication error (Furth, 1969). Thus, an increased blood level of gonadal E_2, which normally helps to stimulate secretion of PRL by the lactotrophs, may result in an autonomous tumor by acting as a growth-stimulating agent (Table 1). The pituitary growth-stimulating action of E_2 can be potentiated by blocking hypothalamic dopaminergic inhibition with a dopaminergic blocking agent, such as haloperidol (Table 1).

Table 1.   Effect of Haloperidol on 17β-Estradiol-Induced Growth of
the Anterior Pituitary (AP) Gland[a]

	Control	HALO	17β-E$_2$	17β-E$_2$ + HALO
AP weight (mg)	7.7 ± 0.2	6.1 ± 0.3	28.7 ± 2.4[b]	39.8 ± 2.6[b]
Total protein (μg)	655.0 ± 54.0	669.0 ± 37.0	3134.0 ± 249.0[b]	2836.0 ± 161.0[b]
Total DNA (μg)	71.0 ± 4.0	70.0 ± 5.0	222.0 ± 19.0[b]	314.0 ± 20.0[b,c]
AP PRL (μg)	12.2 ± 0.8	13.2 ± 1.4	91.2 ± 15.8[b]	91.6 ± 10.9[b]
Serum PRL (ng/ml)	22.4 ± 4.0	19.2 ± 4.1	814.6 ± 105.5[b]	1482.4 ± 138.2[b,c]

[a] Values are mean ± SEM., obtained from 11–20 rats. Ovariectomized female rats of the Fischer 344 strain were decapitated and pituitaries removed after 8 weeks of treatment with 17β-E$_2$, HALO (5 mg/l in 0.1% ethanol drinking water), or both.
[b] Signficantly different from controls and haloperidol ($p < 0.01$).
[c] Significantly different from 17β-E$_2$ ($p < 0.01$).

5.1.   Pituitary Growth Stimulation by Estrogen

Estrogen can stimulate production of PRL by action at two loci: (1) on the hypothalamus where it can influence tuberoinfundibular dopaminergic (TIDA) neurons, and (2) on the AP where it can directly increase PRL production (Meites, 1975). Estrogen can also influence AP function by blocking the PRL "short-loop-feedback" mechanism (Sarkar *et al.*, 1982a), decreasing DA action on the AP (Raymond *et al.*, 1978; Gudelsky *et al.*, 1981), and by increasing mitotic activity (Lloyd *et al.*, 1973), DNA synthesis (Table 1), and thymidine kinase activity (Valotaire *et al.*, 1975).

Ergot derivatives, which are dopaminergic agents, inhibit the release of PRL and decrease pituitary growth, reduce the mitotic index, and inhibit DNA synthesis in the E$_2$-stimulated pituitary (Meites, 1975; Lloyd *et al.*, 1975). Since inhibition of PRL release correlates with inhibition of mitosis in bromocryptine treated rats, PRL cells may have an internal mechanism whereby the cell senses large stores of PRL that can result in inhibition of mitosis (Lloyd *et al.*, 1975). Conversely, hypersecretion of PRL may be associated with increased mitotic division, as is evident after E$_2$ treatment (Table 1; Lloyd *et al.*, 1973; DeNicola *et al.*, 1978). The mechanism of this cellular response is complicated, and may involve calcium and adenylate cyclase-dependent processes, associated with increased hormone release rather than with increased hormone synthesis

(Pawlikowski, 1982). Studies on PRL-secreting pituitary tumors removed from human patients have indicated a significant correlation between the ability of DA to inhibit PRL secretion and inhibition of adenylate cyclase activity (DeCamilli *et al.*, 1980). However, these observations should be interpreted with caution, since DA may not inhibit adenylate cyclase activity in normal lactotrophs of rats and humans (Seeman, 1980).

Estrogen can also influence the growth of lactotrophs by altering the TIDA system. We have obtained evidence that chronic administration of E_2 increased pituitary weight and decreased DA content in the median eminence and in pituitary stalk portal blood (Fig. 2). Thus, synthesis and release of DA by its neurons were reduced after chronic E_2 administration. The decreased release of DA in pituitary stalk portal blood also may be caused by decreased number of functional dopaminergic neurons, since the fluorescent intensity of dopaminergic neurons were diminished after chronic E_2 administration (Fig. 3). These and other studies (Brawer *et al.*, 1978; Casanueva *et al.*, 1982) revealed that part of the E_2 action on development of pituitary tumors is due to degeneration of TIDA neurons, thereby releasing lactotrophs from the inhibitory action of DA.

In contrast to rats, there is no clear evidence that prolonged exposure to E_2 or steroid contraceptive treatments can produce prolacti-

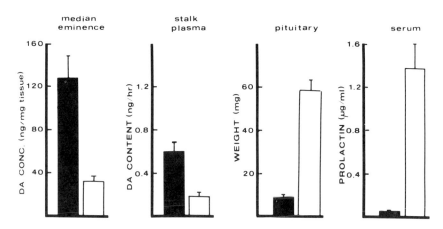

Fig. 2. Effect of chronic 17β-estradiol (E_2) treatment in ovariectomized female Sprague–Dawley rats on median eminence and stalk plasma DA, pituitary weight, and serum PRL. Animals given either an empty (■) or E_2-containing silastic capsule (□), 10 mm in length for 5 months. Values are mean ± SEM., from 6 to 14 rats.

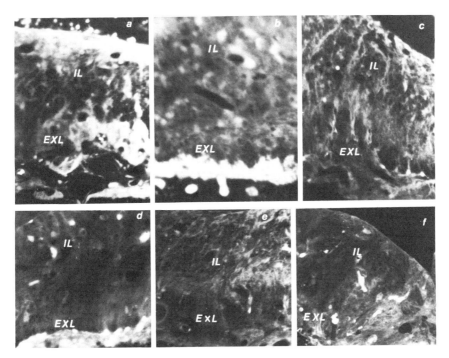

Fig. 3. Fluorescence photomicrographs of coronal sections through the hypothalamus (middle level) of representative female Sprague–Dawley or Wistar–Furth rats bearing or not bearing pituitary tumors (magnification ×240; reduced 53% for reproduction). (a) Normal catecholamine (CA) fluorescence was observed in terminals of the intermediate layer (IL) and external layer (EXL) of the median eminence in young rats (3–4 months). (b and d) Catecholamine fluorescence in the EXL of the median eminence was reduced in a rat bearing an MtT.W_{15} tumor transplant for 4 weeks (4 months), and in an old rat (27 months). (c, e, and f) There was a marked reduction of CA fluorescence in the EXL of the median eminence in a rat bearing an MtT.W_{15} tumor transplant for 8 weeks (5 months), and in rats bearing an *in situ* pituitary tumor occurring spontaneously (27 months), or induced by E_2 (9 months). (From Sarkar *et al.*, 1983c.)

nomas in human subjects (Post *et al.*, 1980). However, the enlargement of the AP and high secretion of PRL during pregnancy are believed to be related to the high levels of E_2 in plasma during this period (Meites, 1981). Estrogen may aggravate an existing pathology of the pituitary in human subjects (El Etreby, 1980). Until more careful investigations and follow-up are performed on human subjects, no definite correlation can be established between chronic E_2 treatment and development of prolactinomas.

5.2. Pituitary Growth Inhibition by Dopamine

As pointed out before, proliferation of lactotrophs may be regulated by an internal mechanism. Any substance which can influence the synthesis and release of PRL may also alter the growth of lactotrophs. Dopamine is a good candidate for a growth-inhibiting agent of lactotrophs, since it can decrease both synthesis and release of PRL from lactotrophs (MacLeod and Lehmeyer, 1974). Also, when the *in situ* pituitary was grafted to another area of the body, secretion of all AP hormones decrease with the exception of PRL (Meites *et al.*, 1977). Lactotrophs in the grafted pituitaries become hyperfunctional (Rennels, 1962; Rossi *et al.*, 1977, 1979). Similarly, a lesion of the medial basal hypothalamus or median eminence, which effectively reduces hypothalamic dopaminergic inhibition, resulted in both hyperplasia and hypertrophy of the lactotrophs (Rossi *et al.*, 1979; Cronin *et al.*, 1982).

Support for the view of DA as a pituitary growth-inhibiting agent comes from studies involving use of agonists and antagonists of DA, and observations on growth of lactotrophs. We have recently observed that when haloperidol (a dopaminergic antagonist), was administered together with E_2, it potentiated growth and DNA synthesis of pituitaries as compared to the action of E_2 alone (Table 1). Conversely, dopaminergic agonists, including ergot derivatives, have been shown to decrease PRL secretion and induce regression of pituitary prolactinomas (Quadri *et al.*, 1972; Quadri and Meites, 1973; Post *et al.*, 1980; MacLeod *et al.*, 1980; Chiodini *et al.*, 1980; Liuzzi *et al.*, 1980), by acting on the DA receptors of lactotrophs (MacLeod and Lehmeyer, 1974; Brown *et al.*, 1976).

5.3. Neurotoxic Action of High Prolactin Secretion on Dopaminergic Neurons

Since a progressive increase of plasma PRL levels was observed in both E_2-induced pituitary tumors and spontaneous prolactinomas in old rats (Meites, 1982), PRL may exert a neurotoxic action on the TIDA system. We have recently found that prolonged elevation of plasma PRL in rats given a subcutaneous (s.c.) transplant of a pituitary "lactotropic" tumor ($MtT.W_{15}$) decreased the number of TIDA neurons. In these rats, we found a decrease of catecholamine (CA) fluorescence intensity in the external layer of the median eminence (Fig. 3), and a reduction of DA content in pituitary stalk portal blood and median eminence (Fig. 4).

Short-term exposure to PRL in rats stimulated DA release into pituitary stalk portal blood (Cramer *et al.*, 1979b; Gudelsky and Porter,

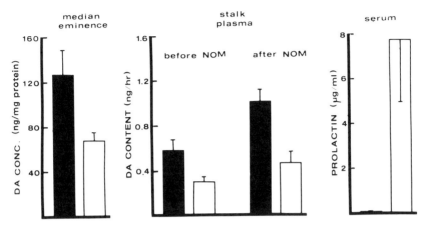

Fig. 4. Effect of hyperprolactinemia on median eminence DA, stalk plasma DA, and serum PRL. Hyperprolactinemia was induced in female Wistar–Furth (W/F) rats by s.c. transplantation of MtT.W$_{15}$ tumor for 6–8 weeks □. Controls were diestrous W/F female rats ■. Stalk blood samples were obtained for a 1-h period before and after injection of a DA-releasing agent, nomifensine (NOM). Values are mean ± SEM from 6–16 rats.

1980), and increased DA release from the median eminence *in vitro* (Sarkar *et al.*, 1982b). This treatment also decreased the size of the *in situ* pituitary and increased median eminence dopamine turnover (Chen *et al.*, 1967; Welsch *et al.*, 1968; Fuxe *et al.*, 1969; Gudelsky *et al.*, 1976). Thus, the action of PRL on dopaminergic neurons depends on its level in the blood and on its duration of action. Acute rises of PRL can stimulate dopaminergic neuronal activity, whereas chronically elevated PRL produces a neurotoxic action on the dopaminergic neurons and reduces the activity of these neurons. High blood levels of PRL may be partly responsible for the reduction of dopaminergic neuronal activity in old rats and in long-term E$_2$-treated rats that develop pituitary tumors.

5.4. Possible Role of Hypothalamic Stimulatory Agents on Pituitary Tumors

Involvement of stimulatory agent from the hypothalamus in the growth of E$_2$-induced PRL-secreting pituitary tumors have been suggested by Welsch *et al.* (1971), who showed that development of pituitary tumors by E$_2$ was greater in the *in situ* site than when transplanted underneath the kidney capsule. This view is also supported by the recent observation that PRL-releasing activity in the hypothalamus was increased in rats bearing E$_2$-induced pituitary tumors (Nakagawa *et al.*,

1980). However, further evidence is needed to substantiate the role of hypothalamic-stimulating agents on pituitary tumorigenesis.

6. Reduction of Hypothalamic Dopaminergic Activity is Associated with Development of PRL-Secreting Pituitary Tumors in Old Rats

Old rats show a high incidence of pituitary adenomas, predominantly involving PRL-secreting cells (Russfield, 1966; Meites, 1981). As indicated earlier, chronically elevated E_2 can produce PRL- and GH-secreting pituitary tumors in rodents, but except for old constant estrous females, E_2 secretion is decreased during aging. This does not rule out a role for E_2 during the many estrous cycles that precede the loss of cyclicity during aging. One possible explanation for the increased incidence of PRL-secreting tumors during aging involves alterations in DA activity. We have recently found that in old rats (24–26 months), with persistently elevated PRL levels, the "short-loop-feedback" action of PRL was diminished (Sarkar *et al.*, unpublished). One possible explanation for this phenomenon is that PRL stimulate TIDA neurons, but in old rats DA release was inadequate or the sensitivity of the pituitary to DA was decreased. A reduction of functional DA neurons in old rats is evident by the decrease in CA fluorescence intensity in the external layer of the median eminence (Fig. 3; Hoffman and Sladek, 1980), and by the depressed secretion of DA in stalk portal blood (Fig. 5).

Studies involving morphological changes in the hypothalamus during aging have been described by Clemens in another chapter of this book. These have indicated a significant loss of cell bodies, axons, and dendrites in the arcuate nucleus. Therefore, the suppressed secretion of DA into the portal blood could be due to reduced synthesis and release of DA, and more importantly, to a reduction in number of functional neurons.

Increased secretion of PRL in old rats may be due not only to a reduction in dopaminergic activity, but also to increased PRF activity in the hypothalamus (Meites, 1982). Increases in serotonin and opioid peptides during aging have been reported in old rats (Simpkins *et al.*, 1977; Steger *et al.*, 1980; Forman *et al.*, 1981), and both of these substances can promote PRL release (Van Vugt *et al.*, 1979; Porter *et al.*, 1980). These substances do not act directly on the AP to induce PRL release, but may inhibit dopaminergic neuronal activity (Van Vugt *et al.*, 1979; Pilotte and Porter, 1980; Kato *et al.*, 1982). These substances also may activate pituitary PRL secretion by increasing the secretion of other hy-

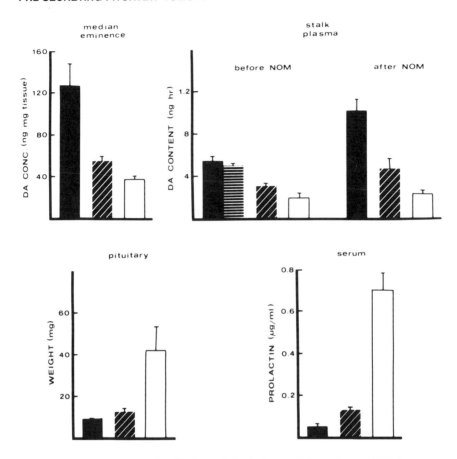

Fig. 5.   Median eminence and stalk plasma DA, pituitary weight, and serum PRL in young (3–4 months) ■, old (24–27 months) ▨, and pituitary tumor-bearing old (26–28 months) □ rats. Animals used were female Sprague–Dawley rats, Stalk blood samples were obtained as in Fig. 4, except in one group of young rats ☰, stalk blood samples were obtained for a 1-h period after saline injection. Values are mean ± SEM, from 5–19 rats.

pothalamic PRL releasing factors into the pituitary stalk portal blood (Porter *et al.,* 1980). Both TRH and VIP have been shown to directly increase pituitary PRL release, and both were shown to be released into the pituitary stalk blood (Tashjian *et al.,* 1971; Eskay *et al.,* 1975; Said and Porter, 1979; Shaar *et al.,* 1979). Involvement of other putative hypothalamic peptides in stimulation of PRL secretion is also possible (Meites, 1977; Neill, 1980; Enjalbert *et al.,* 1982).

In old rats we have recently obtained evidence of histological degeneration of dopaminergic neurons (Fig. 3), and suppression of DA release into pituitary stalk blood (Fig. 5). These were also observed in rats with spontaneously occurring and E_2-induced pituitary tumors (Figs. 2 and 5). Quantitatively, the loss of functional dopaminergic activity was greater in pituitary tumor-bearing rats than in old rats without tumors. Increases in plasma PRL and pituitary weight were also greater in old rats with pituitary tumors than in old rats without pituitary tumors. These observations support the view that DA is a significant inhibitor of PRL release and of growth of PRL cells. Therefore, the progressive decline in TIDA function in old rats is believed to contribute to development of pituitary tumors (Fig. 6).

In human subjects, the etiology of spontaneous pituitary prolactinomas is not clear. Patients with hyperprolactinemia may show reduced TIDA functions (Fine and Frohman, 1978; Müller *et al.*, 1980). A decrease of brain catecholamines in old human subjects has been documented (Robinson *et al.*, 1972; McGeer and McGeer, 1978), but there is no evidence of increased circulating PRL levels in elderly human subjects. The view has been stated that pituitary tumors in human patients may develop autonomously, independently of hypothalamic mechanisms (Daughaday, 1980; Hardy, 1980). However, there is no evidence for such autonomy at present. It is also possible that radiation, or carcinogenic chemicals, can act directly on the pituitary to produce pituitary tumors. Therefore, not all pituitary tumors are necessarily of hypothalamic origin.

7. Use of Ergot Drugs for Producing Regression of Pituitary Tumors

Our laboratory was the first to demonstrate (Quadri *et al.*, 1972) that in rats bearing transplantable PRL- and GH-secreting pituitary tumors ($MtT.W_{15}$), administration of ergot drugs could reduce blood PRL to normal levels and induce regression of these tumors (Fig. 7). Subsequently, ergot drugs were shown to decrease PRL release and induce regression of pituitary prolactinomas in human patients (Nilius *et al.*, 1980). The therapeutic use of ergot drugs to treat patients with PRL-secreting pituitary tumors has become widely accepted (Post *et al.*, 1980).

The suppressive action of ergot compounds on PRL secretion and PRL-secreting tumor growth is believed to be related to their dopaminergic activity. Thus, inhibition of PRL release by ergot alkaloids was prevented by use of dopaminergic antagonists (MacLeod and Lehmeyer, 1974; Caron *et al.*, 1978), and ergot alkaloids were shown to bind to

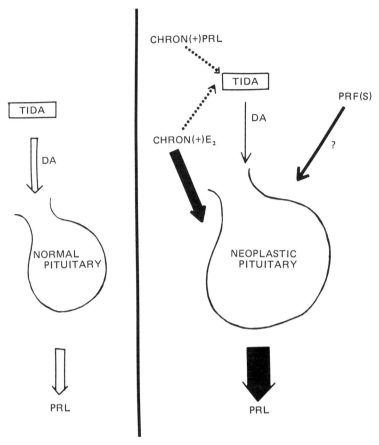

Fig. 6. A schematic diagram showing agents involved in dopaminergic system dysfunc-tion, and a possible mechanism for the development of PRL-secreting pituitary tumors in rats (see text). ⇨ = normal; ➡ = increase; → = decrease; ···→ = neurotoxic. TIDA = tuberoinfundibular dopaminergic system; PRL = prolactin; DA = dopamine; E_2 = estrogen; PRF = PRL-releasing factor; CHRON (+) = chronically elevated.

dopaminergic receptors on the lactotrophs (Caron *et al.,* 1978). Recently, Lamberts and MacLeod (1979) have suggested that the regression of some PRL-secreting pituitary tumors in rats by ergot derivatives, in-cluding ergotamine, are not mediated through a dopaminergic mech-anism, but through their vasoconstrictor action on the blood supply to the tumor. However, ergotamine can reduce DNA synthesis of rat PRL-secreting tumor cells *in vitro* (Prysor-Jones and Jenkins, 1980). Moreover,

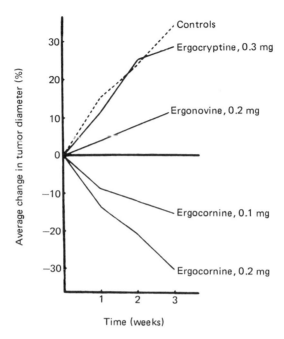

Fig. 7. Effect of 3 ergot drugs on growth of a transplanted pituitary tumor (MtT.W$_{15}$) in rats. The number of animals in each group was as follows: controls, 10; 0.3 mg of ergocryptine, 6; 0.3 mg of ergonovine, 6; 0.1 mg of ergocornine, 6; and 0.2 of ergocornine, 7. (Reproduced from Quadri *et al.*, 1972.)

ergonovine (a relatively weak vasoactive drug), but not ergocryptine (a potent vasoconstrictor), produced regression of PRL-secreting tumors *in vivo* in rats (Quadri *et al.*, 1972; Prysor-Jones and Jenkins, 1980). Reports have appeared recently that *in vitro* cloned pituitary tumor cell lines appear to be unresponsive to DA and to certain known DA agonists (Malarkey *et al.*, 1977). The semisynthetic ergot alkaloid, bromocriptine, appears to produce degradation of PRL in primary cultures of rat pituitary cells after chronic treatment (Dannies and Rudnick, 1980). Hence, the antiproliferative action of some ergot drugs may involve mechanisms other than interaction with DA receptors in the AP.

8. Summary

A decrease in hypothalamic DA activity appears to be associated with development of prolactinomas in rats. In both naturally occurring prolactinomas in old rats and E$_2$-induced PRL-secreting pituitary tumors, TIDA activity was found to be reduced. Haloperidol, a DA antagonist, when given together with E_2, increased the weight of the pituitary of rats more than E_2 alone (Table 1). Lesions of the medial-basal hypothalamus or median eminence, which effectively reduces the activity of hypothalamic DA neurons, resulted in hyperplasia of the lactotrophs in rats (Rossi *et al.*, 1979; Cronin *et al.*, 1982). Furthermore, we have provided evidence here that there is a decline in TIDA function in rats with age, and a similar alteration in TIDA neurons occurs even to a greater extent in old rats with prolactinomas than in nontumor bearing old rats. In human subjects, although a functional decline in TIDA neuronal activity may occur, hypothalamic involvement in development of prolactinomas has not been clearly established.

Although spontaneous prolactinomas in old rats develop in the face of declining gonadal function, the earlier effects exerted by the prolonged combined action of E_2 and PRL during cycling for many months on the TIDA neurons cannot be disregarded, and the subsequent chronic high blood PRL levels in old age may act to augment these earlier effects of E_2 and PRL. During each rat estrous cycle, both E_2 and PRL show a preovulatory surge. Our data strongly indicate that in rats, chronic high blood levels of PRL can produce a neurotoxic action on the TIDA system. It is also probable that the neurotoxic action of E_2 on the TIDA system is mediated at least in part by increasing blood levels of PRL. It is well established that E_2 can increase PRL secretion. Other aging processes also may have a role in producing TIDA dysfunction. Although E_2 can increase PRL secretion in human subjects, E_2 has not been shown to be involved in development of human prolactinomas.

ACKNOWLEDGMENTS. The author's work was supported by NIH research grants CA10771 from the National Cancer Institute, AG00416 from the National Institute on Aging, and AM04784 from the National Institute of Arthritis, Diabetes, and Digestive and Kidney Diseases.

9. References

Axelrod, A. A., and LeBlond, C. D., 1955, Induction of thyroid tumors in rats by a low iodine diet, *Cancer* **8**:339–367.

Besser, G. M., Yed, T., Delitala, G., and Grossman, D. B., 1980, Alteration of prolactin secretion by centrally acting drugs, *Adv. Biochem. Psychopharmacol.* **24**:399–406.

Brawer, J. R., Naftolin, F., Martin, J., and Sonnenschein, C., 1978, Effects of a single injection of estradiol valerate on the hypothalamic arcuate nucleus and on reproductive function in the female rat, *Endocrinology* **103**:501–512.

Brown, G. M., Seeman, P., and Lee, T., 1976, Dopamine-neuroleptic receptors in basal hypothalamus and pituitary, *Endocrinology* **9**:1407–1410.

Bulfield, G., and Nahum, A., 1978, Effect of the mouse mutants testicular feminization and sex reversal on hormone mediated induction and repression of enzymes. *Biochem. Genet.* **16**:743–750.

Caron, M. G., Beaulieu, M., Raymond, M., Gagne, B., Droonin, J., Leftkowitz, J., and Labrie, F., 1978, Dopaminergic receptors in the anterior pituitary gland, *J. Biol. Chem.* **253**:2244–2253.

Casanueva, F., Cocchi, D., Locatelli, V., Flauto, C., Zambotti, F., Bestetti, G., Rossi, G. L., and Müller, E., 1982, Defective central nervous system dopaminergic function in rats with estrogen-induced pituitary tumors, as assessed by plasma prolactin concentrations, *Endocrinology* **110**:590–599.

Chen, C. L., Minaguchi, H., and Meites, J., 1967, Effects of transplanted pituitary tumors on host pituitary prolactin secretion, *Proc. Soc. Exp. Biol. Med.* **126**:317–320.

Chiodini, P. G., Liuzzi, A., Silvestrini, F., Verde, G., Cozzi, R., Marsili, M. T., Horowski, R., Passerini, F., Luccarelli, G., and Borghi, P. G., 1980, Reduction in size of a prolactin-secreting adenoma during long-term treatment with a dopamine agonist (Lisuride), in: *Pituitary Microadenomas* (G. Faglia, M. A. Giovanelli, and R. M. MacLeod, eds.), Academic Press, New York, pp. 413–418.

Clemens, J. A., and Shaar, C. J., 1980, Control of prolactin secretion in mammals *Fed. Proc.* **39**:2588–2592.

Clifton, K. H., 1963, Tumor induction in hypophyseal grafts in radiothyroidectomized mice; hypothalamic-hypophyseal relationships, *Proc. Soc. Exp. Biol. Med.* **114**:559–565.

Clifton, K. H., and Furth, J., 1961, Changes in hormone sensitivity of pituitary mammotropes during progression from normal to autonomous, *Cancer Res.* **21**:913–920.

Cramer, W., and Horning, E. S., 1936, Experimental production by oestrin of pituitary tumours with hypopituitarism and of mammary cancer, *Lancet* **1**:247–249.

Cramer, O. M., Parker, C. R., Jr., and Porter, J. C., 1979a, Estrogen inhibition of dopamine release into hypophysial portal blood, *Endocrinology* **104**:419–422.

Cramer, O. M., Parker, C. R., Jr., and Porter, J. C., 1979b, Secretion of dopamine into hypophysial portal blood by rats bearing prolactin-secreting tumors or ectopic pituitary glands, *Endocrinology* **105**:636–640.

Cronin, M. J., Cheung, C. Y., Weiner, R. I., and Goldsmith, P. C., 1982, Mammotroph and gonadotroph volume percentage in the rat anterior pituitary after lesion of the medial basal hypothalamus, *Neuroendocrinology* **34**:140–147.

Dannies, P. S., and Rudnick, M. S., 1980, 2-bromo-α-ergocryptine causes degradation of prolactin in primary cultures of rat pituitary cells after chronic treatment, *J. Biol. Chem.* **255**:2776–2781.

Daughaday, W. H., 1980, Presidential address 1, in: *Pituitary Microadenomas* (G. Faglia, M. A. Giovanelli, and R. M. McLeod, eds), Academic Press, New York, pp. 1–2.

DeCamilli, P., Spada, A., Beck-Peccoz, P., Moriondo, P., Giovanelli, M., and Faglia, G., 1980, Presence of a dopamine-sensitive adenylate-cyclase in functioning human pituitary adenomas, in: *Pituitary Microadenomas* (G. Faglia, M. A. Giovanelli, and R. M. McLeod, eds.), Academic Press, New York, pp. 165–172.

DeNicola, A. F., and Von Lawzewitsch, I., Kaplan, S. E., and Libertun, C., 1978, Biochemical and ultrastructural studies on estrogen-induced pituitary tumors in F344 rats, *J. Natl. Cancer Inst.* **61**:753–757.

El Etreby, M. F., 1980, The role of contraceptive steroids in pathogenesis of tumors in various experimental animals and in man, in: *Pituitary Microadenomas* (G. Faglia, M. A. Giovanelli, and R. M. MacLeod, eds.), Academic Press, New York, pp. 211–222.

Enjalbert, A., Arahcibia, S., Priam, M., Bluet-Pajot, M. T., and Kordon, C., 1982, Neurotensin stimulation of prolactin secretion *in vitro*, *Neuroendocrinology* **34**:95–98.

Eskay, R. L., Oliver, C., Ben-Jonathan, N., and Porter, J. C., 1975, Hypothalamic hormones in portal and systemic blood, in: *Hypothalamic Hormones: Chemistry, Physiology, Pharmacology and Clinical Uses* (M. Motta, P. G. Crosignani, and L. Martini, eds.), Academic Press, New York, pp. 125–137.

Everett, J. W., 1954, Luteotrophic function of autografts of rat hypophysis, *Endocrinology* **54:**685–690.

Fine, S. A., and Frohman, L. A., 1978, Loss of central nervous system component of dopaminergic inhibition of prolactin secretion in patients with prolactin-secreting pituitary tumors, *J. Clin. Invest.* **54:**973–980.

Forman, L. J., Sonntag, W. E., Van Vugt, D. A., and Meites, J., 1981, Immunoreactive β-endorphin in the plasma, pituitary and hypothalamus of young and old male rats, *Neurobiol. Aging* **2:**281–284.

Furth, J., 1969, Pituitary cybernetics and neoplasia, *Harvey Lect.* **63:**47–71.

Furth, J., and Clifton, K. H., 1966, Experimental pituitary tumors, in: *The Pituitary Gland,* Vol. 2 (G. W. Harris and B. T. Donovan, eds.), Butterworth, London, pp. 460–497.

Furth, J., Ueda, G., and Clifton, K. H., 1973, The pathophysiology of pituitaries and their tumors: methodological advances, in: *Methods in Cancer Research,* Vol. X (H. Busch, eds.), Academic Press, New York, pp. 200–277.

Fuxe, K., Hökfelt, T., and Nelsson, O., 1969, Factors involved in the control of the activity of the tuberoinfundibular dopamine neurons during pregnancy and lactation, *Neuroendocrinology* **9:**257–270.

Gorbman, A., 1949, Tumorous growths in the pituitary and trachea following radiotoxic dosages of I^{131}, *Proc. Soc. Exp. Biol. Med.* **71:**237–240.

Gudelsky, G. A., and Porter, J. C., 1980, Release of dopamine from tuberoinfundibular neurons in pituitary stalk blood after prolactin or haloperidol administration, *Endocrinology* **106:**526–529.

Gudelsky, G. A., Simpkins, J., Mueller, G. P., Meites, J., and Moore, K. E., 1976, Selective actions of prolactin on catecholamine turnover in the hypothalamus and on serum LH and FSH, *Neuroendocrinology* **22:**206–215.

Gudelsky, G. A., Nansel, D. D., and Porter, J. C., 1981, Role of estrogen in the dopaminergic control of prolactin secretion, *Endocrinology* **108:**440–444.

Hardy, J., 1980, Ten years after the recognition of pituitary microadenomas, in: *Pituitary Microadenomas* (G. Faglia, M. A. Giovanelli, and R. M. MacLeod, eds.), Academic Press, New York, pp. 7–14.

Hoffman, G. E., and Sladek, J. R., Jr., 1980, Age-related changes in dopamine, LHRH, and somatostatin in the rat hypothalamus, *Neurobiol. Aging* **1:**27–37.

Ito, A., Moy, P., Kaunitz, H., Kortwright, K., Clarke, S., Furth, J., and Meites, J., 1972, Incidence and character of the spontaneous pituitary tumors in strain CR and W/FU male rats, *J. Natl. Cancer Inst.* **49:**701–711.

Kato, Y., Hiroto, S., Katakami, H., Matslishita, N., Shimatsu, A., and Imura, H., 1982, Effects of a synthetic enkephalin analog on plasma luteinizing hormone and prolactin levels in conscious orchidectomized rats, *Proc. Soc. Exp. Biol. Med.* **169:**95–100.

Lamberts, S. W. J., and MacLeod, R. M., 1979, The inability of bromocriptine to inhibit prolactin secretion by transplantable rat pituitary tumors: Observations on the mechanism and dynamics of the autofeedback regulation of prolactin secretion, *Endocrinology* **104:**65–70.

Lancranjan, I., and Friesen, H. G., 1978, The neural regulation of prolactin secretion, in: *Current Studies of Hypothalamic Function* (W. L. Veale and K. Lederis, eds.), S. Karger, Basel, Switzerland, pp. 131–150.

Liuzzi, A., Chiodini, P. G., Silvestrini, F., Cozzi, R., Oppizzi, G., Botalla, L., and Verde, G., 1980, Effects of neuroactive drugs on growth hormone and prolactin secretion in acromegaly, in: *Pituitary Microadenomas* (G. Faglia, M. A. Giovanelli, and R. M. MacLeod, eds.), Academic Press, New York, pp. 367–382.

Lloyd, H. M., Meares, J. D., and Jacobi, J., 1973, Early effects of stilboestrol on growth hormone and prolactin secretion and on pituitary mitotic activity in the male rats, *J. Endocrinol.* **58:**227–231.

Lloyd, H. M., Meares, J. D., and Jacobi, J., 1975, Effects of oestrogen and bromocryptine on *in vivo* secretion and mitosis in prolactin cells, *Nature* **255:**497–498.

Lu, K. H., Koch, Y., and Meites, J., 1971, Direct inhibition by ergocornine of pituitary prolactin release, *Endocrinology* **89:**229–233.

MacLeod, R. M., and Lehmeyer, J. E., 1974, Studies on the mechanism of the dopamine-mediated inhibition of prolactin secretion, *Endocrinology* **94:**1077–1085.

MacLeod, R. M., Lamberts, S. W. J., Nagy, I., Login, I. S., and Valdengro, C. A., 1980, Suppression of prolactin secretion by the physiological and pharmacological manipulation of pituitary dopamine receptors, in: *Pituitary Microadenomas* (G. Faglia, N. A. Giovanelli, and R. M. MacLeod, eds.), Academic Press, New York, pp. 37–54.

Malarkey, W. B., Groshong, J. C., and Milo, G. E., 1977, Defective dopaminergic regulation of prolactin secretion in a rat pituitary tumor cell line, *Nature* **266:**640–641.

McEuen, C. S., Selye, H., and Collip, J. B., 1936, Prolonged administration of oestrin in rats, *Lancet* **1:**775–776.

McGeer, P. L., and McGeer, E. G., 1978, Aging and Neurotransmitter Systems, *Adv. Exp. Med. Biol.* **113:**41–68.

Meites, J., 1975, Relation of estrogen to prolactin secretion in animals and man, *Adv. Biosci.* **15:**196–208.

Meites, J., 1977, Evaluation of research on control of prolactin secretion, in: *Comparative Endocrinology of Prolactin* (H. Dellman, J. A. Johnson, and D. M. Klachko, eds.), Plenum Press, New York, pp. 135–152.

Meites, J., 1981, Relation of prolactin to development of spontaneous mammary and pituitary tumors, in: *The Prostatic Cell: Structure and Function*, Part B (G. P. Murphy, A. A. Sandbert, and J. P. Karr, eds.), Alan R. Liss, New York, pp. 1–8.

Meites, J., 1982, Changes in neuroendocrine control of anterior pituitary function during aging, *Neuroendocrinology* **34:**151–156.

Meites, J., Simpkins, J. W., Bruni, J., and Advis, J., 1977, Role of biogenic amines in control of anterior pituitary hormones, *IRCS J. Med. Sci.* **5:**1–7.

Mühlbock, O., and Boot, L. M., 1959, Induction of mammary cancer in mice without the mammary tumor agent by isografts of hypophysis, *Cancer Res.* **19:**402–412.

Müller, E. E., Genazzani, A. R., Camanni, F., Cocchi, D., Massara, F., Picciolini, E., Locatelli, V., and Molinatti, G. M., 1980, Neuropharmacologic approach to the diagnosis and treatment of secreting pituitary adenomas, in: *Pituitary Microadenomas* (G. Faglia, M. A. Giovanelli, and R. M. MacLeod, eds.), Academic Press, New York, pp. 347–366.

Nagasawa, H., Chen, C. L., and Meites, J., 1969, Effects of estrogen implant in median eminence on serum and pituitary prolactin levels in the rat, *Proc. Soc. Exp. Biol. Med.* **132:**859–861.

Nakagawa, K., Obara, T., and Tashiro, K., 1980, Pituitary hormones and prolactin-releasing activity in rats with primary estrogen-induced pituitary tumors. *Endocrinology* **106:**1033–1039.

Neill, J. D., 1980, Neuroendocrine regulation of prolactin secretion, in: *Frontiers in Neuroendocrinology*, Vol. 6 (L. Martini and W. F. Ganong, eds.), Raven Press, New York, pp. 129–155.

Nicoll, C. S., and Meites, J., 1962, Estrogen stimulation of prolactin production by rat adenohypophysis *in vitro, Endocrinology* **70:**272–277.

Nilius, S. J., Bergh, T., Lundberg, P. O., Stahle, J., and Wide, L., 1980, Bromocryptine-induced regression of a prolactin-secreting pituitary tumor, in: *Pituitary Microadenomas* (G. Faglia, M. A. Giovanelli, and R. M. McLeod, eds.), Academic Press, New York, pp. 407–412.

Pawlikowski, M., 1982, The link between secretion and mitosis in the endocrine glands, *Life Sci.* **30:**315–320.

Pilotte, N. S., and Porter, J. C., 1980, Concentration of dopamine in pituitary stalk plasma and of prolactin in systemic plasma in rats given 5-hydroxytryptamine, *Soc. Neurosci. Abst.* **6:**(34).

Porter, J. C., Nansel, D. D., Gudelsky, G. A., Reymond, M. J., Pilotte, N. S., Foreman, M. M., and Tilders, F. J. H., 1980, Some aspects of hypothalamic and hypophysial secretion in aging rats, *Peptides* **1:**135–139.

Post, K. D., Jackson, I. M. D., and Reichlin, S., 1980, *The Pituitary Adenoma*, Plenum Publishing, New York.

Prysor-Jones, R. A., and Jenkins, J. S., 1980, Effect of bromocryptine, ergotamine, and other ergot alkaloids on the hormone secretion and growth of a rat pituitary tumor. *J. Endocrinol.* **86:**147–153.

Quadri, S. K., and Meites, J., 1973, Effects of ergocornine and CG603 on blood prolactin and GH in rats bearing a pituitary tumor, *Proc. Soc. Exp. Biol. Med.* **142:**837–841.

Quadri, S. K., Lu, K. H., and Meites, J., 1972, Ergot-induced inhibition of pituitary tumor growth in rats, *Science* **176:**417–418.

Ratner, A., and Meites, J., 1964, Depletion of prolactin-inhibiting activity of rat hypothalamus by estradiol or suckling stimulus, *Endocrinology* **75:**377–382.

Raymond, V., Beaulieu, M., Labri, F., and Boissier, J., 1978, Potent antidopaminergic activity of estradiol at the pituitary level on prolactin release, *Science* **200:**1173–1175.

Rennels, E. G., 1962, An electron microscope study of pituitary autograft cells in the rat, *Endocrinology* **71:**713–722.

Robinson, D. S., Nies, A., Davis, J., Bunney, W. E., Davis, J. M., Colburn, R. W., Bourne, H. R., Shaw, D. M., and Coppen, A. J., 1972, Aging, monoamines, and monoamine-oxidase levels, *Lancet* **1:**290–291.

Rossi, G. L., Probst, D., Panerai, A. E., Gil-Ad, I., Cocchi, D., and Müller, E. E., 1977, Light and electron microscopic studies of thyrotrophin releasing hormone-induced growth hormone and prolactin release in hypophysectomized rats bearing an ectopic pituitary, *J. Endocrinol.* **72:**313–319.

Rossi, G. L., Probst, D., Panerai, A. E., Cocchi, D., Locatelli, V., and Müller, E. E., 1979, Ultrastructure of somatotrophs of rats with median eminence lesions: Studies in basal conditions and after thyrotropin-releasing hormone stimulation, *Neuroendocrinology* **29:**100–109.

Russfield, A. B., 1966, *Tumors of Endocrine Glands and Secondary Sex Organs*, Pub. No. 1332, U. S. Government Printing Office, Washington.

Said, S. I., and Porter, J. C., 1979, Vasoactive intestinal polypeptide: Release into hypophyseal portal blood, *Life Sci.* **24:**227–230.

Sarkar, D. K., Miki, N., Xie, Q. W., Sylvester, P. W., and Meites, J., 1982a, Estrogen can inhibit "short-loop-feedback" action of prolactin on prolactin release, *Soc. Endocrinol.* (*Abst.* 864).

Sarkar, D. K., Gottschall, P. E., Meites, J., Horn, A., Dow, R. C., Fink, G., and Cuello, A. C., 1982b, Uptake and release of ^{3}H-dopamine by the median eminence: Evidence for presynaptic dopaminergic receptors and for dopaminergic feedback inhibition, *Neuroscience* (in press).

Sarkar, D. K., Gottschall, P. E., and Meites, J., 1982c, Damage to hypothalamic dopaminergic neurons is associated with development of prolactin-secreting pituitary tumors, *Science* **218**:684–686.

Schechter, J. E., Felicio, L. S., Nelson, J. F., and Finch, C. E., 1981, Pituitary tumorigenesis in aging female C57BL/6J mice: A light and electron microscopic study, *Anat. Rec.* **199**:423–432.

Seeman, P., 1980, Brain dopamine receptors, *Pharmacol. Rev.* **32**:229–313.

Shaar, C. J., Clemens, J. A., and Dininger, N. B., 1979, Effect of vasoactive intestinal polypeptide on prolactin release *in vitro*, *Life Sci.* **25**:2071–2074.

Simpkins, J. W., Mueller, G. P., Huang, H. H., and Meites, J., 1977, Evidence for depressed catecholamine and enhanced serotonin metabolism in aging male rats: Possible relation to gonadotropin secretion, *Endocrinology* **100**:1672–1678.

Steger, R. W., Sonntag, W. E., Van Vugt, D. A., Forman, L. J., and Meites, J., 1980, Reduced ability of naloxone to stimulate LH and testosterone release in aging male rats; possible relation to increase in hypothalamic met^5-enkephalin, *Life Sci.* **27**:747–753.

Tashjian, A. H., Jr., Barowsky, N. J., and Jensen, D. K., 1971, Thyrotropin releasing hormone: Direct evidence for stimulation of prolactin production by pituitary cells in culture, *Biochem. Biophys. Res. Commun.* **43**:516–523.

Upton, A. C., and Furth, J., 1953, Induction of pituitary tumors by means of ionizing radiation, *Proc. Soc. Exp. Biol.* **84**:255–257.

Valotaire, Y., LeGuellec, R., Kercret, H., Gullaen, G., and Duval, J., 1975, Induction of rat pituitary thymidine kinase: Another physiological response to oestradiol in the male? *Mol. Cell Endocrinol.* **3**:117–127.

Van Vugt, D. A., Bruni, J. F., Sylvester, P. W., Chen, H. T., Ieiri, T., and Meites, J., 1979, Interaction between opiates and hypothalamic dopamine on prolactin release, *Life Sci.* **24**:2361–2368.

Welsch, C. W., Negro-Vilar, A., and Meites, J., 1968, Effects of pituitary homografts on host pituitary prolactin and hypothalamic PIF levels, *Neuroendocrinology* **3**:238–245.

Welsch, C. W., Jenkins, T., Amenomori, Y., and Meites, J., 1971, Tumorous development of *in situ* and grafted anterior pituitaries in female rats treated with diethylstilbesterol, *Experientia* **27**:1350–1352.

Index